Chemical Food Safety

Chemical Food Safety

Dr Leon Brimer

University of Copenhagen

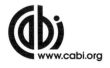
www.cabi.org

CABI is a trading name of CAB International

CABI Head Office
Nosworthy Way
Wallingford
Oxfordshire OX10 8DE
UK

Tel: +44 (0)1491 832111
Fax: +44 (0)1491 833508
E-mail: cabi@cabi.org
Website: www.cabi.org

CABI North American Office
875 Massachusetts Avenue
7th Floor
Cambridge, MA 02139
USA

Tel: +1 617 395 4056
Fax: +1 617 354 6875
E-mail: cabi-nao@cabi.org

A catalogue record for this book is available from the British Library, London, UK.

Library of Congress Cataloging-in-Publication Data

Brimer, Leon.
   Chemical food safety / Leon Brimer.
      p. cm. -- (Modular texts)
   Includes bibliographical references and index.
   ISBN 978-1-84593-676-1 (alk. paper)
1. Food--Toxicology. I. Title. II. Series

RA1258.B75 2010
615.9'54 -- dc22

2101034376

ISBN-13: 978 1 84593 676 1

Commissioning editor: Sarah Mellor
Production editor: Kate Hill

Typeset by SPi, Pondicherry, India.
Printed and bound in the UK by Cambridge University Press, Cambridge.

Contents

Preface

Chemical food safety as an academic discipline deals with all aspects of *chemical risks in food*, which the World Health Organization introduces as follows:

> The contamination of food by chemical hazards is a worldwide public health concern and is a leading cause of trade problems internationally. Contamination may occur through environmental pollution of the air, water and soil, such as the case with toxic metals, PCBs and dioxins, or through the intentional use of various chemicals, such as pesticides, animal drugs and other agrochemicals. Food additives and contaminants resulting from food manufacturing and processing can also adversely affect health.

Chemical food safety has a close relationship to nutrition science, which today has moved on from the classical concepts of avoiding nutrient deficiencies and basic nutritional adequacy to the concept of 'positive' or 'optimal' nutrition. Thus, the research focus of nutrition science has shifted more to the identification of biologically active components in foods that have the potential to optimize physical and mental well-being and which may also reduce the risk of disease. This means that chemical food safety and nutrition science meet around the wide variety of chemical entities present in our food, no matter from which source it comes and no matter its history of production and preparation.

This textbook focuses on the presentation of the subjects and facts necessary to work professionally with chemical food safety.

Chemical risk occurs only if a toxic compound (poison, toxin, toxicant or noxious compound)[1] is present. The fundamental science of poisons is called *toxicology*. Therefore, chemical food safety earlier most often was called *food toxicology*.

Toxicology of course refers to toxicity, which – according to the Organisation for Economic Co-operation and Development (OECD) that has accepted a definition from the United Nations – is 'the ability of a substance to cause poisonous effects resulting in severe biological harm or death after exposure to, or contamination with, that substance'.[2]

The reason to turn to OECD for a definition is that this international organization was the first to develop and launch guidelines for the testing of chemicals with regard to their toxicity.[3]

For food toxicology one could rephrase the definition to become: 'Food toxicology deals with substances found in food that might be harmful to those who consume sufficient quantities of the food containing such substances'.[4]

Notes

[1] The terminology when dealing with toxic compounds is rather blurred. While a toxicant more or less is just another word for a toxic = poisonous substance (a poison), a toxin most often is used to refer to a poison derived from a protein or conjugated protein produced by some higher plant, animal or pathogenic bacterium that is highly poisonous for other living organisms. The term 'a noxious compound' may also be seen although less frequently; the meaning is 'harmful or injurious to health or physical well-being' and is often used in connection with fumes – noxious fumes.

[2] UN (1997) Glossary of Environment Statistics, Studies in Methods, Series F, No. 67. United Nations, New York.

[3] OECD (revised 1993) Guidelines for the Testing of Chemicals, Sections 1–5. http://www.oecd.org/document/22/0,3343,en_2649_34377_1916054_1_1_1_1,00.html (accessed 6 April 2009).

[4] Omaye, S.T. (2004) Food and Nutritional Toxicology. CRC Press, Boca Raton, Florida.

Acknowledgements

I gratefully acknowledge the following persons for good ideas and discussions that either (i) directly during the process of writing this book have been of help and support or (ii) even though taking place before, still have been of significance for the book and its content.

- Professor of International Development Law Morten Broberg, the Faculty of Law, University of Copenhagen, Denmark, for his great knowledge concerning the EU Novel Food legislation and its impact on the possibilities for export of food products from developing countries and to the EU.
- Researcher Linley Chiwona-Karltun, Department of Urban and Rural Development, Swedish University of Agricultural Sciences, Uppsala, Sweden, for her years of educating me about food in Africa.
- Associate Professor M.J.R. Rob Nout, Food Microbiology Laboratory, Wageningen University, Wageningen, the Netherlands, and Professor Federico Federici, Università degli Studi della Tuscia, Viterbo, Italy, for giving me insight into food fermentation and its influence on the characteristics of the final food product.
- Senior Scientific Officer (Toxicology) Jean-Lou Dorne (J-LD), Department CONTAM, EFSA, Parma, Italy; Ulla Bertelsen (UB), CORE Organic Assistant Coordinator, ICROFS (International Centre for Research in Organic Food Systems) and former EFSA employee; Professor Johanna Fink-Gremmels (JF-G), Head of Department and Professor of Veterinary Pharmacology, Pharmacy and Toxicology, Utrecht University, the Netherlands; and Deputy Director-General Jan Alexander (JA), the Norwegian Institute of Public Health, Oslo, Norway. JF-G and JA, both members of the EFSA CONTAM Panel, taught me about risk assessment during my years as a member of the EFSA Work Group on Undesirable Substances in Animal Feed – Section Natural Plant Products. During this period J-LD and UB served as scientific secretaries for the Work Group while JF-G and JA served as heads of the Work Group.

Leon Brimer

1 Food, Nutrition and Food Safety: An Introduction

- Some important differences between the rich and the poor parts of the world or society are discussed.
- We examine the differences in food consumption between children and adults.
- The effects that these differences have on what chemical food security and safety problems we may face are discussed.

1.1 We All Eat and Exercise!

We all eat to stay alive, to enjoy taste and to be together around a table socializing. How much and what we eat affects our health to a great extent.

In poor countries and underprivileged social groups, major problems can be malnutrition and undernutrition. According to the United Nations (UN) Millennium Project (2005), the number of undernourished people in the world has fallen from approximately 1.5 billion in the early 1970s to around 850 million by the 1990s; still a high number, however. More than 200 million of the world's hungry are children, and at present at least 5 million die each year from undernutrition. Insufficient daily food intake can result in protein-energy malnutrition, which may also be associated with micronutrient deficiencies and disease. Thus, iron deficiency alone affects around 2 billion people and vitamin A deficiency at least 100 million children each year. Ironically, in many parts of the rich world, iron overdose is considered a leading cause of poisoning-related injury and death in young children. These children consume iron tablets obtained from a child-resistant container that has been opened by themselves or another child, or left open or improperly closed by an adult.

In the rich world with its effective agricultural sector, food processing industry and distribution networks, other new and hitherto unknown problems have also arisen. Now we get too fat. It started in the USA, where today approximately 127 million adults are overweight, 60 million obese and 9 million severely obese. Thus, obesity (persons with a body mass index (BMI) greater than 30 but less than $40\,kg/m^2$) increased from a prevalence of 14.4% in the period 1976–1980 to 30.5% in the measuring period of 1999–2000. Today we all know that this epidemic is no longer restricted to the USA. This development has given all societies new problems in the form of people suffering from the metabolic syndrome, characterized by a group of metabolic risk factors in one person such as:

- abdominal obesity (excessive fat tissue in and around the abdomen);
- atherogenic dyslipidaemia (blood fat disorders – high triacylglycerols, low HDL cholesterol and high LDL cholesterol – that foster plaque build-ups in artery walls);
- elevated blood pressure; and
- insulin resistance or glucose intolerance (the body cannot use insulin or blood sugar properly).

People with the metabolic syndrome are at increased risk of coronary heart disease and other diseases related to plaque build-ups in artery walls (stroke and peripheral vascular disease) and type 2 diabetes.

The underlying risk factor for this syndrome appears to be abdominal obesity – which again is a result of *high energy intake* and *physical inactivity*, among others.

1.2 But We Are All Different!

From the discussion above it should be obvious that any animal and thereby any human being has nutritional requirements that depend on the level of physical activity. However, other factors such as age, pregnancy (second and third trimester) and general health status also play a role.

According to the new Nordic Nutritional Recommendations of 2004, women between 18 and 60 years of age and weighing around 62 kg require an energy intake of approximately 9.3 MJ day^{-1} (corresponding to 0.15 MJ per kilogram of body weight (BW) per day), decreasing to 8.5 MJ day^{-1} (0.14 MJ kg^{-1} BW day^{-1}) at age 61–74 years, when they have limited physical activity. For women with an active lifestyle, the values are approximately 10.5 MJ day^{-1} (0.17 MJ kg^{-1} BW day^{-1}) at age 18–60 years and 9.5 MJ day^{-1} (0.15 MJ kg^{-1} BW day^{-1}) at age 61–74 years. Men up to 60 years of age with a body weight of around 76 kg require an energy intake of approximately 12 MJ day^{-1} (0.16 MJ kg^{-1} BW day^{-1}) and 13.5 MJ day^{-1} (0.18 MJ kg^{-1} BW day^{-1}) with limited physical activity and for an active lifestyle, respectively. However, when we come to children things change dramatically. Thus, a child between 6 and 13 months of age has an estimated energy requirement of 0.35 MJ kg^{-1} BW day^{-1}; this decreases to 0.33 MJ kg^{-1} BW day^{-1} at age 2–5 years and to 0.31 MJ kg^{-1} BW day^{-1} at age 6–9 years. It should just be mentioned here that 1 MJ is equal to 238 nutritional calories. But what has all this to do with chemical food safety?

1.3 And That Affects Chemical Safety!

Well, first of all we have now learned that small children eat more per kilogram of body weight than do adults. Chemical food safety (food toxicology) as a discipline is dealing with the possible negative influences of chemical compounds on our health and how to reduce/avoid these by combined clever use of risk assessment, risk management and risk communication. The effect(s) of and thereby the risk connected with a given chemical compound – whether a drug or a toxin – on our organism depend(s) on the concentration reached in the different tissues and cells. This again is a function of the amount absorbed from the gastrointestinal tract and the body weight of the individual person. Now imagine that a small child for a certain period is served food that is mostly based on peaches, which babies may begin to eat at any time from 4 to 6 months old. The peaches may be contaminated with one or more pesticides used during the fruit production; for example, the insecticide phosmet, one of the three pesticides most often found on this

fruit in the USA in the period around year 2000. Compared with an adult who eats the same (maybe as a kind of health treatment), the child normally will get higher blood levels as well as tissue concentrations of phosmet, simply because of the fact he/she eats more peach per kilogram of body weight and therefore also more phosmet per kilogram of body weight. The compound inhibits the enzyme acetylcholinesterase in certain nerve junctions (neuronal synapses) resulting in acute intoxication symptoms such as abdominal cramps, convulsions, diarrhoea, vomiting and unconsciousness. For this compound an Acute Reference Dose (ARfD) of 0.045 mg kg^{-1} BW day^{-1} has been internationally agreed upon. The ARfD is defined as 'an estimate of the amount of a substance in food or drinking water, normally expressed on a body weight basis, that can be ingested in a period of 24 h or less without appreciable health risks to the consumer on the basis of all known facts at the time of the evaluation' (FAO/WHO Joint Meeting on Pesticides Residues, 2002). Obviously the child – if very unlucky – more easily risks exceeding this dose.

If we take the example further from phosmet to the so-called *heavy metal* lead, even more factors will be seen to influence what may happen to a child as compared with an adult. Lead was for many years a big pollution problem in the USA and Europe among others due to its occurrence in gasoline for cars (leaded fuel). It was used as an additive to increase the octane number, a measure of the ignition quality of the gasoline. The higher this number, the less susceptible is the gasoline to cause knocking in the engine. Actually, the additive used was the chemical compound tetraethyl lead (TEL), which in the engine was converted to small particles of lead oxides that came out with the combustion. The lead oxides were deposited on the soil as well as on the surface of feed and food crops grown close to busy roads. This gave rise to high lead concentrations in many food products.

Since excessive blood lead is associated with nervous system impairment, including cognitive difficulties and behavioural problems, and at high enough exposures can stunt children's growth and cause permanent brain damage and mental retardation, the use of lead in gasoline has been reduced. The reasons for young children to be the most sensitive to this chemical threat not only include the fact that small children eat more per kilogram of body weight, but also that: (i) the brain is a main target for the toxic effect; (ii) lead can reach the fetus through the mother's blood and already at this stage damage brain development; and (iii) small children typically absorb a higher percentage (around 50%) of the lead ingested compared with an adult person, who typically absorbs less than 10%. So the differences between us influence the risks we meet from chemical compounds in our food (as well as in the environment, in the workplace, etc.).

And just when some of us feel that a specific problem is about to be solved, others may start to face the same problem. Thus, long after a general decline in blood lead levels had been reported from North America as well as Europe, a Chinese study from the city of Shenzhen revealed excessive blood lead levels in two-thirds of the city's children, reflecting what many believed was a problem throughout China's industrialized cities. Researchers with the Chinese Medical Association found that 65% of the 11,348 schoolchildren they tested had concentrations above the safe limit of $10\,\mu g\,dl^{-1}$ set by the World Health Organization (WHO).

Further Reading

Washam, C. (2002) Lead challenges China's children. *Environmental Health Perspectives* 110, A567.

2 The Food Production and Processing Chain

- We look at the production of organic matter as based on photosynthesis.
- Organisms such as plants, animals, fungi, etc. used for food worldwide are discussed.
- The production systems for different food resources (raw materials) are outlined.
- Important chemical food safety issues when dealing with different resources are discussed.
- We give an overview of the processing of food and its consequences for chemical food safety.

2.1 Primary and Secondary Producers of Organic Matter

All living organisms need something to live on; however, what each of the many species does need differs.

In order to describe and understand ourselves and our environment or maybe even predict incidents, risks or developmental trends in our nearby surroundings or in nature as such, we divide the environment into so-called *spheres*. As human beings we are, together with our husbandry, members of the *biosphere* of planet Earth. The other spheres are made up by the *geosphere*, the *hydrosphere* and the *atmosphere* (Fig. 2.1). The biosphere includes the terrestrial and aquatic biota: the viruses, the bacteria, the fungi, the plants and the animals. While the viruses do not have a metabolism of their own, being multiplied inside and by the cells of living organisms, all other members of the biosphere consist of cells, have a metabolism and, as such, need something to live on.

The bacteria are so-called *prokaryotes* with no membrane separating the DNA-containing area from the rest of the cell, while the fungi, plants and animals are all *eukaryotes*. This fundamental difference in cell structure is not, however, defining the most fundamental difference when it comes to the need for something to live on. In this respect, across the boundary between prokaryotes and eukaryotes, we divide organisms into the groups of *autotrophs* and *heterotrophs*.

The autotrophic species (from the Greek *autos* = self and *trophe* = nutrition, related to *trephein* = to make solid) are the only organisms that make new complex organic matter, that all organisms need, from simple inorganic carbon in the form of carbon dioxide or bicarbonate. As such they are also called *primary producers*. In terms of the production of organic matter the most important group of autotrophic organisms is the plants. Plants are responsible for most of the fixation of inorganic carbon into organic form (sugar) by the process of photosynthesis:

$$6CO_2 + 6H_2O + \text{light (energy)}$$
$$\rightarrow C_6H_{12}O_6 + 6O_2 \text{ (simplified summary)}$$

Plants in this respect include algae (micro-algae as well as seaweeds) and all terrestrial plants; i.e. the spore plants (e.g. mosses, liverworts, horsetails and ferns) and the seed-bearing plants (including the gymnosperms such as the pines and all of the angiosperms).

However, some bacteria, i.e. prokaryotes, also conduct photosynthesis as just described. These organisms form the group of cyanobacteria, also known as blue-green algae, found in the marine environment as well as in freshwater and even in hypersaline inland lakes. The cyanobacteria are important primary producers in many areas of the ocean.

In addition to the light-dependent autotrophic organisms, some species of bacteria derive energy from oxidizing inorganic compounds such as hydrogen sulfide and at the same time fixing inorganic carbon

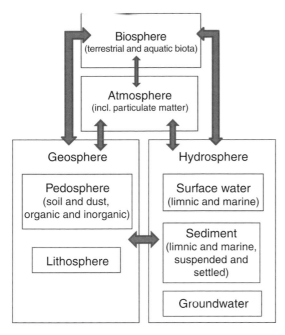

Fig. 2.1. A schematic presentation of the spheres and their interactions.

into organic compounds (carbohydrates). These so-called *chemoautotrophic organisms* are also primary producers, although of very little importance.

In summary, the autotrophs are the real producers in a food chain, while some of the heterotrophic species use (e.g. fungi) or consume (e.g. herbivorous animals) plants as their source of organic compounds for growth, body maintenance and energy. Other heterotrophic animals – the carnivores – consume herbivorous animals for the same purposes. All heterotrophic organisms, through their catabolic reactions to produce energy, have a key role in recycling carbon to carbon dioxide:

$$C_6H_{12}O_6 + 6O_2 \rightarrow 6CO_2 + 6H_2O$$
$$+ \text{(chemical 'cell' energy)}$$

As recyclers the heterotrophic organisms are also called *secondary producers*.

When a heterotrophic organism absorbs organic compounds from the intake of another organism some of these are used directly. Examples are the essential amino acids, the vitamins and the essential fatty acids. Others are degraded either to carbon dioxide and water to form energy (see above) or to basic building blocks needed for the formation of new organic compounds needed by the organism.

2.2 Food Raw Materials

As human beings we are omnivorous organisms, i.e. we eat plants (primary producers) as well as products from secondary producers (animals) such as meat, eggs and milk in order to nourish our body. After production or gathering of the raw materials these are further processed into different kinds of intermediate products (e.g. in order to reduce weight prior to transport or to obtain a prolonged shelf-life) or ready-to-eat foods/dishes. In the following sections, we look a little further into the different groups of raw food materials worldwide.

Terrestrial plants

Most of the food consumed for the necessary human energy production worldwide originates from terrestrial plants. Rice (*Oryza sativa*) is the world's most important food source and helps feed about half the globe's people. Close to this comes wheat(s) (*Triticum aestivum* and other *Triticum* spp.) of which about 70% of the world production is used directly for human consumption, while maize (corn; *Zea mays*), although close to double in world production compared with each of the two other grains, follows on only in third place since close to 60% is used for animal feeds and an increasing amount also goes to the production of bioethanol. Other plant commodities of major importance for human energy intake include the starch-rich tubers of Irish potato (*Solanum tuberosum*), cassava (*Manihot esculenta*), yam (includes a number of *Dioscoria* spp.) and sweet potato (*Ipomoea batatas*).

Locally, other commodities may be of major importance as the main staple food. Thus, a number of traditional cereals such as sorghum ('grain sorghum', 'milo'; *Sorghum bicolor*), finger millet ('ragi', 'wimbi'; *Eleusine coracana*), teff ('tef'; *Eragrostis tef*), white fonio ('fonio', 'acha', etc.; *Digitaria exilis*), kodo millet ('kodon', 'creeping paspalum', 'ditch millet', etc.; *Paspalum scrobiculatum*) and pearl millet ('bulrush millet', 'babal', 'bajra'/'bajira'; *Pennisetum glaucum*) are of great importance in different parts of Africa, while the pseudocereals quinoa (*Chenpodium quinoa*) and amaranth (*Amaranthus cruentus*) are produced in the Americas from where they originate (as well as in Asia when it comes to amaranth).

Some of the starch-rich tubers mentioned above, such as the root tuber of cassava, have a very low content of protein as well as of a number of the vitamins and essential fatty acids needed for adequate human nutrition. With respect to protein supply, a large number of different beans, peas and lentils (pulses) of the plant family *Fabaceae* (= *Leguminosae*) play a particularly important role worldwide. When restricting ourselves to terrestrial plants, vitamins are also supplied by a number of other vegetables as well as fruits.

With plants it is important to remember that mankind uses nearly all the different plant organs as parts of prepared human foods, although some mostly in the form of spices. Examples are immature seeds (green peas), seeds (cereal grains, beans, sunflower seeds), newly sprouted seeds (bean sprouts), seedlings (cress), whole mature fruits (grapes/raisins), whole immature fruits (haricot verts, okra), pericarps (the fruit wall; capsicum fruits/sweet pepper), flower buds (capers), flowers ('stuffed' flowers of courgette), flower stigmas (saffron), immature inflorescences (broccoli grown for the edible immature flower panicles), inflorescences (artichoke: the fleshy lower portions of the involucral bracts and the base of *Cynara cardunculus* known as the 'heart'), leaves (lettuce, cassava leaves, cabbages, etc.), leaf stalks (celery sticks), stems/young shoots (asparagus, bamboo shoots), barks (cinnamon), rhizomes/rootstocks (Irish potato is a tuberous rhizome) and roots (cassava).

With regard to the chemical food safety of meals prepared from the different plant raw materials as briefly touched upon above, problems may arise for example from: mycotoxins in cereals; the level of selenium in maize (e.g. from the US states of Dakota, North Dakota, Missouri and Kansas); the level of glycoalkaloids in Irish potato; the level of cyanogenic glycosides and their degradation products in cassava root products; the toxic non-protein amino acids or trypsin inhibitors in different pulses; the residues of pesticides in a number of crops; the toxic haemolysis in individuals deficient in the enzyme glucose-6-phosphate dehydrogenase (G6PD) after intake of faba beans (broad bean/horse bean); or the diarrhoea, failure to thrive and fatigue as symptoms of coeliac disease in individuals showing gluten intolerance but still eating wheat, a cereal crop which – although supplying much of the world's dietary vegetable protein and food – still presents this risk to one in about 100 to 200 people.

Animals

Animals for food are a very varied selection of species belonging to different phyla (the first subgrouping) of the animal kingdom, Animalia. Typically, different cultures/ethnic groups use different species, due to both different local resource availability and different tradition. Thus, to give examples on the great diversity: the use of insects as food seems to be a major phenomenon mainly in the Far East (e.g. China and Thailand); the guinea pig is eaten as a source of meat mostly in the Andes region of South America; Eskimo communities in Greenland and elsewhere traditionally use seals and whales as important sources of meat; and fish and seabirds are major types of food at the North Atlantic Islands. Also frogs are widely eaten in the form of frogs' legs; annual imports were estimated at about 8000 t in 2001 in the European Union (EU) member states and 30,000 t throughout the world. Frog consumption is an ancient tradition in most wetland areas. France has the highest European consumption of frogs.

On a worldwide perspective, however, a limited number of mammal and bird species (phylum Chordata) are dominating the animal production for food. The mammals include: pigs (*Sus scrofa domesticus* = *Sus scrofa* = *Sus domesticus*); a number of ruminants such as different types of cattle (*Bos primigenius*), the yak (*Bos grunniens*), the domestic Asian water buffalo (*Bubalus bubalis*), goats (*Capra aegagrus hircus*), sheep (*Ovis aries*) and camels/dromedaries (e.g. *Camelus dromedarius*); and also rabbits (seven different genera) including the species European rabbit (*Oryctolagus cuniculus*) and the cottontail rabbits (genus *Sylvilagus*). The birds (poultry) used for human consumption include: the chicken (*Gallus gallus*, sometimes *Gallus gallus domesticus*); the domesticated goose (*Anser anser domesticus*, a domesticated grey goose); ducks including domesticated ducks descended from both the mallard (*Anas platyrhynchos*) and the Muscovy duck (*Cairina moschata*); and finally the domesticated turkey, descended from the wild turkey species *Meleagris gallopavo*.

To the mammals and birds being used as food sources already mentioned should be added fish, bivalves (scallops, clams and oysters), shrimps, crayfish, crabs and lobsters. Fish, bivalves and shrimps include marine as well as freshwater forms. Until relatively recently, most of these species were gathered/caught through fishing activities. However, today a very significant amount of shellfish (a culinary and fisheries term for those aquatic invertebrate animals that are used as food, i.e. various species of molluscs, crustaceans and echinoderms) and fish is produced through farming. Using the Scottish waters as an example, the following shellfish species are commonly cultivated at farms: common mussel (*Mytilus edulis*), Pacific oyster (*Crassostrea gigas*), native oyster (*Ostrea edulis*), scallop (*Pecten maximus*) and queen scallop (*Chlamys opercularis*). The Atlantic salmon (*Salmo salar*) is by far the dominating fish species produced by farming with a world total annual production of about 1.25 million t, of which Norway farmed about 570,000 t in 2006.

From different animal types and species obviously different parts/organs are used, also depending on tradition and religion. With regard to the amounts consumed, for the majority of species the muscular meat definitely contributes the most. However, to this should be added, in particular, the liver and the kidneys. Due to the many changes made since 1989 in order to control bovine spongiform encephalopathy (BSE; commonly known as mad-cow disease) and to avoid transfer to human beings of the infectious agent (prions) that may cause brain disease (i.e. Creutzfeldt–Jakob disease, an incurable degenerative neurological disorder that is ultimately fatal), brain tissues are rarely eaten today. In addition to the parts of animals consumed as food, eggs and milk must also be remembered as important food resources.

For products of animal origin, chemical food safety can be threatened in a number of ways. Pig kidneys and livers may contain high concentrations of the nephrotoxic mycotoxin ochratoxin A (OTA; from feed); milk may contain the carcinogenic metabolic product aflatoxin M_1 (AFM$_1$) formed from the genuine mycotoxin aflatoxin B_1 if present in the feedstuff used; and fatty fish (such as salmon) may contain mercury, dioxins and the so-called *dioxin-like polychlorinated biphenyls* (PCBs) in concentrations that may impair health, the compounds being biomagnified through the food chain that leads to the food eaten by the salmon. Bivalves may contain toxic levels of a number of different algal toxins concentrated by the shellfish as a result of their filter feeding.

Fungi (and lichens)

Fungi are eukaryotic heterotrophic organisms possessing a chitinous cell wall. The majority of fungal species grow as multicellular filaments called hyphae, forming a mycelium. Some fungal species grow as single cells, however. Yeasts, moulds and mushrooms are examples of fungi. The term 'mushroom' is used here in a broad sense to include members of the group *Basidiomycota* that produce fruiting bodies and some *Ascomycota* that do the same. The fruiting bodies are the parts we use as food resources.

Until the 1970s, the use of fungi as a component in food in Europe was more or less restricted to one cultivated species, *Agaricus bisporus* (the button mushroom), supplemented with a relatively restricted use of a number of collected wild edible mushrooms. The cultivation of the button mushroom started in Paris around 1650, but it took several centuries before the production spread and intensified to the present level, where the button mushroom is the most cultivated fungus in the world. In Asia and particularly China, Japan and neighbouring countries, the use of fungi for food is better established and cultivation of a number of species started much earlier. Thus, the shitake (or forest) mushroom (*Lentinus edodes*), the paddy straw mushroom (*Volvarilla volvacea*), the ear fungus (*Auricularia auricular* and *Auricularia polytricha*) and enoki (*Flammulina velutipes*) were all produced by one or another form of cultivation long ago. Actually, the cultivation of shitake was reliably recorded from China 800 years ago.

All of the above-mentioned species belong to the *Basidiomycota*, while the most sought-after delicacy among the fungi, the truffles, belongs to *Ascomycota*. The truffles include the black truffle (*Tuber melanosporum*) and the white truffle (*Tuber mangatum*). Truffles live in close mycorrhizal association with the roots of specific trees. Their fruiting bodies grow underground. The gathering of truffles has been recorded as far back as 1600 BC. Around the year 2000 the world market price of the black truffle was about US$2000 kg^{-1}. The highly appreciated flavour of the truffle is directly related to its aroma. The chemicals necessary for the odour to develop are created only after the spores are mature enough for release, so they must be collected at the proper time or they will have little taste. This is the only sure indication that the mushrooms are ready to be harvested. Until 1972 all truffles were collected as wild with the aid of female pigs or truffle dogs, which are able to detect the strong smell of mature truffles beneath the surface of the ground. Since then some success has been seen for truffle production by means of the establishment of plantations of various species of oaks and hazel trees, which are inoculated with the truffle mycelium.

increase production for economic reasons, in Zambia and Malawi – taken as examples – the introduction of disease- and pest-resistant varieties of the starch root crop cassava during the 1990s has meant an average annual increase in production of 6 and 8%, respectively. Smallholders thereby have doubled their cash returns, and subsistence farmers have enjoyed increased food security.

The production of crops for sale and intended for widespread distribution through a commercial processing and distribution chain, i.e. the private farmer/farmer community living from the money earned on the production, is the next step, which we call *commercial agriculture* (or farming). At this point, it becomes more profitable for the land-owner to specialize in one or a few particular crops due to economies of scale. Emphasis on capital formation and technological development, as opposed to natural resource utilization, is an important difference compared with the situation for small-scale farmers. The use of fertilizers, pesticides and other agricultural chemicals is today an integrated component of such productions, if they are not part of the slowly growing commercial sector of organic agriculture.

Commercial farming becomes *industrial agriculture* as production size grows and the ownership becomes different from the daily managing of the production. Often technological/scientific, general economic and political aspects, such as how to obtain large-scale subsidies from the state or in Europe from the EU, become important factors determining what is produced and how. Innovation in agricultural machinery and farming methods, genetic technology, the active creation of new markets for the products, the application of patent protection to genetic information and a focus on global trade are characteristics of this production form. In general one can say that the large-scale production of genetically modified crops (i.e. genetically modified organisms, GMOs) for some productions adds greatly to the already mentioned commercial farming characteristics such as an integrated use of agricultural chemicals.

Concerning the chemical food safety of plant-based food products coming from each of the different production systems described, the following generalizations can be made. Products from subsistence/smallholder farming are consumed only by the producing family or a limited number of persons nearby living. No control except for their own is available and food scarcity may reduce the possibility of discarding crops or products thereof. Risks are mostly from mycotoxins as well as from toxic and anti-nutritional substances naturally inherent in the plants. Pollution chemicals coming from soil, air or the water used for irrigation/processing can also be a problem depending on the local environment. A naturally high content of, in particular, certain metals and metalloids in soil or water may furthermore give rise to non-safe levels of such elements in plant crops, examples being selenium (intoxications described from Venezuela, China and the USA) and arsenic (Bangladesh). Raw products from commercial farming may in addition contain residues of pesticides used before the production (e.g. to clear soil for weeds), during the growth period (e.g. to protect the crop against insects or fungi or to combat weeds), applied to surfaces of empty, clean stores (e.g. to help reduce the risk of pests moving into stored grain) or admixed with grain bulks to offer protection from infestation. The latter practice is becoming more and more restricted by legislation worldwide.

When looking at plant production it is only natural these days to also touch upon the question of whether there is any difference in the overall carbon dioxide economy in organic versus conventional modern farming. In general the differences seem to be small, if any. This is due to the fact that the yield per unit area from organic farming typically is around 60% that of intensive farming, which depends on fertilizers. The production and transportation of these to the place of use, on the other hand, have some substantial costs when it comes to carbon dioxide.

Terrestrial animals

The production of terrestrial animals for food, as well as of products of animal origin such as eggs and milk, is today taking place under just as diverse conditions as described for plant products. Especially for cattle and a few other ruminants produced for meat, one can moreover distinguish between intensive as opposed to extensive production. The major differences found with regard to chemical food safety originate from farmers' different use of veterinary drugs for the treatment of diseases and for preventive control of parasites such as fleas, ticks or mites on the animal's skin or in its ears. Both may give rise to drug residues in the animal products. The need for veterinary drugs depends on the form of production, with more intensive production with many animals per unit area and high productivity (e.g. litres of milk per animal per year) most often resulting in a more frequent use of medication. Other aspects are the possibility of carry-over of toxic compounds from feedstuffs. These may be natural plant constituents, persistent organic compounds from pollution or fraud in the feed production, or they may be due to fungal infection of feed. An example of the first mentioned is gossypol from the use of cottonseed meal, which may be found in edible parts such as muscle and offal of ruminants and poultry. Dioxins and dioxin-like PCBs may reach meat products (meat/fat) from industrial oils added to feed (by accident or as fraud), while fungal infection of feed plants may result in animal exposure to mycotoxins such as OTA (stored in the kidneys, liver or meat) or aflatoxins (in the milk). Ruminants and horses exposed during their entire lifespan to cadmium present in pastures may, in distinct regions with a high cadmium content, end up with an undesirable cadmium accumulation, particularly in the kidneys. Frequent consumption of kidney tissue from such older animals, as well as the frequent consumption of liver and kidneys from wildlife, may contribute significantly to the overall human exposure.

During the last decades, growth-promoting hormones (GPHs) have been used to increase the weight gain of cattle, especially in the USA. In 2005, 32.5 million cattle were slaughtered to provide beef for US consumers and it is believed about two-thirds of American cattle raised for slaughter today are injected with hormones to make them grow faster. However, such use is not permitted in Europe because of concerns about possible health risks from residues in the meat and other edible parts of these animals. This has resulted in intense disputes between the USA and the EU. In 2007, the European Food Safety Authority (EFSA) re-evaluated this subject. EFSA concluded that, while more sensitive analytical techniques have been developed to identify and quantify the presence of GPHs, these techniques have not been widely used. Hence, there still was a lack of data on the type and amount of GPH residues in meat upon which to make a quantitative exposure assessment. Consequently, EFSA did not find it possible to assess the significance of the large-scale use of hormones in relation to many epidemiological studies that indicate a correlation between eating red meat and certain hormone-dependent cancers.

Water-living organisms

The water-living organisms produced for food purposes by farming represent a diverse collection of fish, bivalves and, for example, crayfish (crawfish) as stated above. While the major fraction of bivalves and fish is now farmed in the sea (salt water), today the USA harvests more than 45,000 t (100 million lb) of crayfish per annum produced in freshwater ponds. The crayfish industry has become specialized, i.e. more and more crayfish are being processed, the tail meat frozen and shipped to other locations, including Europe. Over 90% of crayfish cultured in the USA comprise either red swamp crayfish (*Procambarus clarkii*) or white river crayfish (*Procambarus acutus*).

Water quality is of course of major importance for the chemical (as well as microbiological) food safety of farmed water-living animals. Thus, fatty fish especially may concentrate toxic lipophilic substances such as methylmercury, DDT (dichloro-diphenyltrichloroethane), dioxins and dioxin-like PCBs, while a number of bivalves can concentrate the metals lead and cadmium and the metalloid arsenic. Likewise, crabs can accumulate arsenic if living in contaminated waters. However, luckily the arsenic accumulated in both bivalves and crabs is mostly of organic nature (90–95%) such as arsenobetaine and arsenocholine, considered to be much less toxic than inorganic arsenic compounds. In fish farming a number of antibiotics such as metronidazole, olaquindox, oxolinic acid, oxytetracycline, streptomycin, sulfadiazine, tetracycline, tiamulin and tylosin are used, either legally or illegally. This makes it important to observe risks for residues as well as for their potential to cause adverse effects on the aquatic environment. Oxolinic acid thus has been shown to be relatively toxic to the daphnia *Daphnia magna*.

2.4 Collection, Hunting and Fishing

Even though deliberate production of plants, animals and fungi today dominates as the source of the food supply more or less worldwide, we must not forget that collection of wild plants and fungi, hunting and fishing each still has its role in the food supply.

Collection of wild plants and fungi first of all presents the risk of picking the wrong (i.e. unintended) species. This can – and sometimes does – lead to acute intoxications, some of which are fatal. However, for the fungi the threat posed by poisonous and lethal species is often overstated. Incidents of poisoning and deaths are few and far between compared with the regular and safe consumption of wild edible species, but publicity and cultural attitudes continue to fuel an intrinsic fear of wild fungi in some societies. This is more commonly found in developed countries and has undoubtedly led to the general belief that global use of wild edible fungi is small in scale and restricted to key areas. However, wild edible fungi are collected for food and to earn money in more than 80 countries according to the Food and Agriculture Organization of the United Nations (FAO) in their 2004 publication *Wild Edible Fungi: A Global Overview of Their Use and Importance to People.*

Fish is a vital source of food. According to FAO statistics from 1997, it is man's most important single source of high-quality protein, providing approximately 16% of the animal protein consumed by the world's population. It is a particularly important protein source in regions where livestock is relatively scarce. According to the same analysis, fish supplies less than 10% of the animal protein consumed in North America and Europe, but 17% in Africa, 26% in Asia and 22% in China. In the year 2000 FAO estimated that about 1 billion people worldwide relied on fish as their primary source of animal protein. Although fish farming has increased, still the major part of fish brought to the market for food is coming from capture fisheries. Depending on the waters in which the fish have been living and are captured, such 'wild fish' may or may not contain unhealthy concentrations of a number of chemical compounds such as methylmercury, dioxins and other persistent organic pollutants (POPs).

2.5 Processing: An Overview

At least some food raw materials may be eaten as they are, i.e. 'raw'. However, as human beings we often process our raw foods. Processing may be in order to obtain: (i) something more easy to digest; (ii) something more delicious; (iii) something with a longer shelf-life (less perishable); or (iv) something more safe. Since extending the shelf-life of food is part of the purpose of processing we often combine things, talking about 'food processing and preservation technologies'. Especially for highly perishable raw materials of plant origin (some fruits and vegetables), the term *postharvest technology* tends to cover parts of what we in a broader perspective call 'food processing and preservation'.

In general we divide our methods of processing into a number of so-called *unit operations*. However, depending on the professional role and educational background of the person, different authors classify and name these operations in varied ways. Often one talks about *primary processing* focusing on the conversion of raw materials to food commodities, milling being an example that can lead from the raw material of a cereal to the food commodity flour. The *secondary processing* in this terminology is the conversion of ingredients into edible products, baking being an example.

Some of the most common unit operations used in the modern food industry include:

- size reduction – grinding, cutting, emulsification;
- mechanical separation – sieving, filtration, centrifugal separations, sedimentation/flotation;
- mixing;
- drying/dehydration/evaporation;
- thermal processing – cooking, blanching, pasteurization, baking, roasting/frying, canning, (hot) smoking;
- cold preservation – refrigeration (chilling), freezing;
- contact equilibrium processes – extraction/washing, crystallization, membrane separations, distillations;
- irradiation; and
- fermentation.

For each unit operation the industry has today developed a large number of different processing equipments. Thermal processing and cold preservation both are examples of *heat exchange processes*. For these we can mention a number of generalized equipment examples such as:

1. Continuous-flow heat exchangers (e.g. cooling of milk in a pipe heat exchanger).
2. Jacketed pans (heating of soup in a jacketed pan).
3. Heating coils immersed in liquids (in some food processes, e.g. for the boiling of jam, quick heating

is required in a jacketed pan and thus a helical coil may be fitted inside the pan and steam admitted to the coil).

4. Scraped surface heat exchangers (typically for products of higher viscosity, i.e. in the freezing of ice cream and the cooling of fats during margarine manufacture).

5. Plate heat exchangers (for low-viscosity liquids such as milk).

Processing and storage – chemical food safety

The lack of processing and inefficient/wrong processing can lead to the risk of a chemically unsafe food, for example, the formation of myco-toxins in non-efficiently dried raw materials or non-properly processed commodities or end products. Processing, on the other hand, will most often result in safer products, although it also can lead to the formation or transfer of toxic substances resulting in unsafe end products. A few examples may be given as follows:

- Mechanical separation (sieving/floating): fungicide treatments are generally not recommended to control ergot (attack of the fungus *Claviceps purpurea* on rye, *Claviceps fusiformis* on pearl millet, *Claviceps paspali* on dallis grass or *Claviceps africana* on sorghum). If ergot occurs in the form of toxic sclerotia harvested with the grain, efforts focus on removing them by sieving or by soaking contaminated seed in brine to float off sclerotia.

- Size reduction (cutting and milling): the starch-rich tuberous root of cassava (*M. esculenta*) contains cyanogenic glycosides. Upon disintegration of the root tissue these are degraded to release a mixture of two principal toxic substances, cyanohydrins and hydrogen cyanide. The final content of these toxicants depends on the original content of cyanogenic glycosides and the subsequent processing steps.

- Thermal processing (frying/roasting-grilling): during high-temperature processing of meat a number of different compounds can be formed, many of which are well proven to be mutagenic and carcinogenic. Thus, heterocyclic aromatic amines (HAAs) have been shown to induce tumours at various organ sites in experimental animal studies, and high levels of dietary intake of HAAs have been associated with increased cancer risk in humans. These HAAs are formed in meat on heating from precursors such as amino acids, reducing sugars and creatine or creatinine.

- Contact equilibrium processes (extraction): (i) a number of legume seeds, especially certain beans such as lima bean (*Phaseolus lunatus*) and runner bean (*Phaseolus coccineus*) contain levels of lectins as well as certain oligosaccharides that call for extraction (overnight) and cooking (discarding the cooking water) to avoid stomach problems such as diarrhoea, vomiting and flatulence; (ii) the production of a number of food additives of natural origin involves extraction with organic solvents. Thus, *cassia gum*, a food additive made from the seed endosperm of *Cassia obtusifolia* or *Cassia tora* and used as a thickener and gelling agent (E499), is produced by a process involving extraction of cathartic (and therefore unwanted) anthraquinones using isopropanol. Hence, the content of isopropanol allowed in the final product is regulated.

Production machinery and packaging materials may also give rise to contamination of food products. A conveyer belt or other moving parts thus can risk contaminating foods with lubricants, which is why many food industries use only those lubricants approved for food contact e.g. by NSF International (a not-for-profit, non-governmental organization in the USA). Finally, packaging materials such as plastic and rubber polymers may release a number of low-molecular-weight compounds such as plasticizers (of which some may have oestrogenic or anti-androgenic effects) into foods.

2.6 Conclusion

Health-impairing chemical compounds may enter food at a number of different points of the food production and processing chain as illustrated in Fig. 2.2 for plant products. If we look at animal products, plant contaminants as well as toxic natural plant constituents may enter from feedstuffs while residues of veterinary drugs used during the production is another possibility to be aware of.

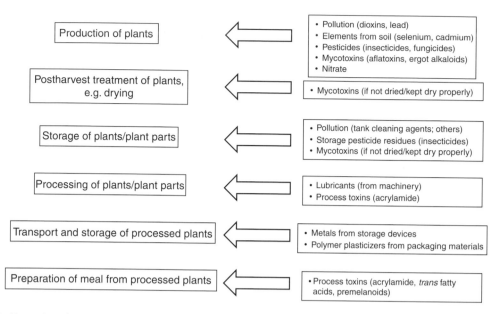

Fig. 2.2. Examples of entrance points for different toxic food contaminants during the production from plant to plate.

Further Reading

Herrchen, M. (2006) Pathways and behavior of chemicals in the environment. In: Duffus, J.H. and Worth, H.G.J. (eds) *Fundamental Toxicology*. RSC Publishing, Cambridge, UK, pp. 238–256.

Wilkinson, M. (2006) Ecotoxicity – effects of toxicants on ecosystems. In: Duffus, J.H. and Worth, H.G.J. (eds) *Fundamental Toxicology*. RSC Publishing, Cambridge, UK, pp. 257–272.

3 Unwanted Chemical Substances

- The important difference between compounds and elements with regard to their fate in organisms and the environment is discussed.
- The different possible chemical identities/structures of unwanted substances are described.
- The different possible origins of unwanted substances are discussed.

3.1 Introduction

Chemical substances unwanted in food may have many different origins and possess very different chemical structures.

Our planet is made up of a number of *elements* distinguished by their atomic number, i.e. by the number of protons in the nucleus (Table 3.1). Common examples of elements are iron, lead, silver, gold, hydrogen, carbon, nitrogen and oxygen. In total, 94 elements occur naturally on Earth. Eighty elements have stable isotopes, namely all elements with atomic numbers from 1 (hydrogen) to 82 (lead), except numbers 43 and 61, which are technetium and promethium (a lanthanide), respectively. Elements with atomic numbers of 83 or higher (bismuth and above) are inherently unstable and undergo radioactive decay but are nevertheless found in nature, either surviving as remnants of the primordial stellar nucleosynthesis which produced the elements in the solar system or else produced as short-lived daughter isotopes through the natural decay of uranium and thorium. Bismuth is generally considered to be the last naturally occurring stable, non-radioactive element in the periodic table; however, it is actually slightly radioactive, with an extremely long half-life.

The elements may be present as such, examples being the solid metal of sodium, the liquid metal of mercury, one of the different (solid) forms of carbon (graphite, diamond or amorphous carbon) or the gases chlorine, oxygen and hydrogen; or they may form *chemical compounds*. Excluding the elements chemical compounds are pure chemical substances consisting of two or more different elements. Examples of the latter are sodium chloride ($NaCl$, also known as 'salt'), carbon dioxide (CO_2) which we all exhale, ethanol (CH_3CH_2OH, commonly known as 'alcohol') and methylmercury (shorthand for the monomethylmercuric cation CH_3Hg^+, sometimes written as $MeHg^+$). As a positively charged ion, methylmercury combines with anions. In this form it becomes so lipophilic that it can bioaccumulate (long-term exposure) in the fat of fish and other marine organisms to make them toxic.

Chemical compounds can undergo *transformation/degradation* to other compounds. This may be a result of physical conditions such as high temperature or irradiation. For example, degradation caused by irradiation can be UV photolysis as observed for many compounds under high solar light intensity or transformation/degradation following food irradiation, i.e. the process of exposing food to ionizing radiation to destroy microorganisms, bacteria, viruses or insects that might be present. Changes in molecular structure can also be a result of *chemical reactions* such as hydrolysis of glycosides (see later) under the influence of acidic or alkaline conditions, oxidation or reduction. Chemical transformation/degradation can happen without any influence of enzymes or living organisms, but may also be a result of metabolism after contact with or absorption by a microorganism, plant or animal. An example of the latter could be the metabolic transformation and degradation of alcohol in a man who

Table 3.1. The periodic system of the elements (excluding the lanthanides and actinides).

Period	1	2	3	4	5	6	7	8	9	10	11	12	13	14	15	16	17	18
																		Group
1	H																	He
2	Li	Be											B	C	N	O	F	Ne
3	Na	Mg											Al	Si	P	S	Cl	Ar
4	K	Ca	Sc	Ti	V	Cr	Mn	Fe	Co	Ni	Cu	Zn	Ga	Ge	As	Se	Br	Kr
5	Rb	Sr	Y	Zr	Nb	Mo	Tc	Ru	Rh	Pd	Ag	Cd	In	Sn	Sb	Te	I	Xe
6	Cs	Ba		Hf	Ta	W	Re	Os	Ir	Pt	Au	Hg	Tl	Pb	Bi	Po	At	Rn
7	Fr	Ra		Rf	Db	Sg	Bh	Hs	Mt	Ds	Rg	Cn						

has been drinking a glass of wine. The first step in the metabolism of alcohol is the oxidation of ethanol to acetaldehyde catalysed by alcohol dehydrogenase containing the coenzyme NAD^+ ($CH_3CH_2OH + NAD^+ \rightarrow CH_3CH=O + NADH + H^+$). The acetaldehyde is further oxidized to acetic acid and finally to carbon dioxide and water through the citric acid cycle. A number of metabolic effects from alcohol are directly linked to the production of an excess of acetaldehyde.

While chemical compounds thus may 'disappear', it is very important to realize that the elements always stay with us and thus may re-enter the food chain after being excreted. A good example is the very toxic metal mercury.

The exact mechanisms by which mercury enters the food chain may vary among ecosystems. Some bacteria play an important early role. Bacteria that process sulfate (SO_4^{2-}) in the environment take up mercury in its inorganic form and convert it to methylmercury through metabolic processes. The conversion of inorganic mercury to methylmercury is important because its toxicity is greater and because organisms require considerably longer to eliminate methylmercury. The methylmercury-containing bacteria may be consumed by the next higher level in the food chain, or the bacteria may excrete the methylmercury into the water where it can quickly adsorb on to plankton, which are also consumed by the next level in the food chain. Because animals accumulate methylmercury faster than they eliminate it, animals consume higher concentrations of mercury at each successive level of the food chain. Small environmental concentrations of mercury can thus readily accumulate to potentially harmful concentrations of methylmercury in fish, fish-eating wildlife and people.

Methylmercury that has been excreted back into the environment may for example be degraded by reaction with ·OH as formed in sunlit surface waters, the products being Hg^{2+} and Hg^0. These forms of inorganic mercury may now re-enter the ongoing circle to be methylated again.

Also the macroscopic aquatic plant water spinach (*Ipomoea aquatica*), which is a popular vegetable in tropical regions, has been demonstrated to be able to form methylmercury; since the young shoots of this plant make a delicious and very appreciated vegetable, consumption may contribute to human health problems.

3.2 Why Unwanted?

Chemical compounds and elements can be unwanted in food (and feed) products for several different reasons.

- They may affect the taste and smell (olfactory characteristics). This is the case for example with compounds characteristic of rancid fatty products, i.e. different products of hydrolysis and oxidation of lipids based on unsaturated fatty acids. To avoid the formation typically we add antioxidants to products prone to this kind of degradation. Another example is the indole compound 3-methylindole (skatole; Fig. 3.1) formed by and concentrated in the meat of boars. The compound is a degradation product of the amino acid tryptophan. In very low concentrations it has a floral smell which, however, becomes faecal and very unpleasant at higher concentrations. For this compound a threshold value of 0.2 ppm has been set by many pig meat producers in order to be able to sell the meat. In many pig production systems male piglets are castrated in order to avoid this problem.

- They may reduce the intestinal absorption of for example important minerals such as calcium, magnesium, iron and zinc. This is the case for phytic acid (inositol hexakisphosphate, IP_6; or phytate when in salt form), which is the principal storage form of phosphorus in many plant tissues, especially bran and seeds. In cereal products minerals are bound by phytic acid, for which reason phytic acid is historically considered to have a negative effect on health. However, phytic acid also functions as an antioxidant in the stored food product by chelating iron ions and therefore a certain amount of phytic acid is desirable.

- They may degrade vitamins before these can be absorbed. This is the case for the thiaminases. Thiaminases are enzymes found in a few plants and the raw flesh and viscera of certain fish and shellfish. When ingested these enzymes split thiamine (vitamin B_1) and render it inactive (Fig. 3.2).

- They may be toxic (poisonous). In the rest of this book the toxic compounds are those that we focus on, although the so-called *anti-nutritional compounds* (factors) – to which the two above-mentioned examples of phytic acid and thiaminase belong – are also dealt with further.

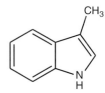

Fig. 3.1. Skatole (3-methylindole).

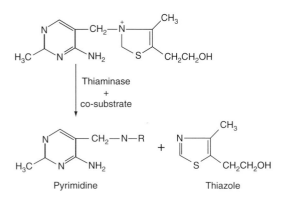

Fig. 3.2. The degradation of thiamine by thiaminase.

3.3 Elements and Inorganic Compounds

Metals and metalloids

Metals are elements that in general show good electric and thermal conductivity, high lustre and density, and the ability to be deformed under stress without cleaving. However, there are metals that have relatively low density, hardness and melting points; these (the alkali and alkaline earth metals) are in general very reactive and therefore are rarely encountered in their elemental, metallic form. Metals are usually inclined to form cations through electron loss. The metals may occur in the elementary state, as oxides or salts with different counterions (examples are Cl^-, NO_3^-, SO_4^-, PO_4^{3-}), or they may – in plants or animals – be bound (chelated) to more complex counterions such as phytate (see above) or special metal-binding proteins biosynthesized by animal tissues, an example being metallothionein, which binds cadmium in the liver. In addition some metals form parts of so-called *organometallic compounds* (see section 3.5 below).

A number of metals are essential to our body, i.e. included in the group of elements also called 'dietary minerals'. The essential metals are calcium, copper, iron, magnesium, manganese, molybdenum, potassium, sodium and zinc.

Also cobalt is essential, but as a part of vitamin B_{12} (cyanocobalamin), which is biosynthesized by bacteria in the environment and absorbed as such. Chromium appears to have a beneficial role in the regulation of insulin action, in metabolic syndrome and in cardiovascular disease. There is growing evidence that chromium may facilitate insulin signalling, and chromium supplementation therefore may improve systemic insulin sensitivity. Tissue chromium levels of subjects with diabetes are lower than those of normal control subjects, and a correlation exists between low circulating levels of chromium and the incidence of type 2 diabetes. Controversy still exists, however, as to the need for chromium supplementation.

Metalloids are elements showing properties of both metals and non-metals. Some of the metalloids, such as silicon and germanium, are semiconductors. This means that they can carry an electrical charge under special conditions. This property makes metalloids useful in computers and calculators. The following elements are generally considered metalloids: boron, silicon, germanium, arsenic, antimony, selenium and tellurium. The two metalloids arsenic and selenium both occur at very different levels in the soil crust when looking at their distribution worldwide and as, we shall see later, this has food safety implications. Of the metalloids only selenium seems to be essential for the human organism, although discussions are ongoing concerning a role for boron.

Taking selenium as an example of a metalloid, this element (melting point 217°C, boiling point 685°C, density 4819 kg m^{-3}) occurs in a number of oxidation states which include compounds formed with oxygen, sulfur, metals and/or halogens, namely as selenates (Se^{6+}; example Na_2SeO_4), selenites (Se^{4+}; Na_2SeO_3), selenides (Se^{2-}; Na_2Se) and as elemental selenium (Se^0). In environmental samples selenium can exist in inorganic as well as organic species (methylated compounds; selenoamino acids, selenoproteins and their derivatives). Inorganic selenium species thus can be transformed into volatile compounds such as dimethylselenide $(CH_3)_2Se$ through microbial action. In general, selenium speciation (Table 3.2) in soil and water is strongly affected by the oxidation state and pH of the soil/water environment. Organic selenium species are more frequently found in biological systems. In the living body, in contrast to metal–protein complexes, selenium is not bound by coordination but forms covalent C–Se bonds and is present in the form of either selenocysteinyl (SeCys) or selenomethionyl

Table 3.2. Examples of molecular species of selenium.

Selenium species	Acronym	Formula
Inorganic species		
1. Selenite (selenous acid salt)	Se(IV)	SeO_3^{2-}
2. Selenate (selenic acid salt)	Se(VI)	SeO_4^{2-}
Amino acids		
3. Selenocysteine	SeCys	$HSeCH_2CH(NH_2)COOH$
4. Se-methylselenocysteine	MeSeCys	$CH_3SeCH_2CH(NH_2)COOH$
5. Se-allylselenocysteine	AllSeCys	$CH_2=CHCH_2SeCH_2CH(NH_2)COOH$
6. Se-propylselenocysteine	PrSeCys	$CH_3CH_2CH_2SeCH_2CH(NH_2)COOH$
7. Selenocystine	SeCys$_2$	$HOOC(NH_2)CHCH_2Se-SeCH_2CH(NH_2)COOH$
8. Selenohomocystine	SeHoCys$_2$	$HOOC(NH_2)CHCH_2CH_2Se-SeCH_2CH_2CH(NH_2)COOH$
9. Selenomethionine	SeMet	$CH_3SeCH_2CH_2CH(NH_2)COOH$
10. Se-methylselenomethionine	MeSeMet	$(CH_3)_2SeCH_2CH_2CH(NH_2)COOH$
11. Selenoethionine	SeEt	$CH_3CH_2SeCH_2CH_2CH(NH_2)COOH$
Selenomium species		
11. Trimethylselenonium ion	TMSe	$(CH_3)_3Se^+$
12. Dimethylselenonium propionate ion	DMSeP	$(CH_3)_2Se^+CH_2CH_2COO^-$

(SeMet) residues. The SeCys residues are incorporated into proteins according to the corresponding UGA codon. Selenium compounds with SeCys residues are defined as selenoproteins and participate in redox reactions as the active centre of selenoenzymes. Selenium in the form of SeMet residues is incorporated without a specific codon and the selenium-containing proteins act as the biological pool of selenium.

Both non-essential and essential metals can be toxic, depending on the dose. The difference between the two groups is that, for the essential metals (as well as for other essential elements that can cause intoxications at high dose levels), we have a life window between the lowest intakes to prevent deficiency syndromes and the highest acceptable to prevent intoxication (Fig. 3.3).

Later we describe in detail the toxicology related to a number of metals and metalloids of importance for food chemical safety. These will include cadmium, chromium, copper, iron, lead, mercury and tin (metals), as well as arsenic, boron and selenium (metalloids).

Non-metallic elements

Of non-metallic elements of major concern for chemical food safety we find just fluorine. The mineral fluorspar (= fluorite), consisting mainly of calcium fluoride, was described in 1530 by Georgius Agricola for its use as a flux, i.e. a compound used to promote

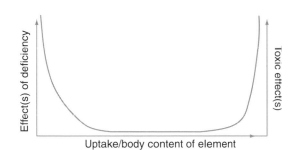

Fig. 3.3. An example of a life window for an essential element.

the fusion of metals or minerals. Fluorine forms a single bond with itself in elemental form, resulting in the diatomic F_2 molecule. F_2 is an extremely reactive, poisonous, pale yellowish brown gas. Inorganic compounds of fluoride, including sodium fluoride (NaF), are used in toothpaste to prevent dental cavities by direct treatment and added to some municipal water supplies for the same reason, a process called water fluoridation. Black tea (based on the plant *Camellia sinensis*) has a high content of fluoride, which has led to safety evaluations concerning the possible consequences of a high intake of this product.

3.4 Organic Compounds

Organic compounds in general are made up of carbon atoms linked to each other in chains as supplemented with hydrogen (e.g. CH_3-CH_3, ethane), but often can incorporate oxygen and nitrogen into the skeleton. Nitrogen is a key atom in a number of very strongly physiologically active natural organic compounds, such as a high number of alkaloids and several hundred non-protein amino acids known from a number of plants. Substitutions can include atoms of a number of other elements such as sulfur, phosphorus, chlorine, fluorine and iodine. The halides will often be found in organic compounds of natural origin as biosynthesized by marine organisms, although some important toxins that may cause food safety problems such as the mycotoxin OTA contain chlorine.

Biologically formed organic compounds

A large number of the organic compounds that we discuss during the course of this book are of biological origin. These include: a large number of toxic compounds naturally inherent in plants used for food; compounds formed by fungi attacking our crops or covering our food products with mould (mycotoxins); algal toxins whether found in algae or in different types of shellfish which have accumulated these natural compounds through their filter feeding; and tetrodotoxin from puffer fish; just to mention a few. Pathogenic microorganisms (bacteria) are not covered in this book. However, one should note this does not mean that they do not form toxins. Actually pathogenic bacteria generally inflict damage to a host organism through the synthesis of toxins rather than by massive cell invasion. Virulence is a measure of the capacity of these toxins to harm host cells. Bacterial toxins are normally categorized into *exotoxins*, which are released from the progenitor (e.g. botulinum toxin, which has a median lethal dose (LD_{50}) of 0.000025 μg in the mouse), and *endotoxins*, which generally are lipopolysaccharide in nature, associated with the outer cell envelope of Gram-negative bacteria and show an approximate LD_{50} of 400 μg in the mouse. The endotoxins of food and waterborne enteric bacteria are often designated *enterotoxins*.

Anthropogenic organic compounds

Human activity on Earth has resulted and is still resulting in a large number of organic compounds now used in our daily life spreading into the environment. Thus, the global annual production of chemicals increased from about 1 million t in 1930 to 400 million t in 2001. In the late 1960s the EU decided to produce a list of all chemicals (chemical entities) on the European market. The published list of compounds marketed between 1 January 1971 and September 1981, entitled the *European Inventory of Existing Commercial Chemical Substances* (ELINCS), was produced by the European Chemicals Bureau (part of the European Commission's Joint Research Centre in Ispra, Italy). The list includes 100,106 substances, most of which are organic in nature!

Recognizing that most of these compounds have never been tested for their biological effects and pressed by the facts that: (i) the incidence of, for example, testicular cancer in young men; and (ii) of allergies has increased significantly over the last decades; and (iii) links have been reported between reproductive and developmental effects and endocrine-disrupting substances in wildlife populations, the EU decided that new legislation concerning the control of chemicals in our environment was needed. Hence, a white paper, entitled *Strategy for a future Chemicals Policy* (Commission of the European Communities, Brussels, 27.2.2001, COM (2001) 88 Final), was produced. The white paper led to a continuous political process, which ended with the approval of the REACH (Registration, Evaluation and Authorisation of Chemicals) legislation (about 700 pages) in 2007. During the next 11 years, the newly established European Chemicals Agency in Helsinki shall evaluate all chemicals on the European market.

With these facts in mind it should not be difficult to understand that the structural pallet of anthropogenic organic compounds is indeed very broad. However, the number of compounds deliberately produced for the market is one thing; quite another is all the compounds that are formed as a result of, for example, degradation during combustion in incinerators and as side products during chemical processes.

Synthesized compounds

Industry synthesizes a high number of organic compounds for use in all sectors of our modern communities worldwide. Examples of use are as pesticides, drugs, cosmetics and toiletries, packaging materials, building materials and food additives. While food additives clearly end up in foods, it is also important to understand that most of the other compounds ultimately can – and most often will – find their way into the food chain. An example is plastic softeners used in food packaging materials that diffuse into food products.

Organic components of pollution

Pollution has many faces. Of course chemical pollution is not only made up of organic compounds; in particular, close to mining activities as well as other production facilities handling inorganic compounds in great amounts, severe inorganic pollution may also occur. Another example is the distribution along busy roads of lead oxides from the combustion of TEL in gasoline, as discussed earlier in Chapter 1. However, pollution by organic compounds deserves special attention for several reasons.

Organic pollution may consist of: (i) organic compounds produced for marketing and use, whether in industrial sectors other than chemical, in agriculture or by individual consumers; and (ii) intermediate products formed for example during a chemical synthesis. Compounds may leak continuously from badly designed (open) production facilities or from the waste handling at any later step after production. Compounds that have reached the market will often escape into the environment during waste handling or due to loss from more complicated equipments that face a breakdown, such as a refrigerator leaking cooling liquid. Organic pollution may, however, also consist of 'new' organic compounds formed during waste handling (especially by combustion in incinerators) or as a result of a general human activity such as just heating your own house.

A very good example of a class of compounds that have been and may be formed and spread to the environment in many different ways is the so-called *dioxins*. These are very toxic organic compounds that have already been mentioned several times and are dealt with in detail later in this book (see Chapter 20). Dioxins were identified for the first time as unwanted side products (impurities) from the synthesis of the very effective herbicide 2,4,5-T (2,4,5-trichlorophenoxyacetic acid), intensively used in the 1960s to kill broadleaved weeds in fields for the production of cereals. By this activity dioxins were spread to the fields together with the pesticide. The same herbicide was also used by the US Army, which sprayed it over Vietnamese forests during the Vietnam War (also known as the Second Indochina War, September 1959 to April 1975) to defoliate the trees in order to better be able to identify the North Vietnamese and Vietcong soldiers

hiding there. This activity led to a very heavy pollution with dioxins in certain provinces of Vietnam. Also, dioxins were spread in Italy around a pesticide production plant in the Italian town of Seveso (July 1976) when parts of the plant exploded. As time went by, research gradually showed that dioxins were also formed as a result of the burning of mixed waste materials, such as for example mixtures containing a wide range of different organic compounds together with the plastic (polymeric material) PVC (polyvinyl chloride). This observation led to legislative initiatives in many countries to reduce the formation of dioxins in incinerators by controlling the burning temperature to be higher than 800°C. Today dioxins are found all over the world, even far away from any incidents of accidental spot pollution or more widespread continuous leakage to the environment. This is due to the fact that these compounds are indeed very persistent (to both biological and non-biological degradation) and can be spread by the wind to places very distant from their production. With these characteristics the dioxins add themselves to the growing group of POPs which may be found everywhere. This is what makes organic pollutants so interesting and important to be aware of in a chemical food safety context.

3.5 Organometallic Compounds

Some organometallic (and organo-metalloid) compounds have already been mentioned. These are methylmercury, several different selenium-containing organic compounds such as dimethylselenide and selenoamino acids, and TEL. In general what makes these compounds of special interest is that they often prove to have different characteristics concerning absorption and distribution, and therefore also toxic profiles, with respect to the effects seen for the elemental metals and metalloids or their inorganic salts.

Thus, TEL for the leading of gasoline is a purely man-made synthetic compound which can be absorbed through the skin, a characteristic of interest mostly for work hygiene. However, it also (as described) gives rise to pollution with lead oxides ingested with feed and food. In contrast, methylmercury is biosynthesized by microorganisms, a fact not well known to mankind when we started synthesizing it in our laboratories for use as a fungicide. This use led, among others, to a fatal intoxication of many Iraqi people in the 1970s from the intake of grains meant for sowing but used for making bread instead. The grains had been surface treated with methylmercury to prevent fungal attack after being sowed and before sprouting. Gradually we stopped producing this and a number of other mercury-based fungicides, while other research during the same decades disclosed that nature itself actually produces methylmercury, and that this accumulates in for example fatty fish at a high trophic level. This latter fact is why many national food authorities today do not recommend that pregnant women eat too much of these products. Also, for the toxic metalloid arsenic, organometallic compounds are of interest to look at (as we shall see in Chapter 18).

3.6 Conclusion

To conclude this chapter we can – just as an appetizer – again take a look at mercury. Only for mercury is substantial absorption of the elemental metal, as such, seen under normal conditions. Thus, mercury vapour is readily absorbed into the bloodstream from the alveoli in the lungs, while absorption of the fluid metal when ingested is very restricted. Elemental mercury so absorbed from the lungs may pass the blood–brain barrier and affect the central nervous system (CNS), as may organometallic mercury (e.g. methylmercury). In contrast, inorganic mercury compounds mostly affect the kidneys. In general metals are absorbed from the intestines as ions if the salts ingested are water soluble to present the ions in the intestines.

Further Reading

Cope, W.G. (2004) Exposure classes, toxicants in air, water, soil, domestic and occupational settings. In: Hodgson, E. (ed.) *Modern Toxicology*, 3rd edn. John Wiley & Sons, Hoboken, New Jersey, pp. 33–48.

Herrchen, M. (2006) Pathways and behavior of chemicals in the environment. In: Duffus, J.H. and Worth, H.G.J. (eds) *Fundamental Toxicology*. RSC Publishing, Cambridge, UK, pp. 238–256.

Wilkinson, M. (2006) Ecotoxicity – effects of toxicants on ecosystems. In: Duffus, J.H. and Worth, H.G.J. (eds) *Fundamental Toxicology*. RSC Publishing, Cambridge, UK, pp. 257–272.

4 The Production and Processing Chain in Food Safety

- A number of examples are presented to give an idea of how a processing chain can look.
- Depending on the raw material and unit operations involved in the processing, potential contaminants vary.
- Raw materials in examples include cereals, root crops, grapes, pig liver, chicken meat and milk.
- Feed contaminants may be carried over to meat-based products.

4.1 Introduction

This chapter outlines the full production from plant to plate of a small number of ready-to-eat food products. For each the purpose is to point to stages in the production where unwanted chemical substances can enter the product or be formed in the product. Such a critical analysis of the full production chain for potential hazards actually is the basis for the development of what we will learn to know later as a full HACCP (Hazard Analysis Critical Control Points) plan. Each of the compounds or compound classes mentioned here is dealt with in detail, i.e. concerning their origin, way(s) into food and their toxicity, later in this book.

4.2 From Plant to Processed Plant-based Food

From cereals to crisp bread

Crisp bread is a baked cereal-based product originating in the Scandinavian region (Denmark, Finland, Iceland, Norway and Sweden). It is flat and very dry and will keep fresh for a long time if stored under dry conditions. Traditionally, crisp bread was made from wholemeal rye flour, salt and water only. Today, a lot of varieties are produced commercially, some of which are leavened with yeast or sourdough and contain wheat flour, spices and/or seeds such as sesame seeds. In the traditional unleavened crisp bread, bubbles are introduced mechanically (e.g. using rolling pins) or today by kneading the dough under pressure in an extruder. The sudden drop in pressure then causes water to evaporate, creating bubbles in the dough. Crisp bread is rolled out very thinly and baked at relatively high temperatures. Unwanted chemical substances in the final product here could include pesticide residues introduced by the flour(s), mycotoxins occurring in the flour(s) used and acrylamide formed during the baking process.

To exemplify the possibilities for the occurrence of pesticide residues let us for a while look to the UK. UK flours were tested twice for pesticide residues by the government authorities within the period between January 2000 and June 2005. The total number of samples tested was 72, which included six organic samples. Of these samples, 47 were white wheat flour, 24 were wholemeal or brown flour and one organic sample was of rye flour. The pesticides found were chlormequat (in 77% of the samples), pirimiphos-methyl (14%) and glyphosate (11%). Eighteen per cent of the samples had more than one pesticide residue. However, it should be strongly emphasized that in these two surveys no sample of flour had a residue that was above the legal limit.

The occurrence of residues was strongly dependent on the type of flour; thus:

- the proportion of samples in which chlormequat was found was higher for wholemeal/ brown flour than for white flour;
- the mean concentration of chlormequat in wholemeal/brown flour was more than twice that found in white flour;

- there were seven glyphosate occurrences, all of which were in wholemeal or brown flour;
- there were nine pirimiphos-methyl occurrences, seven of which were in wholemeal or brown flour; and
- 13 samples contained more than one pesticide, 11 of which were wholemeal or brown flour.

With regard to mycotoxins, both OTA and the so-called *trichothecenes* often contaminate cereals under temperate growth conditions. However, since we are dealing here with a product often based on rye, it is only natural to mention that rye especially can be contaminated by the toxic schlerotia of the fungus *Claviceps purpuria* 'ergot'. These contain the toxic so-called *ergot alkaloids*. A survey from 2008 including 24 unknown rye flour samples from Danish mills showed that these contained on average 46 mg of total alkaloids per kilogram, with a maximum content of 234 mg kg^{-1}. The most common ergot alkaloids found were ergotamine and ergocryptine.

The carcinogenic and neurotoxic substance acrylamide can be formed during heat processing of starch-rich food products in particular. In addition to starch the presence of the amino acid asparagine also seems to be crucial for the reaction, leading to the formation of acrylamide. At the present time intense research and development activities are ongoing in order to reduce the resulting concentration in the final marketed products. Crisp bread is one of the products in which acrylamide concentrations have been found to be high relative to many other generally consumed food products. This has prompted industries to develop methods to reduce this content. As an example one can mention the commercialization of an asparaginase by the international enzyme producer Novozymes. Company trials carried out in its bakeries and in industry showed that this product, Acrylaway®, can reduce acrylamide by up to 90% in crisp bread. Also, the company states that no changes in the taste and appearance of the crisp bread occur.

From cassava roots to 'garri' ('gari')

'Garri' is a fermented dry food product with a long shelf-life produced after harvest of the very perishable, starchy tuber cassava root, from the plant *Manihot esculenta*. Cassava roots form the staple food (source of energy) for approximately 800 million people worldwide. The plant originates in the Amazonian region of South America, but today cassava is grown in all tropical regions nourishing hundreds of millions in Africa and elsewhere. 'Garri' is made from cassava tubers that have been peeled, washed and grated to produce mash. Different methods exist for the further processing. In one of these the mash is put into a non-waterproof bag and allowed to ferment for 1 or 2 days, while weights are placed on the bag to press the water out. During this part of the processing pH is decreasing as a result of lactic acid fermentation, which gradually becomes dominating. The fermented dewatered mash is then sieved (or sifted) and roasted by heating in a bowl. During the roasting palm oil may be added to produce so-called 'yellow garri' instead of the white quality. The resulting dry granular 'garri' can be stored for long periods and used in several ways, such as to make 'eba', a pastry made by soaking 'garri' in hot water, or 'kokoro', a common snack food in Nigeria made from a paste of maize flour mixed with 'garri' and sugar and deep-fried.

Cassava contains in all its parts the compounds linamarin and lotaustralin, which liberate the toxic chemical entity hydrogen cyanide (HCN) upon processing and chewing. The glucosides are stored in the plant cell, while a β-glucosidase (linamarase) able to hydrolyse these is bound to the cell wall. When the plant tissues are damaged as a result of chewing/processing, the linamarase comes into contact with the glucosides and the process of degradation takes place. Linamarin and lotaustralin thus are *cyanogenic glucosides* and their degradation to HCN involves cyanogenic intermediates in the form of cyanohydrins (α-hydroxynitriles). Together the glucosides, the cyanohydrins and HCN – all of which are toxic – may be termed *cyanogens*. The toxicity seen after consumption includes acute poisoning, which can be fatal. Also some studies have shown a strong association between a monotonous diet on insufficiently processed cassava and the CNS disease konzo, which gives rise to walking disabilities. Konzo mostly affects women of childbearing age and children over 2 years of age and is persistent in, for example, Mozambique and Tanzania.

Cassava cultivars are classified as sweet (cool) or bitter depending on whether the tubers may be eaten without any prior processing or not. The bitter taste of the tubers has been shown to correspond with higher levels of linamarin (and lotaustralin). Cassava is the only domesticated staple crop for which a significant part of the edible production is toxic. In areas where cassava is a main staple crop, bitter and toxic cultivars often are preferred, whereas sweet (cool) cultivars abound in areas where cassava plays a secondary staple role.

All cassava-consuming societies have developed and adopted effective processing methods to reduce the potential toxicity of the root tubers upon consumption. Of these methods the production of 'garri' is among the most effective, giving rise to a safe and easy-to-store product with a long shelf-life. The reduction of the original content of cyanogenic glucosides in the roots during the production of 'garri' is due to: (i) the grating, which brings together the linamarase and the glucosides to start hydrolysis; (ii) the dewatering, where most of the remaining glucosides together with the HCN formed leave the mash; and (iii) the roasting, during which the remaining cyanohydrins and HCN leave the product by evaporation.

'Garri' is produced commercially in many countries in West Africa and exported to most European countries among others.

From grapes to wine

Several moulds can develop on grapes. These include *Botrytis cinerea*, which is responsible for the disease 'grey root', and species of *Alternaria*, *Cladosporium*, *Fusarium*, *Aspergillus* and *Penicillium*. Analysis conducted in 1997 and 1998 showed that wines could contain significant levels of the mycotoxin OTA, a nephrotoxic substance leading to irreversible damage of the kidneys, as can cereals, coffee, beer and cocoa. OTA is synthesized by *Aspergillus* and *Penicillium* species. Experiments in France in 2001 proved that *Aspergillus carbonarius* was the absolute most important source of OTA formation in grapes. The fungus establishes itself at a very early stage of the development of the grapes on the wine plant. It penetrates into the berry through already existing skin damage and starts its OTA production.

Today we know that for several groups of European consumers cereals are responsible for the main OTA burden (45–50% of average intake), while wine is responsible for the second largest contribution (10–20% of average intake). According to several analyses carried out in Europe since the middle of the 1990s, certain wines and grape juices at that time contained up to $10\,\mu g$ OTA l^{-1}. Within France it has been demonstrated that Mediterranean wines are more affected by OTA than wines from

other regions. Similarly, broader surveys have shown that wine produced in Europe varies in incidence and concentration of the toxin OTA, higher contents being found in wines from southern regions, increasing in the order white < rosé < red. Later investigations of wines produced in Chile and Argentina have indicated that these may contain lower levels.

4.3 From Plant to Animal Products

From feed to pig liver pâté

In modern agriculture most pigs are produced using very effective methods of reproduction and extremely intensive methods ensuring optimal growth rates. The composition of the feedstuff with regard to nutrients varies according to the animal's age; however, the single components used to obtain the desired composition also vary depending on the prices of the different raw materials.

Barley is often used as a component in the feeding of pigs. The mycotoxin OTA produced by *Aspergillus* and *Penicillium* fungi is a common contaminant of barley and may occur in unacceptable levels in cool wet conditions, as reported for example from the state of Alberta, Canada. OTA produces depressed appetite and reduced growth rate in pigs. At concentrations greater than 5 to 10 ppm, a number of conditions may arise such as impaired kidney function, necrosis of lymph nodes and fatty liver changes.

Barley by-products are alternative feeding supplies for animal production including swine feed. In a recent survey from Brazil, maize, brewers' grains (barley by-product) and finished swine feed samples were collected from different factories. Fungal counts were higher than 2.8×10^4 CFU g^{-1}. *Fusarium*, *Aspergillus* and *Penicillium* genera were isolated at high levels. About 25% of the isolates produced from 9 to $116\,\mu g$ OTA kg^{-1} *in vitro*. Maize samples (44%) were contaminated with $42–224\,\mu g$ OTA kg^{-1}. Finished feed (31%) and brewers' grains samples (13%) were contaminated with $36–120\,\mu g$ OTA kg^{-1} and $28–139\,\mu g$ OTA kg^{-1}, respectively.

The feeding of pigs with OTA-contaminated material for finishing before slaughter may lead to the development of so-called *porcine mould nephrosis*. The kidneys are swollen and pale. This condition must be recognized during meat inspection at the slaughterhouse, since the liver especially will also contain unacceptably high levels of this nephrotoxic substance. Since OTA is also relatively stable towards heat treatments, such carry-over from feedstuffs to the pig liver will also mean a risk for contamination of highly processed food products made from liver, for example, pig liver pâté produced industrially in high amounts in certain countries.

From feed to chicken meat

Chickens may be kept on the basis that they find their food themselves by pecking around the farm or they may be produced using much more intensive setups. Especially in certain regions of the world a substantial part of their feed could be cottonseed or cottonseed press cakes (meal) from the expression of cotton oil. Cotton plants (*Gossypium* spp.) are grown in dry climates at temperatures between 11 and 25°C in Asia and Africa as well as in North and South America, and are used for production of the raw material for cotton cloth and cottonseed oil. The total annual production of cotton in 2007/2008 was about $46{\times}10^6$ t from about 35 million ha, principally in the People's Republic of China and India (31 and 23% of the global production, respectively).

When the fibres have been removed, the seeds undergo further processing to remove the oil by crushing and/or solvent extraction. The remaining meal is used as a feed material because of the high protein content. However, non-processed whole cottonseeds, as well as processed cottonseed meal, may contain large amounts of free gossypol, which may cause adverse and toxic effects if used as a

feedstuff. Gossypol is an intensely yellow compound that is insoluble in water and soluble in organic solvents and fats. Because of the presence of the polyhydroxylated aromatic aldehyde moieties in the molecule, gossypol exhibits complex tautomerism (Fig. 4.1), which influences its chemical reactions. The two forms (+)-gossypol and (−)-gossypol generally coexist in the cotton plant, usually with a slight predominance of the (+)-form.

Gossypol shows a variety of biological actions. Signs of gossypol toxicity are similar in all animals and include laboured breathing and anorexia. Acute toxicity has been shown in the heart, lung, liver and blood cells, resulting in increased erythrocyte fragility. Post-mortem findings include generalized oedema and congestion of lungs and liver, fluid-filled thoracic and peritoneal cavities, and degeneration of heart fibres. Reproductive toxicity is seen particularly in males, where gossypol affects sperm motility, inhibits spermatogenesis and depresses sperm counts. Ruminants are less sensitive to gossypol than non-ruminants.

The presence of gossypol has been demonstrated in muscle tissue from broilers fed cottonseed-derived materials. In 2008 EFSA published a risk assessment on possible problems with the occurrence of gossypol in feedstuffs. The assessment showed that gossypol concentrations in tissues from broiler chickens fed a diet containing the maximum permitted level of free gossypol in cottonseed meal and the maximum recommended inclusion rate (2.5%) in feed for poultry (30 mg kg^{-1}) will mean that average human consumers can occasionally be

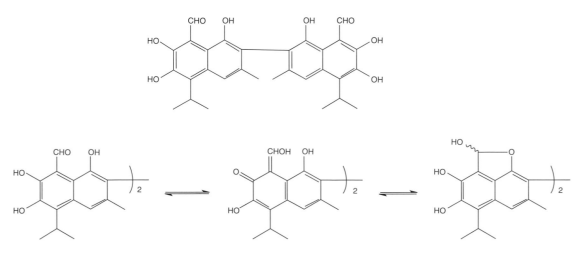

Fig. 4.1. Tautomeric forms of gossypol.

exposed to 0.0036–0.036 mg gossypol kg^{-1} BW day^{-1}, whereas for high consumers occasional exposure would range from 0.01 to 0.06 mg kg^{-1} BW day^{-1}. This is not regarded as being a problem. However, the risk assessment also states that 'in some developing countries, live stock is to a large extent fed with cottonseed products with high levels of gossypol and its transfer to edible tissues might represent a hazard for human health'.

From feed to dairy products (yoghurt)

Man has been making yoghurt for at least 4500 years. The name is derived from the Turkish word *yoğurt*, and is related to *yoğurmak* = to knead and *yoğun* = dense or thick. Today it is a common food product throughout the world, a nutritious dairy product rich in protein, calcium, riboflavin, vitamin B$_6$ and vitamin B$_{12}$. Yoghurt is produced by bacterial fermentation of milk. Fermentation of the milk lactose produces lactic acid, which acts on milk protein to give yoghurt its texture and its characteristic tang. Yoghurt is produced using a culture of two bacteria, *Lactobacillus delbrueckii* subsp. *bulgaricus* and *Streptococcus salivarius* subsp. *thermophilus*.

Unwanted chemical substances in the final product here could include the mycotoxin AFM$_1$. In the EU legislation that sets the maximum accepted levels for unwanted substances in feedstuffs, the lowest level found is that for the mycotoxin AFB$_1$ in feedstuffs for dairy cows. This is due to the fact that this extremely toxic and strongly carcinogenic compound is metabolized by the cow to form the almost as toxic compound AFM$_1$, of which a fraction is excreted into the milk. Hence, we immediately see that a well-functioning control for the occurrence of aflatoxins in feedstuffs as well as in raw milk is crucial.

4.4 From Water Quality to Shellfish Dish

Water quality is important for the final quality of the shellfish (molluscs and crustaceans) that live and grow in the water. Thus, shellfish accumulate arsenic present in the water and furthermore they may contain toxic levels of a number of different algal toxins (marine biotoxins) concentrated as a result of their filter feeding. The latter is the reason why state/regional authorities can close fishing/production areas if an algal bloom is occurring or if the level of such algal toxins has been found to be too high in shellfish from the area.

4.5 Conclusion

A thorough understanding of the existing interrelationships in the overall production chain from plant to plate or meat to meal is crucial for the success of our work to ensure a good chemical food safety situation.

Further Reading

Parker, R. (2003) *Introduction to Food Science*. Delmar-Thomson Learning, Albany, New York.

Singh, B.P. (ed.) (2010) *Industrial Crops and Uses*. CABI Publishing, Wallingford, UK.

Varnam, A.H. and Sutherland, J.P. (1995) *Meat and Meat Products: Technology, Chemistry and Microbiology*. Chapman & Hall, London.

5 Introduction to ADME (Absorption, Distribution, Metabolism and Excretion)

- Here we define the term xenobiotic.
- We define an outer surface with regard to our body.
- We further define the terms absorption, distribution, metabolism and excretion.
- Finally we look at the definitions of local versus systemic poisoning/intoxication.

Our daily activities at home, in our neighbourhood and at work constantly brings us into contact with a large number of chemical substances. Some of these are well known to our body, such as the mixture of gases we breathe and call 'air', the water we swim in and the amino acids that the proteins in our food are degraded into before being absorbed into the bloodstream. Others are foreign to our body such as the plant alkaloid caffeine present in the coffee and tea we drink during the day and the polycyclic aromatic hydrocarbon (PAH) benzo[a]pyrene formed through pyrolysis (decomposition of a substance by heat) in the engine of our car, present in the smoke from our cigarette and maybe on the surface of the steak we have grilled a little too much.

While our body has distinct routes for the uptake, distribution, interconversion (metabolism) and excretion of the chemical compounds that make up our cells and tissues, things are different when it comes to foreign compounds. Such compounds we often term *xenobiotic compounds*, or in short just *xenobiotics*. This definition includes both natural and man-made compounds; others prefer to restrict the term to man-made compounds only.

No organism on Earth can risk being able to deal only with its own constituents. This is due to the fact that, although the barriers which protect an organism from the outside world are astonishingly effective, they are not perfect. Animals (including man) are protected by the skin, the mucous membranes in the eyes, nose and mouth, bronchioles and lungs, and by the surfaces that our mechanically degraded food meets in the stomach and the intestines. As we immediately understand from this, no chemical compound has entered our body before it has penetrated one of these barriers; thus, the gut surface with its villi and microvilli is also an outer surface of our body.

All of the barriers mentioned have several functions besides being barriers. The understanding of this is crucial when analysing the possibilities for a given compound to pass a given barrier. Thus, the skin has sweat glands and hair follicles, structures that can be entrance ports; the pulmonary alveoli – of which each human lung contains about 300 million, each wrapped in a fine mesh of capillaries covering about 70% of its area – are specially designed to allow effective gas exchange; and the surface of the small intestine is designed to allow uptake of nutrients essential to our survival.

A toxic substance can act locally at the site of exposure. Thus, an acidic or alkaline solution can irritate or corrode the skin or a mucous membrane, while several salts of different metals such as copper and lead can cause cell necrosis in the intestines upon ingestion. The latter effect is due to the action of the metal ions binding to thiol (–SH) groups in enzymes essential to the function of the borderline cells. When discussing chemical food safety we are lucky only to have to focus on the oral intake of xenobiotic substances and the effects that may follow such an intake. Hence, the following discussion looks at the possible local effects on the gastrointestinal tract and the effects caused by the substance after its absorption into the bloodstream and further distribution to intercellular and/or intracellular spaces throughout the body.

The term *absorption* describes the process of the transfer of the parent compound from the gastrointestinal tract into the general circulation. However, it should be noted that a number of chemicals will be metabolized or transformed during this passage, so that little parent compound may reach the general circulation. After absorption the element or compound can act directly on one or more of the blood components. For example, this can be by binding to the cell membrane of erythrocytes (red blood cells), thereby destabilizing them and shortening their lifespan. Such a mechanism of toxicity is known for the heavy metal lead and for a number of natural plant constituents grouped under the name of saponins. However, apart from such local effects on the elements of the circulating blood, the mere presence of a compound in the blood normally does not lead to a toxic response; one exception is the binding of carbon monoxide to haemoglobin, which causes poisoning.

A compound absorbed in the stomach or in the small intestine is led by the portal vein directly to the liver where it may be partly or fully metabolized to another compound, the so-called *first-pass effect*. However, for most compounds a substantial fraction will pass the liver with its genuine structure intact and enter systemic circulation. In contrast, compounds absorbed already in the oral cavity enter the general circulation directly. An example

of a toxic compound easily absorbed from the oral cavity is the plant alkaloid nicotine, a weak base with a pK_a of 8.5.

Apart from the poisonous effects caused directly to the blood, to be poisonous systemically in a broader sense the toxic compound must leave the vascular space and enter the intercellular or intracellular spaces or both. Movement through membranes is required for this *distribution* to the various tissues of the body, including the target sites for toxicity of the compound in question. This transport of the absorbed compound can broadly be divided into transcellular and paracellular processes (Fig. 5.1).

When a compound has reached a specific tissue and the cells characterizing this tissue, it either may leave it again relatively soon with the bloodstream or it may be stored to a great extent. The latter is the case for fluorine and lead in bone and for a number of highly lipophilic compounds such as the POPs, which include the old insecticide DDT and the dioxins in the fat deposits of the body.

Animals have developed a number of general biochemical routes for the *metabolism* (transformation) of xenobiotics entering the body. All cells have a metabolizing capacity; however, the liver is by far the most important player in this game. In general we divide the process of metabolism into the phase I reactions, i.e. the reactions caused by oxidative and reductive enzymes, and the phase II reactions, which include a number of

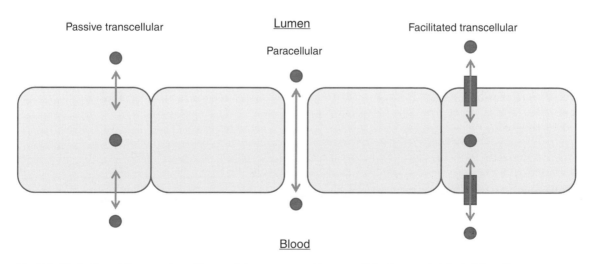

Fig. 5.1. Illustration of the meaning of transcellular as opposed to paracellular transport. Adapted from Tozer and Rowland (2006).[1]

reactions where conjugative enzymes metabolize the compounds by attaching (conjugating) a more polar molecule to the original toxin or one of its phase I metabolites, thereby increasing the water solubility. While the metabolism is meant to detoxify and ease the excretion of a compound, sometimes the general tools available for the organism are not sufficient. Thus, some compounds are transformed into much more toxic molecular species; this is the case, for example, for the mycotoxin AFB_1 that often occurs in nuts and groundnuts but also in different cereals, especially maize (corn) grown in tropical regions.

The final removal of a xenobiotic compound from the body is the result of the two processes of metabolism and *excretion* working together. A compound may remain totally unchanged, i.e. 100% is excreted unmetabolized, or it may be excreted as a mixture of the original compound together with one or more metabolites. For very many compounds and their metabolites excretion is mainly by filtration into the pre-urine formed by the kidneys (renal excretion). However, other routes of excretion exist. Thus, a number of compounds are secreted by the liver into the bile and from there into the small intestine. While some are reabsorbed here (enterohepatic circulation), others such as the toxic plant constituents termed cardiac glycosides are excreted with the faeces without being reabsorbed. Also a compound or its metabolites may be excreted by the pulmonary route, i.e. with the expired air. This is seen for selenium, which in certain cases and to a certain degree may be excreted by the pulmonary route as dimethyl-selenide. Other compounds are to a smaller or greater degree excreted with sweat or lost together with dead skin cells.

Already here during the introduction to ADME it is important to stress that both the intestinal absorption (with respect to the degree of absorption) and the metabolism of many compounds differ between species. This is important to be aware of when selecting an animal species for a toxicity test if the result is intended for extrapolation to man, as is often the case.

Note

[1] Tozer, T.N. and Rowland, M. (2006) *Introduction to Pharmacokinetics and Pharmacodynamics – The Quantitative Basis of Drug Therapy*. Lippincott Williams & Wilkins, Philadelphia, Pennsylvania.

Further Reading

Craig, C.R. and Stitzel, R.E. (2004) *Modern Pharmacology with Clinical Applications*. Lippincott Williams & Wilkins, Philadelphia, Pennsylvania.

Hodgson, E. (ed.) (2004) *Modern Toxicology*, 3rd edn. John Wiley & Sons, Hoboken, New Jersey.

6 Absorption and Distribution of Chemical Compounds

- Different routes of exposure and corresponding absorption are presented.
- Mechanisms of absorption after consumption are described.
- Mechanisms of distribution and the result are discussed.

6.1 Exposure and Absorption Routes

Concentrating on one specific compound which could, for example, be a phthalate, we can ask ourselves from where and in which situations we are exposed to this compound, the level of exposure and the route of absorption in each case.

Phthalates such as butylbenzylphthalate (BBP), dibutylphthalate (DBP), bis(2-ethylhexyl) phthalate (DEHP), di-isononylphthalate (DINP) and di-isodecylphthalate (DIDP) are widely used as plasticizers in various polymers (e.g. PVC). Such soft PVCs are found in a range of consumer products including wall and floor coverings, furnishings, car interiors, clothing, plastic pipes and toys. In addition phthalates are also applied to paints and lacquers, adhesives and sealants, and printing inks. Since the phthalates are not chemically bound in the polymers, migration or emission of the phthalates from the product to the environment is likely to occur and the phthalates are thereby widespread in the environment.

The phthalates can be absorbed upon inhalation, by the oral route and through the skin (dermal absorption). For example, sheets of PVC film containing 40% (w/w) DEHP applied on the shaved back of rats gave rise to an absorption rate of $0.24\,\mu g$ DEHP cm^{-2} h^{-1}. This scenario is by no means unrealistic since three out of four disposable examination gloves investigated in a Danish study contained phthalates with contents between 23 and 42% (w/w). Other phthalates may have different dermal absorption rates; DIDP is absorbed through the skin about ten times less than DEHP.

Knowing that sealants softened with phthalates could be used in jars for baby food (whether allowed or not), that phthalates could be found in toys that a small child licks and that phthalates can be inhaled from the air as coming from wall or floor coverings, the Danish Veterinary and Food Administration in 2003 made an estimation of the human exposure to selected phthalates. As an example taken from the report, Table 6.1 shows that a child aged 6–12 months is estimated to be exposed to and absorb DEHP by the dermal, the pulmonary and the oral routes.

In the next section we discuss only oral absorption, but with the example just discussed in mind it is important always to analyse whether a person or a population is or may be exposed by other routes and from other sources than food and beverages.

6.2 Oral Intake and Absorption

General mechanisms of absorption

Upon oral intake a chemical compound can be absorbed from the oral cavity (as already mentioned for nicotine in Chapter 5), the stomach, the small intestine and/or the large intestine. In general the process of absorption is one of passing the membrane between the gastrointestinal lumen with its contents and the lumen of the blood vessels. Such a membrane is made up of one or more layers of cells, meaning that passing through a cell or filtering through a pore between two cells is what the molecule must do in order to be 'absorbed'. The general cell membrane (plasma membrane) consists of a phospholipid bilayer

Table 6.1. The combined oral, inhalatory and dermal exposure to bis(2-ethylhexyl)phthalate via all evaluated pathways for children aged 6–12 months.

	Exposure ($\mu g\ kg^{-1}\ BW\ day^{-1}$)		
	Oral	Inhalation	Dermal
Toys	200.3	–	9.0
Baby food	23.5	–	–
Indoor air	–	1.9	–
Via environment (maximum local)	50.0	–	–
Via environment (measured local)	1.7	–	–
Via environment (measured food)	13.0	–	–
Total	273.8	1.9	9.0

in which protein molecules and cholesterol are embedded. Both globular and helical proteins traverse the bilayer. The 'tails' of α-helix proteins exposed on the outer surface of the cell membrane may have oligosaccharide side chains attached (Fig. 6.1).

Absorption from the stomach

The stomach has a rich blood supply and its contents are in close contact with the epithelial lining of the gastric mucosa. Due to these factors the stomach is a potential site for absorption even though the primary function is not absorption. The low pH of the gastric contents (pH 1–2) can dramatically affect the degree of ionization of a compound with acidic or basic properties, however. Thus, a weak base such as most alkaloids (e.g. caffeine) will be highly protonated in the gastric juice, and consequently absorption across lipid membranes of the stomach will be slow. Due to the fact that stomach emptying time can vary depending on the volume of ingested material, type and viscosity of the meal, body position

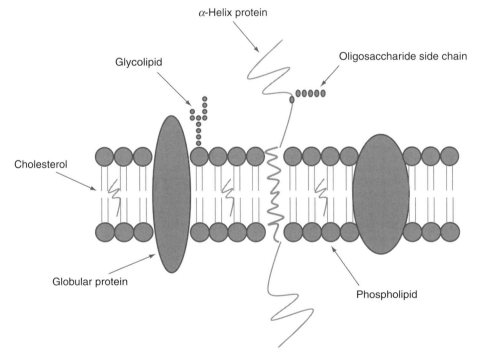

Fig. 6.1. The plasma membrane: overview of the general structure.

and others factors, the extent of gastric absorption will vary between and within persons.

Absorption from the small intestine

The intestine may be broadly divided into the small and the large intestine as separated by the ileocaecal valve. The epithelial lining of the small intestine is composed of a single layer of cells called enterocytes. The intestinal surface area, which in the small intestine is very high due to the occurrence of many villi and microvilli, decreases per unit length from the duodenum and to the rectum. Active and facilitated transport systems as well as proteolytic and metabolic enzymes are distributed variably along

the intestine as such, most often in restricted regions. Most absorption of xenobiotics occurs in the proximal jejunum, i.e. in the first one to two metres, in an adult human being. Since food intake (volume and nature) can affect the intestinal transit time, food already, for this reason, may have an influence on the total absorption (absorption fraction) of a given xenobiotic compound. This is especially true for slowly dissolved compounds ingested as particles.

The transport of compounds across the membrane can occur by mechanisms such as: (i) active transport; (ii) facilitated transport; (iii) ion-pair transport; (iv) endocytosis; (v) filtration; and (vi) diffusion (Fig. 6.2).

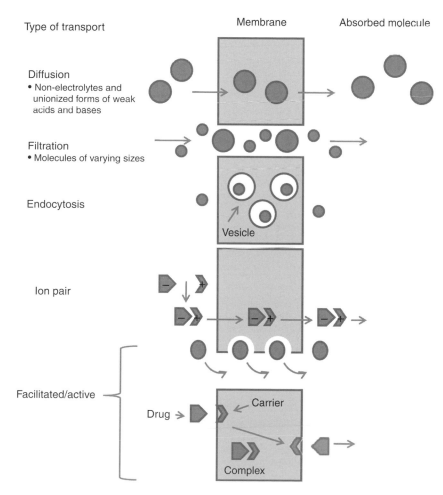

Fig. 6.2. Schematic overview of the different mechanisms of transport across membranes. Adapted from Craig and Stitzel (2004).[1]

Absorption and Distribution of Chemical Compounds

- *Active transport*: active transport refers to the energy-dependent movement of compounds across membranes, often against their concentration gradient. Active transport requires energy in the form of ATP. According to one model for active transport, the molecule combines with a specific mobile carrier on one side of the membrane. The complex formed then diffuses to the other side of the membrane and dissociates. Compounds that inhibit energy production such as cyanide and fluoride will impair active transport.
- *Facilitated transport*: this form of transport also takes advantage of a protein carrier-mediated mechanism that shows saturability and selectivity. However, since the movement is from regions of higher to regions of lower concentration, no energy is needed – the driving force is the concentration gradient itself.
- *Ion-pair transport*: in order to explain the absorption of highly ionized compounds such as certain sulfonic acids and quaternary ammonium compounds from the gastrointestinal tract, a so-called ion-pair transport, where the compound combines reversibly with such endogenous compounds as mucin in the gastro-

intestinal lumen and diffuses through the lipid membrane, has been postulated.
- *Endocytosis*: in endocytosis the cell takes up the molecule inside a vesicle derived from the plasma membrane.
- *Filtration*: filtration depends on the existence of aqueous channels in the membrane. The hypothetical diameter of these pores has been determined as around 7 Å. This allows small hydrophilic compounds of molecular weight less than 100 (e.g. ethylene glycol) to filter through the membrane along a pressure/concentration gradient.
- *Diffusion*: it is generally believed that most toxicants and drugs pass through membranes (including those of the intestinal epithelial lining) by passive diffusion of the unionized moiety. The diffusion occurs down their concentration gradient and the rate of diffusion depends on the lipid–water partition coefficient. This being said, it must however be emphasized that recent intensive research concerning the oral absorption of a number of drugs has disclosed that some actually are actively absorbed or pass the membrane facing the intestine lumen by facilitated transport

Box 6.1. Facilitated transport of drugs – and maybe toxins?

The compound called gaboxadol (Fig. 6.3) was developed as a potential new active agent in 'sleeping tablets' by Lundbeck and Merck. In March 2007 the companies cancelled work on the drug, according to them due to safety concerns and the failure of an efficacy trial. The compound acts on the γ-aminobutyric acid (GABA) system. Intensive research has shown that this compound is transported through the first cell membrane of the intestinal epithelium by the PAT1 transporter. PAT1 is an amino acid transport protein that facilitates uptake not only of small neutral amino acids

such as glycine, proline and alanine, but also of some amino acid-like compounds such as the osmolytes sarcosine, betaine and taurine and the neurotransmitter GABA, and actually also some other drugs, namely D-cycloserine (syn. oxamycin, a broad-spectrum antibiotic) and vigabatrine (an antiepileptic drug).

PAT1 is a proton-coupled amino acid transporter, meaning that every time it moves one molecule across the membrane it also transports one proton the same way. This is quite unusual since most other characterized transporters of amino acids or neurotransmitters are coupled to the transport of sodium or chloride ions.

After proteins eaten have been hydrolysed in the intestine to small peptides they are transported across the intestinal wall and into the bloodstream by the human intestinal proton-coupled oligopeptide transporter hPEPT1. This has been shown also to transport penicillins and cephalosporins.

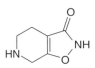

Fig. 6.3. Gaboxadol.

(Box 6.1). Of course, such knowledge opens the question of whether some toxins today believed to passively diffuse are also taken up this way; only time will show.

Absorption from the large intestine

Relatively little absorption occurs from the large intestine due to both a considerably smaller surface area and the fact that the content is relatively more solid in nature, which impedes diffusion of a compound from the content to the mucosa.

Degradation of compounds in the digestive tract

A number of toxic compounds may start to undergo structural changes in the gastrointestinal tract.

A classic example is the conversion of the artificial sweetener cyclamate, a white crystalline compound that is about 30 times sweeter than sucrose, to cyclohexylamine. As a commercial sweetener cyclamate is the sodium or calcium salt of cyclamic acid (cyclohexanesulfamic acid; Fig. 6.4). The sweetener is banned in the USA but allowed in the EU (E952) with its main uses being beverages (400 mg l^{-1}) and certain solid foods (250–1000 mg kg^{-1}). This use is based on an EU Acceptable Daily Intake (ADI) of 7 mg kg^{-1} BW, as calculated in a risk assessment that takes into account the possible effects of the cyclohexyl amine formed. Cyclohexylamine can induce testicular atrophy and a number of studies have shown that different individuals form more or less cyclohexylamine depending on their intestinal microflora.

Other important examples can be found within the group of toxic glycosides of plant origin. Glycosides can be hydrolysed to their aglycone (genin) and sugar part(s). Such hydrolysis is favoured in the lower part of the intestines including the large intestine, where a number of microorganisms may posses the ability to hydrolyse a given glycosidic toxin. Examples of such compounds and the possible consequences of their hydrolysis include the following:

- Cyanogenic glycosides, which are present in a number of plant raw materials used in food and for condiments and beverages, such as bitter almond, seeds of apricot and peach, flaxseed, bamboo shoots, lima beans, and the tuberous roots and leaves of cassava. Upon hydrolysis of the cyanogenic glycosides, α-hydroxynitriles (cyanohydrins) are formed. Under the near-to-neutral pH in the terminal part of the digestive tract, these spontaneously degrade to release the toxic constituent HCN, which is absorbed.
- Vicine and convicine occurring in the faba bean (*Vicia faba* L.). The aglycones (divicine, isouramil) of these glucosides are absorbed in the intestine after hydrolysis has taken place. This can facilitate the development of haemolytic anaemia (favism) in individuals who have a (genetically determined) deficiency with regard to the enzyme G6PD.
- Cycasin present in the seeds of *Cycas* spp. can be converted to its aglycone, methylazoxymethanol. This compound is hepatotoxic and can induce demyelination with axonal swelling in the spinal cord and tumours. Cycasin occurs exclusively in the cycads, a relict group of ancient gymnosperms. The seeds of different *Cycas* spp. were traditionally eaten in Australia and on some neighbouring islands such as Guam.

Local effects of compounds on the digestive tract

A number of metal ions can irritate and corrode the intestinal mucosa as already mentioned in Chapter 5. In addition, some classes of organic compounds, mostly naturally occurring plant constituents, possess the ability to change the absorptive characteristics of the digestive tract, the small intestine in particular. These include the saponins and the lectins (phytohaemagglutinins; PHAs).

- Saponins (from the Latin *sapo* = soap) are low-molecular-weight secondary plant constituents containing either a tetracyclic steroidal or a

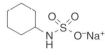

Fig. 6.4. Sodium cyclamate.

pentacyclic triterpenoid aglycone and one or more sugar chains. The compounds can form a stable foam (as can soap) in aqueous solutions. Traditionally, saponins were used as detergents, piscicides (fish poisons) and molluscicides (mollusc poisons), in addition to an industrial application as surface active agents. If present in food, saponins may cause toxic effects by a general membrane-disrupting property, which includes pore formation by an unknown mechanism. Thus, an investigation in young rats of the effect of the saponins from *Madhuca* spp. (used in feed) found toxicity to the absorptive cells of the intestinal mucosa, especially those near the tips of the villi. The concomitant intestinal inflammation caused an increased mucoid secretion from the goblet cells. At higher inclusion rates in the diet, the damage extended to deeper layers of the intestine.

- Lectins (PHAs) are sugar-binding proteins which are highly specific for their sugar moieties. They typically play a role in biological recognition phenomena involving cells. A number of detrimental effects of PHA on gut microbiota and physiology, such as reduced growth rates, loss of body weight, diarrhoea and epithelial hyperplasia, have been demonstrated in several animal species. Among food items, beans in particular are rich in PHAs. Several incidents of food poisoning have been reported after the intake of raw or little processed (red) kidney beans. PHAs such as those from red kidney bean have been reported to dose-dependently induce bacterial overgrowth in the intestine, which is associated with weight loss, malabsorption and villus damage. It has been suggested that PHAs increase the turnover of epithelial cells, promoting the expression of mannosylated receptor glycans on the gut surface and thus leading to increased adhesion and subsequent proliferation of mannose-sensitive type 1-fimbriated *Escherichia coli*.

6.3 Organ, Tissue and Cell Distribution of Compounds

When a xenobiotic compound has been absorbed into the bloodstream the process of distribution within the body starts immediately.

Distribution within the blood components

Nearly all compounds found in the vascular compartment are bound reversibly with one or more of the macromolecules in plasma. These plasma proteins include albumin, globulins, transferrin, caeruloplasmin, glycoproteins, and α- and β-lipoproteins. Acidic compounds often bind to albumin, while basic compounds frequently bind also to other plasma proteins such as different lipoproteins and to α_1-acid glycoprotein (α_1-AGP). The overall degree of protein binding has been investigated thoroughly for many drugs, which is why we know that it may vary to a great extent (Table 6.2).

Some compounds and elements distribute in an even more complicated manner within the blood. The toxic heavy metal lead is a very good example. It was observed relatively early on that lead distributes approximately 1:100 if one looks at the distribution of total lead between plasma and erythrocytes, respectively. That is, 99% of blood lead is bound to the erythrocytes. Of the about 1% in plasma, most is bound to albumin. Of the 99% in the erythrocytes most is found intracellularly bound to haemoglobin, in equilibrium with a very low concentration in the cell cytosol. However, observations of a high fragility of erythrocytes from workers exposed to lead resulted in further investigations of the erythrocyte membrane by electron microscopy and X-ray diffraction. The investigation showed that lead also binds to this membrane and that lead particles adhered to the external and internal surfaces of the human erythrocyte membrane can be observed, as can a disturbance of the lamellar organization of the membrane.

Table 6.2. The overall degree of protein binding of different drugs when occurring in the blood.

Compound (all drugs and all organic compounds)	Protein binding (approx. %)
Diemal	5
Digoxin	20
Fenemal	20
Sulfadiazin	40
Tiomebumal	65
Salicylic acid	70
Sulfametizol	85
Diazepam	96
Sulfadimetoxin	99

Distribution from the blood to other tissues and organs

The extent of protein binding will influence the distribution as well as excretion (rate of elimination), since only the unbound fraction can diffuse through the capillary wall, produce its systemic effects, be metabolized and be excreted. But to start we take a look at the distribution.

The rate at which a xenobiotic compound may enter (or leave) a specific tissue is governed by two main factors: (i) the ability of the compound to cross cell membranes; and (ii) the blood flow to the tissue in question (perfusion). Highly water-soluble compounds will in general distribute relatively slowly into the cells of body organs and tissues such as liver and muscle owing to their slow transfer from plasma and into these cells. The cells of the adipose tissue will not be a target for accumulation of such compounds. On the other hand, highly lipid-soluble chemical compounds may rapidly cross cell membranes. For such compounds this means that we often see the phenomenon that they rapidly accumulate (distribute to) the well-perfused tissues such as liver, muscle and lung, after which the compounds gradually redistribute to finally end up in the adipose tissue, which has a more restricted blood flow but the ability to store the compound 'dissolved' in the fatty matrix (Fig. 6.5).

The rate of the initial distribution can change, especially with changes in blood flow through an organ. Significant changes in perfusion are especially seen for the muscles (and the lungs) depending on the degree of physical activity. An overview of blood perfusion rates in adult humans are given in Table 6.3.

Certain compounds distribute to and accumulate in certain tissues to a high degree, as already mentioned. Thus, many lipophilic substances such as chlorinated pesticides (e.g. DDT) and pollutants (dioxins/PCBs), as well as metallo-organic compounds like methylmercury, sometimes may be found in very high concentrations indeed in the adipose tissue and/or in the lipid structures of the nervous system. For lead, strontium and fluorine, bone is the major site for storage. The storage is due to an exchange adsorption reaction between the toxic ions in the interstitial fluid and the hydroxyapatite crystals of bone mineral. Similarities in ion size and charge between F^- and OH^- mean that fluoride may replace hydroxyl,

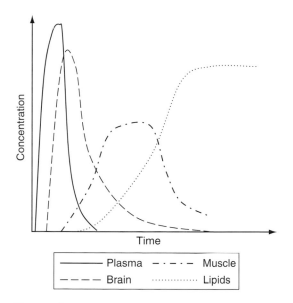

Fig. 6.5. Concentration of thiomebumal in different organs/tissues after intravenous injection as a function of time.

while calcium may be replaced by lead and strontium.

In general, toxicants stored in the adipose tissue or in the bone matter are of no great concern from a toxicological point of view. However, the plasma concentration of DDT or other stored lipophilic substances may suddenly rise sharply as a result of a rapid mobilization of fat following starvation. In this case, symptoms of acute intoxication may appear. Likewise, the ions stored in bone matter may be released by dissolution of bone crystals through osteoclastic activity.

While the occurrence of relatively high concentrations of lipophilic toxicants in the adipose tissue under normal conditions may not give rise to immediate concern, the situation is different when we talk about accumulation of such compounds in the peripheral and/or CNS.

The barriers

Three physiological barriers of major importance to the actual distribution of chemical compounds to specific organs exist. These are: (i) the blood–brain barrier; (ii) the placental barrier; and (iii) the blood–testis barrier. The barriers are different in structure and therefore must be dealt with separately.

Table 6.3. An overview of the blood perfusion rates in adult humans.

Tissue	Blood flow (l min⁻¹)	Perfusion rate (ml 100 g⁻¹ tissue min⁻¹)
Adipose	0.25	3
Brain	0.75	55
Heart	0.25	84
Kidney	1.23	350
Liver	1.55	85
Lung	5.40	400
Muscle	0.80	5
Skin	0.40	5

The blood–brain barrier

In contrast to the general situation, the capillary endothelial cells in the brain are tightly joined, leaving no or only few pores between the cells. This means that the capillary membrane between the plasma and the brain cells is much less permeable to water-soluble substances than is the membrane in other tissues. The toxicant has to pass through the capillary endothelium itself. A lack of vesicles in these cells further reduces their transport ability. Only compounds with a high lipid–water partition coefficient can penetrate this membrane, and compounds that are partly ionized will penetrate at considerably slower rates. A very good example is the toxic compound methylmercury, which enters the brain readily, in contrast to inorganic mercury compounds that cannot pass. In accordance with this pattern of distribution, methylmercury exerts its toxicity mainly to the CNS while the inorganic species of mercury are toxic to the kidney.

The placental barrier

The placental barrier impedes the transfer of toxicants to the fetus. The blood vessels of the fetus and the mother are separated by a number of tissue layers that collectively constitute the placental barrier. Actually this barrier differs anatomically between various animal species. In some species there is only one layer between fetal and maternal blood, while other species have up to six layers. Highly polar compounds do not pass the barrier readily while substances that are lipid-soluble cross with relative ease in accordance with their lipid–water partition coefficient and degree of ionization. As an example of a food-relevant compound for which the transfer is impeded one can look at the food colourant amaranth (Red No. 2), which is banned in the USA but allowed in Canada and the EU. For this compound the concentration in fetal blood is less than 0.1% that in the maternal blood. In contrast, the concentration of methylmercury may be higher in the developing fetal brain than in the maternal blood due to the facts that: (i) as a lipophilic compound, it can pass the placental barrier; and (ii) the fetal blood–brain barrier is less effective than the fully developed barrier.

The blood–testis barrier

The blood–testis barrier is not as easy to define morphologically as the two other barriers just mentioned. However, studies indicate that the barrier lies beyond the capillary endothelial cell and is most likely to be found at the specialized Sertoli–Sertoli cell junction. Evidence also is present for a special transporter protein, i.e. an ATP-dependent multidrug transporter efflux called 'the permeability glycoprotein' (Pgp), to be part of the barrier and its effect on different compounds.

6.4 Conclusion

Depending on the molecular structure and, in turn, the chemico-physical characteristics of a compound, it may or may not be absorbed after ingestion. The absorption fraction may vary depending on age (e.g. lead), on other compounds eaten simultaneously and even on the nutritional status of the individual. Some compounds may be degraded/metabolized in the intestines, examples being the artificial sweeteners cyclamate (already mentioned) and aspartame plus other compounds discussed above. Such a metabolism may result in the formation of either fewer or more toxic compounds. Depending on the same chemico-physical characteristics including molecular size and lipophilicity/hydrophilicity, a compound may either stay in the blood or be distributed to one or more organs and tissues within organs.

Note

[1] Craig, C.R. and Stitzel, R.E. (2004) *Modern Pharmacology with Clinical Applications*, 6th edn. Lippincott Williams & Wilkins, Philadelphia, Pennsylvania.

Further Reading

Klaassen, C.D. (2008) *Casarett & Doull's Toxicology: The Basic Science of Poison*, 7th edn. McGraw-Hill, New York, New York.

Lu, F.C. and Kacew, S. (2009) *Lu's Basic Toxicology: Fundamentals, Target Organs, and Risk Assessment*, 5th edn. Informa Healthcare, New York, New York.

Niesink, R.J.M., de Vries, J. and Hollinger, M.A. (1996). *Toxicology: Principles and Applications*. CRC Press, Boca Raton, Florida.

Tozer, T.N. and Rowland, M. (2006) *Introduction to Pharmacokinetics and Pharmacodynamics – The Quantitative Basis of Drug Therapy*. Lippincott Williams & Wilkins, Philadelphia, Pennsylvania.

Table 7.1. Overview of reactions catalysed by the cytochrome P450 (mixed function oxidase) system.

Type of reaction	Example
Aliphatic oxidation	n-Propylbenzene $\rightarrow$ 3-phenylpropan-1-ol
Aromatic hydroxylation	Naphthalene $\rightarrow$ naphthalene-1,2-epoxide $\rightarrow$ 1-naphthol + 2-naphthol
Epoxidation	The pesticide aldrin $\rightarrow$ dieldrin
Oxidative deamination	Amphetamine $\rightarrow$ phenylacetone
Oxidative N-dealkylation	Dimethylacetamide $\rightarrow$ monomethylacetamide
O-dealkylation	p-Nitroanisole $\rightarrow$ p-nitrophenol
S-dealkylation	Methitural $\rightarrow$ formaldehyde + S-demethyl methitural
N-oxidation	Trimethylamine $\rightarrow$ trimethylamine oxide
N-hydroxylation	Aniline $\rightarrow$ phenylhydroxylamine
P-oxidation	Diphenylmethylphosphine $\rightarrow$ diphenylmethylphosphine oxide
Sulfoxidation	Methiocarb $\rightarrow$ methiocarb sulfone
Desulfuration	Replacement of S by O in the insecticide parathion $\rightarrow$ paraoxon

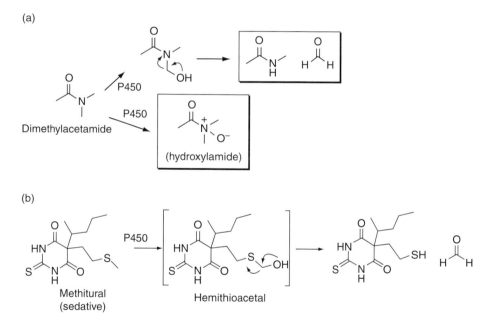

Fig. 7.1. (a) Alkyl amides are metabolized by oxidative N-dealkylation (top) or N-oxidation (bottom). Both reactions are catalysed by cytochrome P450. Here the example of dimethylacetamide is shown. (b) Oxidative S-dealkylation is not as common as the analogous oxidative N- or O-dealkylation but does occur as shown here for the drug methitural.

named FMO1–5. As with the cytochrome P450 enzymes, the FMOs are also located in the endo-plasmic reticulum, making up the so-called *micro-somes* upon subcellular fractionation.

The mechanism is that one oxygen atom from O_2 is incorporated into the substrate. A flavine hydroper-oxide is the putative intermediate in the process. This is attacked by the substrate nucleophile (Fig. 7.2).

FMO3 is the most important and is abundantly expressed by many tissues but mainly by the liver. The level of liver expression is around 60% that of cyto-chrome P4503A4. FMO1 is the main FMO found in the kidney, while FMO2 is found in the lungs. Several mutations coding for inactive FMO3 exist, resulting in an inability to metabolize endogenously generated trimethylamine to its N-oxide. Trimethylamine is then exhaled unchanged and is responsible for 'fish odour syndrome' in its sufferers.

The regional distribution in male Sprague–Dawley rat liver and kidney of FMO isoforms 1, 3 and 4 was

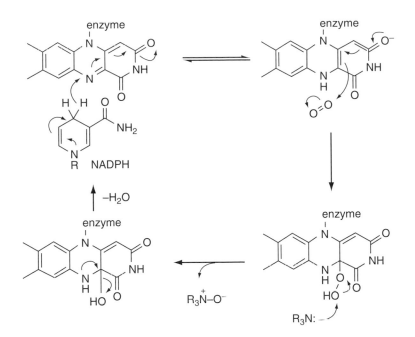

Fig. 7.2. The reaction mechanism for monooxidation of an amine as catalysed by a flavin-containing monooxygenase enzyme.

investigated recently. In the liver, the highest concentrations of FMO1 and FMO3 were detected in the perivenous region and decreased in intensity towards the periportal region. FMO4 in contrast was detected with the opposite lobular distribution. In the kidney, the highest concentrations of FMO isoforms 1, 3 and 4 were detected in the distal tubules. FMO1 and FMO4 were also detected in the proximal tubules with high activity in the brush borders, whereas less FMO3 was found in the proximal tubules.

Examples of substrates that have been shown to be oxidized by FMOs are inorganic compounds/ions such as HS⁻, I⁻ and CNS⁻, organic nitrogen-containing compounds including acyclic and cyclic amines, organic sulfur compounds including thiols, disulfides and dithiocarbamides, and also certain selenium-containing compounds such as selenides and selenocarbamides.

Epoxidation and epoxide hydrolysis

As already described, cytochrome P450 hydroxylates aliphatic and aromatic compounds. While alkyl side chains of aromatic compounds are easily oxidized to alcohols, epoxides of aromatic rings are intermediates in aromatic hydroxylations. These may be very reactive indeed and thereby more toxic – especially when it comes to mutagenicity by binding to DNA – than the original compound. The organism tries to overcome such toxicity by intermediates, although not always with 100% success. Released epoxides thus are hydrolysed to form alcohols. As an example, the microsomal epoxide hydrolase (EPHX1) metabolizes such epoxides of PAHs, i.e. of carcinogens found in cigarette smoke and in fried or smoked food, and is in general the key enzyme involved in the hydrolysis of epoxides formed from xenobiotics. It has wide substrate specificity with a high apparent affinity. However, the turnover of substrate by the enzyme is low. Non-synonymous variants of EPHX1 at Tyr113His (exon 3) and His139Arg (exon 4) are associated, respectively, with low (113His) and high (139Arg) activity. Studies in humans have shown that EPHX1 variants (polymorphisms) at codons 113 and 139 associated with high enzymatic activity appear to increase risk for colorectal adenoma, particularly among recent and current smokers.

Polymorphisms also exist for many of the *CYP* genes, giving rise to persons with very low activity (poor metabolizers) and others with high activity (extensive metabolizers) of these enzymes. Apart from the polymorphism the activity of these genes depends on species. This has very clearly been shown using the barbiturate sleeping time as an indicator for metabolism. Estimation of sleeping time is used (*in vivo* experiments) as a measure of changed metabolism due to exposure to chemicals. Age and gender may also have an influence on metabolism and it has been shown that females have higher activity than males in some strains of mice and pig. Environment, food and drugs may also change the metabolism. It is known that environmental contaminants such as PAHs induce the activity of *CYP1A*, and alcohol induces the activity of *CYP2E1*. Furthermore, people treated with blood thinners are asked not to eat grapefruits because they induce the metabolism of the drug; protein and lipid intake also influences metabolism as a reduction in metabolism is seen after a low intake of protein and a high intake of lipids.

Before we turn to the hydrolysis and reduction reactions it must also be mentioned that alcohol dehydrogenase (ADH; containing the coenzyme NAD⁺) catalyses the transformation of alcohols to aldehydes or ketones. ADH has a broad specificity. The carbonyl compounds formed are in general more toxic and, due to their higher lipophilicity, not easily excreted. As an example, acetaldehyde formed from ingested and absorbed ethanol is further oxidized by acetaldehyde dehydrogenase to acetic acid, which may combine with coenzyme A to form acetyl coenzyme A, the major substrate for the Krebs cycle. The first step, catalysed by ADH, is the rate-limiting step in that the second reaction, acetaldehyde oxidation, occurs much more quickly. The first step in the metabolism of ethanol is:

$$CH_3CH_2OH + NAD^+ \rightarrow CH_3CH{=}O + NADH + H^+$$

Hydrolysis of esters and amides

Mammalian tissues contain a large number of non-specific esterases (and amidases). These are involved in the hydrolysis of toxicants containing ester-type bonds. The esterases are either cellular constituents and in this case mostly located in the soluble cell fraction, or they are contained in the plasma. Four broad classes can be distinguished:

- acetylesterases – hydrolyse esters of acetic acid;
- arylesterases – hydrolyse aromatic esters;
- carboxylesterases – hydrolyse aliphatic esters; and
- cholinesterases – hydrolyse esters of the alcohol choline.

Esterases are the target of deliberate poisoning by nerve gases like Sarin and Tabun and others and of accidental human poisoning by pesticides like parathion, paraoxon, malathion and many others. These compounds are all organophosphates which inhibit the cholinesterase acetylcholinesterase, present in the endplate (the neuromuscular junction) and in the synapses where acetylcholine is the neurotransmitter (= cholinergic synapses).

Reduction

Reductions are not very common as phase I reactions catalysed by human enzymes. However, a number of toxic compounds do undergo reduction in the intestines as catalysed by microorganisms. Among the few examples of reductions catalysed by mammalian enzymes we find the reduction of the nitro group by the membrane-bound (microsomal) nitroreductase system as seen in the conversion of nitrobenzene via nitrosobenzene to phenylhydroxylamine and finally aniline (Fig. 7.3).

7.3   Phase II Reactions

In phase II, enzymes catalyse the transformation of both parent xenobiotics and phase I metabolites such as those described already. Phase II reactions involve the attachment of a generally polar, readily available *in vivo* molecule to a susceptible functional group. In most cases this renders the resulting (final) metabolite more hydrophilic, i.e. increases the water solubility, thereby permitting more rapid excretion. Many phase II enzymes consist of multiple isoforms as also seen for the cytochrome P450 enzymes; however, in general the phase II enzymes are less well characterized in this respect. The most important phase II reactions conjugate the toxicant to glucuronic acid, glutathione, a sulfate group or an acetyl moiety. However, conjugation to an amino acid is also seen, as is methylation, the latter being the exception from the general rule of increasing the polarity.

The enzymes catalysing these processes, in contrast to the *CYP* isoenzymes, are not all present in the endoplasmic reticulum and thereby in the microsomal fraction, as shown in Table 7.2.

As shown in Table 7.2, microsomes can catalyse the glucuronidation and part of the glutathione

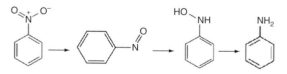

Fig. 7.3. The reduction of nitrobenzene to aniline.

Table 7.2. The cellular location of the different phase II enzymes (microsomes representing the endoplasmic reticulum).

Conjugation reaction	Cellular location
Glucuronidation	Microsomes
Sulfation	Cytosol
Glutathione	Cytosol, microsomes
Acetylation	Mitochondria, cytosol
Methylation	Cytosol
Amination	Mitochondria, cytosol

conjugations and the cytosol can catalyse the sulfation, methylation, acetylation and part of the glutathione conjugations. The mitochondria also play a role in these reactions as they contain enzymes that can carry out part of the acetylation and amination reactions. An overview of the reactions is shown in Fig. 7.4.

The glucuronic acid and the glutathione conjugations in particular are of major importance when it comes to phase II metabolism of toxic xenobiotic compounds (Fig. 7.4).

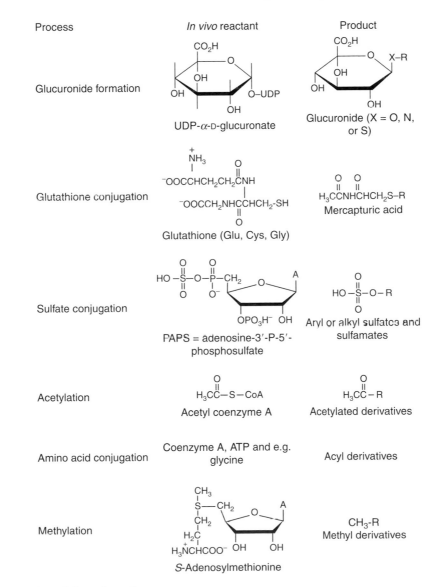

Fig. 7.4. An overview of phase II reactions.

Glucuronide formation and glucuronosyl transferases

Glucuronidation occurs mostly in the liver, the kidneys and the intestinal mucosa. Glucuronosyl transferases (UGTs) conjugate the toxicant (or its phase I metabolites) with glucuronic acid through the establishment of an ether, ester or amide bond. At least eight UGTs are expressed in humans, of which probably the most important (exhibiting a broad substrate specificity) is the isoform named UGT2B7. Glucuronides are the most common conjugates of toxicants, and most products are excreted in the bile.

Typically the product of a glucuronidation (as well as other conjugations) is physiologically inactive; however, exceptions do exist. Thus, morphine-6-glucuronide is around 50 times as potent an analgesic as morphine itself. But let us look into the formation of a glucuronide in a little more detail.

In order to form a glucuronide, first UDP–glucuronic acid (UDPG) must be synthesized by activating and oxidizing glucose, i.e. glucose → UDPG, via the following reactions:

$$\text{Glucose} + \text{ATP} \rightarrow \text{G-6-P} + \text{ADP}$$

$$\text{G-6-P} \rightarrow \text{G-1-P}$$

$$\text{G-1-P} + \text{UTP} \rightarrow \text{UDPG} + \text{PP}_i$$

$$\text{PPi} \rightarrow 2\text{P}_i$$

where G-6-P is glucose-6-phosphate, G-1-P is glucose-1-phosphate, PP_i is inorganic pyrophosphate and P_i is inorganic phosphate. Note that the hydrolysis of PP_i drives the reaction, since it is very favourable, and the product of the previous reaction is removed. These reactions take place in the cytosol.

Secondly, conjugation by glucuronosyl transferase now takes place on the endoplasmic reticulum, mostly via reaction with hydroxyls in aliphatic and aromatic alcohols, carbonyl groups and, occasionally, with nitrogen and sulfur in amines and sulfhydryls. Generally we see S_N2 reactions, so the α-UDPG yields a β-glucuronide. Examples are shown in Fig. 7.5.

Glutathione conjugation

Glutathione is a tripeptide (γ-glutamylcyteinyl-glycine). It is used in cells as a recyclable antioxidant

Example 1 Conjugation of phenol gives an *acetal* glucuronide, phenyl-β-D-glucuronide:

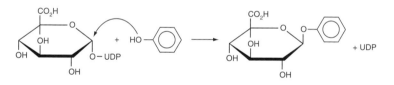

Example 2 Conjugation of benzoic acid gives an ester glucuronide, benzoyl-β-D-glucuronide:

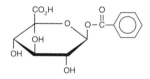

Examples with nitrogen and sulfur include (i) conjugation of aniline to give phenylamino-β-D-glucuronide and (ii) conjugation of 2-mercaptobenzothiazole to give benzothiazole-2-thio-β-D-glucuronide:

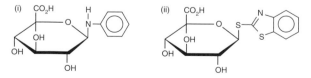

Fig. 7.5. Examples of conjugations catalysed by glucuronosyl transferases.

Example 1 Glutathione S-transferase:

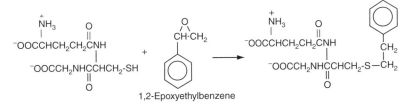

1,2-Epoxyethylbenzene

Example 2 γ-Glutamyltranspeptidase:

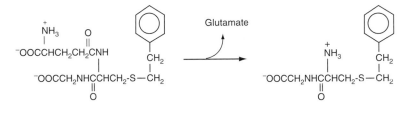

Glutamate

Example 3 Cysteinyl glycinase:

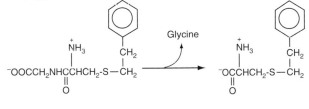

Glycine

Example 4 N-acetyl transferase:

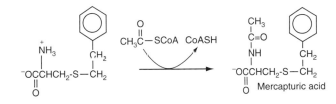

Mercapturic acid

Fig. 7.6. Examples of glutathione conjugation.

as well as a conjugating agent. When used in conjugation it is initially conjugated by a glutathione S-transferase, or sometimes as a simple chemical reaction. Generally the conjugation occurs as a nucleophilic attack by the –SH group on a reactive electrophilic centre of epoxides, aromatic halogens, unsaturated aliphatic moieties and nitro groups as shown in the examples in Fig. 7.6. Conjugation is often followed by metabolic cleavage of the peptide to leave only the cysteinyl residue, which may then be acetylated to give a mercapturic acid.

Not all glutathione derivatives are further metabolized; some may be excreted as is. However, if the derivative is excreted via the bile, it may be metabolized by the gut fauna and the toxin may be reabsorbed. Glutathione is of special importance as it deactivates the very reactive phase I epoxides. These may react with proteins, lipids and DNA in the cell. This may cause a decrease in enzyme activity, degradation of the cell membrane or induction of mutations in the DNA.

Others

Compounds that may be sulfate conjugated are most often aliphatic and aromatic alcohols and aromatic amines; compounds that may be acetylated are primary aromatic amines, hydrazine, sulfonamides and some aliphatic amines.

Amino acid conjugations take place between the amino acid glycine or glutamine and aromatic carboxyl acids, aryl acetic acids and aryl-substituted acryl acids.

A low intake of carbohydrates may induce conjugation activities, which may result in a decrease in reactive oxygen species (ROS).

7.4   Conclusion

After absorption and distribution any xenobiotic compound may undergo a number of different molecular changes. This can often be schematically described as a sequence consisting of a phase I reaction such as an oxidation or reduction followed by a phase II reaction where a generally polar moiety is attached to a functional group of the phase I metabolite. For a given xenobiotic compound administered to an animal species, we may find either that no metabolism whatsoever occurs or a situation where several different phase I metabolites are formed, catalysed by different enzymes. Each of these formed metabolites is then either excreted or conjugated with one of the moieties described above.

Further Reading

Fenton, J.J. (2002) *Toxicology: A Case-Oriented Approach*. CRC Press, Boca Raton, Florida.

Klaassen, C.D. (2008) *Casarett & Doull's Toxicology: The Basic Science of Poison*, 7th edn. McGraw-Hill, New York, New York.

Lu, F.C. and Kacew, S. (2009) *Lu's Basic Toxicology: Fundamentals, Target Organs, and Risk Assessment*, 5th edn. Informa Healthcare, New York, New York.

Niesink, R.J.M., de Vries, J. and Hollinger, M.A. (1996) *Toxicology: Principles and Applications*. CRC Press, Boca Raton, Florida.

Tozer, T.N. and Rowland, M. (2006) *Introduction to Pharmacokinetics and Pharmacodynamics – The Quantitative Basis of Drug Therapy*. Lippincott Williams & Wilkins, Philadelphia, Pennsylvania.

8 Excretion of Chemical Compounds and their Metabolites

- The different routes of excretion are defined.
- The two major routes, i.e. the urinary and the biliary, are briefly described.
- Some basic information about the function of the kidneys and the formation of bile is provided as a background to ease the understanding of the mechanisms of excretion.

8.1 Introduction

After absorption and distribution a xenobiotic compound is eliminated from the different parts (organs and tissues) of the organism. The elimination is a combination of the already described metabolism and different processes of excretion, taking care of both the genuine xenobiotic compound and its metabolites (including conjugates).

Excretion may be: (i) with the urine; (ii) with the bile, which is excreted into the content of the small intestines and thereby leaves the body with the faeces; (iii) with the exhaled air; (iv) with the sweat; or (v) as constituents in hair, nails and dead skin cells.

8.2 Urinary Excretion

The kidneys produce the urine and are the primary organ of removal for most toxicants. This is especially true for those xenobiotics and metabolites/conjugates that are water-soluble and not volatile.

The kidney produces urine through an overall process that involves *glomerular filtration*, tubular secretion and *tubular reabsorption* of small molecules and water. But what do these words mean?

Glomerular filtration of compounds

The kidneys, of which we have two, directly receive approximately a quarter of the cardiac blood output. This is filtered in the so-called glomeruli of the kidneys, meaning that for an average adult person

around 180 litres of blood is filtered per day. The nephron is the functional unit, responsible for the actual filtration of the blood. A sketch of the structure of the central parts of a kidney may be seen in Fig. 8.1.

There are about 1 million nephrons in the cortex of each human kidney and accordingly also about 1 million glomeruli. The total length of the capillaries in a single glomerulus is about 1 cm, making up a total of nearly 20 km for all 2 million glomeruli. The total surface area of all glomerular capillaries in a normal healthy human being is approximately 6000 cm², the total filtration surface area being around one-tenth, i.e. 500 cm². The filtration process is due to the fact that the glomerular capillaries have large pores (up to around 70 nm) and thus allow most non-polymeric (i.e. low molecular weight) substances – including toxicants – to pass. The average molecular weight limit for filtration is around 60,000 Da. This molecular size corresponds to an effective molecular radius of 20 Å easily being ultra-filtered, while compounds for which this radius approaches 40 Å tend to be filtered at very slow rates.

Due to the size limits the described filtration applies only to the non-protein-bound form of a low-molecular-weight compound, and so the concentration of a given xenobiotic in the glomerular filtrate will approximate the free concentration in plasma. Charged substances are usually filtered at slower rates than neutral compounds even when their molecular sizes are comparable, as demonstrated for sulfated dextrans as compared with neutral

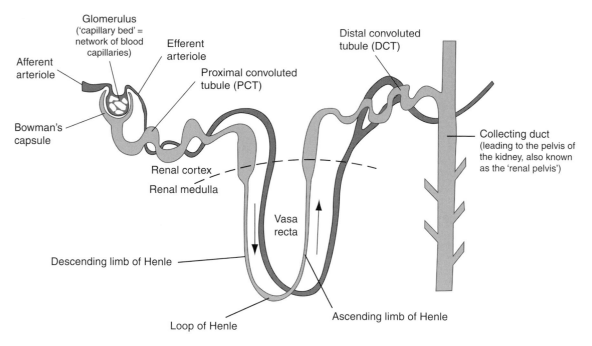

Fig. 8.1. The structure of a kidney nephron. Adapted from IvyRose Holistic web page.[1]

dextrans. The restriction to filtration of charged molecules, particularly anions, is probably due to an electrostatic interaction between the filtered molecule and fixed negative charges within the glomerular capillary wall.

Reuptake and active secretion of compounds

Of the aforementioned around 180 litres of filtrate formed daily, only approximately 1.5 litres is excreted as urine. The remainder is reabsorbed during its passage through the nephrons. Thus, the ultrafiltrate collected in the Bowman's capsule runs into the proximal tubule, through the loop of Henle and into the distal tubule. During this passage a number of processes determine which xenobiotics we find in the urine and in what concentration:

- Substances may diffuse back across the tubular membrane and re-enter the circulation. As water is gradually reabsorbed an increased concentration of the xenobiotic occurs in the luminal fluid of the tubule, thus facilitating passive diffusion back into the blood. In particular, toxicants with a relatively high lipid–water partition coefficient will re-enter the blood circulation by this

mechanism. The back diffusion occurs primarily in the distal tubule and in the collecting duct.
- Some substances are reabsorbed by active transport systems found primarily in the proximal tubules. Such active reabsorption happens in particular for important endogenous substances such as ions, glucose and amino acids.
- The proximal tubules hold two independent systems for active secretion of compounds from the blood and into the luminal fluid of the tubule. One system transports organic anions, the other organic cations. Both systems can be saturated, and one substrate may compete with the transport of another. This has been demonstrated by the fact that one drug can decrease the overall rate of secretion of another. Examples of non-physiological compounds (xenobiotics) that are substrates for active tubular excretion are given in Table 8.1.

One of the factors which affect the resulting excretion of compounds in the urine is the urinary pH. If a compound which is filtered or diffuses into the tubular fluid is ionized at the pH of that fluid, it will not be reabsorbed into the bloodstream by passive diffusion.

Table 8.1. Compounds secreted by renal tubular systems.

Organic anion transport	Organic cation transport
Aminohippuric acid	Atropin
Furosemide	Cimetidine
Penicillin G	Morphine
Salicylate	Quinine

The influence of age

The kidneys are incompletely developed at birth. Neonates and infants thus have a lower glomerular filtration rate than adults even when corrected for body surface area. This means, among other things, that a number of compounds such as penicillin and tetracycline are excreted more slowly. Thus, the clearance of penicillin in infants is only around 20% of that seen for older children. While this enhances the toxicity of the compounds, renal immaturity also can reduce toxicity. This is the case for certain toxicants that normally are subject to active uptake (active tubular reabsorption) in the kidneys after first being filtered into the pre-urine in the glomeruli. Since the active reuptake mechanism(s) are not fully developed in the kidneys of the newborn, such compounds become less toxic.

8.3   Biliary Excretion

The formation of bile

Besides its already described role as the most important site of metabolism of xenobiotic compounds (Chapter 7), the liver also possesses the unique and vital function of producing and secreting bile into the gallbladder. From here the bile is released into the lumen of the duodenum upon intake of a meal rich in lipids. When chyme from an ingested meal enters the small intestine, acid and partially digested fats stimulate the secretion of cholecystokinin and secretin. These enteric hormones have important effects on the secretion and flow of bile. Thus, cholecystokinin once released stimulates contractions of the gallbladder and common bile duct, resulting in delivery of bile into the gut. Secretin is secreted in response to acid in the duodenum. Its effect on the biliary system is that it stimulates biliary duct cells to secrete bicarbonate and water, which expands the volume of bile and increases its flow out into the intestine.

The human liver secretes about 1 litre of bile daily. Bile is a complex aqueous secretion composed of about 95% water and endogenous constituents including bile salts, phospholipids, bilirubin (a porphyrin breakdown product of haem from the haemoglobin in erythrocytes) and cholesterol. Bile salts are the major organic solute in bile and are necessary for the emulsification and digestive absorption of dietary lipids. In man the most important bile acids are cholic acid, deoxycholic acid and chenodeoxycholic acid. Prior to secretion by the liver, they are conjugated with one of the amino acids glycine or taurine. This conjugation increases their water solubility, thus preventing passive reabsorption once secreted into the small intestine. As a result, the concentration of bile acids in the small intestine can stay high enough to form micelles and solubilize the dietary lipids as described.

Excretion of compounds in the bile

Bile also serves to eliminate potentially harmful compounds. Since the bile is secreted into the intestine, compounds that are excreted into the bile consequently are usually eliminated in the faeces. Factors that affect biliary excretion are especially charge and molecular weight. Thus, compounds of high polarity (anionic and cationic), conjugates of compounds bound to plasma proteins and compounds with molecular weights greater than about 300 are favoured when we talk about biliary excretion. Glutathione and glucuronide conjugates also have a high probability of being excreted into the bile. Excretion into the bile is often, although not always, an active process. There are three specific transport systems, one for neutral compounds, one for anions and one for cations. The influence of molecular weight on the relative excretion by the urinary as opposed to the biliary route is exemplified in Table 8.2.

Reuptake and enterohepatic circulation

A compound excreted via the bile into the intestine comes into contact with the gut microflora. Here the bacteria may metabolize the excreted compound; this is seen for glucuronide conjugates for example, which in this way can be hydrolysed to the more lipid-soluble aglycone, which in turn can be reabsorbed from the intestine into the portal venous blood supply and so return to the liver. This process is known as *enterohepatic recirculation*

Table 8.2. Effect of molecular weight on the route of excretion of biphenyls by the rat.

Compound	Molecular weight	Percentage of total excretion	
		Urine	Faeces
Biphenyl	154	80	20
4-Monochlorobiphenyl	188	50	50
4,4′-Dichlorobiphenyl	223	34	66
2,4,5,2′,5′-Pentachlorobiphenyl	326	11	89

and may increase the toxicity of a compound. Also, the gut microflora may metabolize a compound to a more toxic constituent, which again can be reabsorbed and cause systemic toxicity. An example of this latter mechanism is the hepatocarcinogen 2,4-dinitrotoluene.

8.4   Other Routes of Excretion

Other routes of excretion include the pulmonary (excretion via the lungs) and excretion in mother's milk. An example of pulmonary excretion is the excretion of a volatile metabolite of certain selenium compounds, i.e. of dimethylselenium. Excretion into milk is of importance when discussing chemical food safety in two ways: (i) compounds may be excreted into the milk of cows (or other lactating animals) and subsequently ingested by humans (e.g. lead, the mycotoxin AFM_1 or dioxins); or (ii) they can be excreted into the mother's milk and thereby feed the newborn directly. Lipophilic compounds such as PCBs and different persistent organochlorine pesticides (which were used intensively in the 1950s and 1960s) reach a higher level in the milk than in the blood plasma of the mother because of the higher fat content in the milk.

8.5   Conclusion

Excretion of xenobiotic compounds may be diverse, taking many different routes and even showing reuptake with the consequence of an enhanced toxicity – a mechanism actively used, for example, in the design of certain currently used rodenticides with an anticoagulant effect such as bromadiolone and brodifacoum. These compounds antagonize vitamin K, which interferes with the normal synthesis of coagulation proteins (factors I, II, VII, IX and X) in the liver, and thus adequate amounts are not available to convert prothrombin into thrombin.

Note

[1] IvyRose Holistic (not dated) The Structure of a Kidney Nephron. Ivy Rose Ltd, Chalgrove, UK; available at http://www.ivy-rose.co.uk/HumanBody/Urinary/Urinary_System_Nephron_Diagram.php

Further Reading

Klaassen, C.D. (2008) *Casarett & Doull's Toxicology: The Basic Science of Poison*, 7th edn. McGraw-Hill, New York, New York.

Lu, F.C. and Kacew, S. (2009) *Lu's Basic Toxicology: Fundamentals, Target Organs, and Risk Assessment*, 5th edn. Informa Healthcare, New York, New York.

Niesink, R.J.M., de Vries, J. and Hollinger, M.A. (1996) *Toxicology: Principles and Applications*. CRC Press, Boca Raton, Florida.

Tozer, T.N. and Rowland, M. (2006) *Introduction to Pharmacokinetics and Pharmacodynamics – The Quantitative Basis of Drug Therapy*. Lippincott Williams & Wilkins, Philadelphia, Pennsylvania.

9 Toxicokinetics

- In this chapter we define toxicokinetics and toxicodynamics.
- We get an outline of the general mechanisms and principles behind the description of kinetics.
- We look at simple mathematical models to describe the concentration versus time relationship of xenobiotics.

9.1 Introduction

In the preceding chapters we have had a look at the mechanisms of absorption, distribution, metabolism and excretion of xenobiotics, together often abbreviated as ADME. What is left is to: (i) understand the concentration–time relationship for a compound and its metabolites in different target and non-target organs (toxicokinetics); (ii) classify important mechanisms of toxicity on the cellular, subcellular and molecular levels; and (iii) look at tools for the description of the concentration–effect (dose–response) correlation for a given toxicant and its effect(s).

In the toxicological (and pharmacological) literature we work with a concept called *toxicodynamics* (*pharmacodynamics*). Unfortunately, the definition of this varies depending on the author. This text uses a definition of toxicodynamics (and its relationship to *toxicokinetics*) as outlined by Heinrich-Hirsch *et al.* (2001) (Fig. 9.1). As seen from Fig. 9.1, the mechanisms of toxicity on the cellular, subcellular and molecular levels here are part of the toxicodynamics. All of these subjects will therefore be treated together in Chapter 10 on toxicodynamics.

9.2 Toxicokinetics – General Mechanisms and Principles Behind Descriptions of Kinetics

The blood concentration over time (a first view)

When we think of and talk about blood concentrations we must remember what has already been discussed concerning the distribution of a given compound within the different blood compartments. Thus, a compound may occur freely dissolved in the water phase or bound to different plasma proteins and/or to some of the cellular components of the blood. We thus can determine and talk about the whole blood concentration, the plasma concentration and the serum (blood liquid without fibrin) concentration of the compound. In this chapter, in general we refer to blood concentrations as plasma concentrations.

Depending on the route of administration/absorption, the relationship between (i) the time, as measured from the exposure onset (administration), and (ii) the observed blood concentration looks different for a given compound. We know a lot about such relationships from numerous studies on drugs and drug candidates as well as on pesticides, especially among non-drug agents. Studies have been performed using different animal species and even humans. Figure 9.2 shows a theoretical example of how different the time–blood concentration curve may look for a given compound even when we assume an overall fraction of absorption of 100%.

It is important here to stress that for another compound the picture could be different. Thus, we do have examples of compounds with a very quick uptake after oral administration, especially if the compound is absorbed from the oral cavity or the (empty) stomach.

The maximum concentration reached for each of the resulting plasma curves is determined, among other things, by the total volume in which

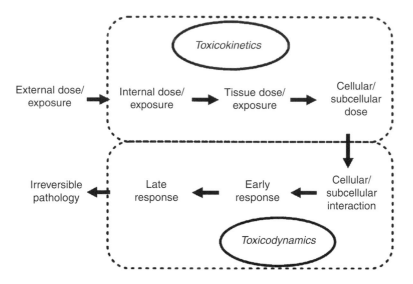

Fig. 9.1. Schematic representation of toxicokinetics and toxicodynamics. Irreversible pathology may be part of toxicodynamics. With permission from Elsevier; adapted from Heinrich-Hirsch *et al.* (2001).[1]

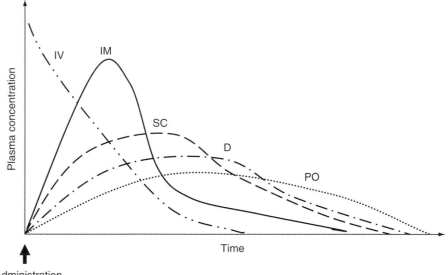

Fig. 9.2. Plasma concentration as a function of time after intravenous injection (IV), intramuscular injection (IM), subcutaneous injection (SC), or dermal (D, percutaneous) or oral (PO, per os) administration of a hypothetical compound with an absorption fraction of 100%.

the amount of compound absorbed (and not yet eliminated) to the circulation initially is distributed in the organism. In most cases this is equal to the volume of blood and of the extracellular water in direct equilibrium with the circulating blood. Later distribution to, for example, body fat deposits or into bones may take place.

Each of the curves shown in Fig. 9.2 actually represents the sum of input and output, i.e. the absorption to the bloodstream and the elimination (metabolism + excretion) from the blood. This is further illustrated in Fig. 9.3a and b on a linear and semi-logarithmic coordinate system, respectively.

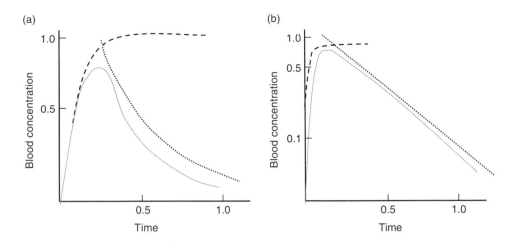

Fig. 9.3. The origin of the blood concentration–time curve (——) as the sum of input (- - -) and output (· · ·) in linear coordinates (a) and semi-logarithmic coordinates (b).

Absorption as well as elimination will normally be the result of several simultaneously ongoing processes; however, we can still often mathematically approximate – and hence describe – the picture seen by using either a so-called *zero-order model* or *first-order model*. In many cases both absorption and elimination can be described reasonably as first-order processes. As shown in Fig. 9.3b, a semi-logarithmic plot (logarithmic with respect to the concentration) in this case will result in a graphically linear representation of the decrease in concentration versus time.

First-order reactions (kinetics)

A first-order chemical (biochemical) reaction is one in which the rate of the reaction depends on the concentration of only one reactant, and is proportional to the amount of this reactant. Said in another way, this means that a constant fraction of the xenobiotic is: (i) absorbed to circulation; or (ii) eliminated from the body per unit time.

Why this order of reaction and hence *kinetics* (= the mathematical description of the reaction as time goes on) can often be used for both absorption and elimination processes can be understood if one looks at a few examples:

● Consider the absorption of a compound by simple diffusion through the membrane separating the gut content and the blood flow. In this case the area over which such diffusion can take place is large and no competition occurs between the individual molecules of the xenobiotic compound

in question. Hence, the uptake is dependent only on the amount (concentration) of the compound, since: (i) the rate of passive diffusion (= absorption) will be a function of the concentration gradient over the membrane; and (ii) this in turn will be determined by the amount of still non-absorbed compound because the absorbed fraction on the other side of the membrane will be removed quickly by the bloodstream.

● When the concentration of the xenobiotic in plasma declines with time and the rate of the elimination also slows, the elimination process most probably can be described as first-order elimination. This is characteristic of a compound that is primarily eliminated by the renal route. The healthy kidney has a high capacity for elimination and so the rate is determined not by the kidney, but by the concentration of the toxicant. A well-studied example is the alkali metal lithium. Lithium has been used in medicine since the 1870s. Initially it was used to treat depression, gout and neutropenia, and for cluster headache prophylaxis. However, the US FDA banned the use of lithium because of fatalities in the 1940s but lifted the ban in 1970. Presently, lithium is used as maintenance treatment of bipolar disorder (manic depression). Lithium poisoning occurs frequently, since it is used in a population at high risk for overdose. Furthermore, lithium has a relatively narrow therapeutic index that predisposes patients on chronic lithium maintenance treatment to poisoning with relatively minor changes in medications or health status.

Toxicokinetics

Mathematically, a first-order reaction for elimination can be described by the following equation:

$$C(t) = C(0) \times e^{-kt}$$

The fate of the equation when transforming it using the natural logarithm (ln = log$_2$) is as follows:

- $\ln C(t) = \ln(C(0) \times e^{-kt})$
- $\ln C(t) = \ln(C(0)) + \ln(e^{-kt})$
- $\ln C(t) = \ln C(0) + (-kt \times \ln(e))$
- $\ln C(t) = \ln C(0) + (-kt \times 1)$
- $\ln C(t) = \ln C(0) - kt$

The last equation clearly represents a straight line with the slope of $-k$ (k is denoted the *rate invariable* or the *rate constant*) in a semi-logarithmic plot of concentration (C) versus time (t), as already shown in Fig. 9.3b.

The influence of the rate constant on the curves

The rate invariable (k) for the absorption and elimination (metabolism + excretion), respectively, determines the actual shape of the curves. As we have seen, the ascending part of the plasma concentration curve is a result of the rate of absorption being greater than the rate of elimination. At the maximum these two are identical, while the elimination is dominating when we look at the descending part. Strictly speaking this only applies to one-compartment systems, which we will come back to.

The influence on the blood concentration–time profile of the value of k for absorption and elimination is illustrated in Fig. 9.4a and b, respectively.

It was mentioned earlier that in other cases we see reactions (especially of metabolism) that follow so-called zero-order kinetics. If we take elimination as the example, zero-order elimination is characterized by the double linear plot of concentration versus time being a straight line. This means that the rate of elimination is not influenced by the concentration. The toxicant is eliminated at a constant rate irrespective of whether there are small or large amounts of it. This is characteristic of hepatic elimination, the route of elimination for non-polar molecules. The rate of zero-order elimination depends on the availability of hepatic enzymes and these are limited. At enzyme saturation, which often occurs at low concentration of the toxicant, the rate is maximal. The concentration of metabolizing enzyme, not the concentration of toxin, is the major factor in setting the rate of elimination.

The elimination of alcohol (ethanol = ethyl alcohol) in man represents still another type of kinetics. At high concentrations the rate of

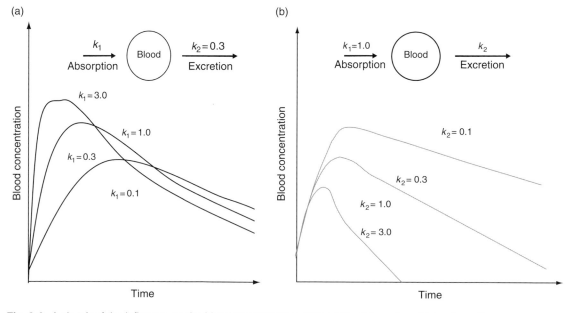

Fig. 9.4. A sketch of the influence on the blood concentration–time profile of the value of k for absorption (a) and elimination (b).

elimination is dictated by the concentration of the fully saturated enzyme (in this case, ADH). At these concentrations zero order prevails and elimination is not related to the concentration; the elimination rate is constant. At a certain concentration, the amount of alcohol is too low to saturate ADH. Beyond that point the reaction rate is a function of the concentration of alcohol. The rate becomes first order.

The organ and tissue concentrations over time

Up until now we have been looking only at the immediate distribution in the blood and extracellular water. However, as already discussed in Chapter 6, gradually lipophilic compounds especially distribute to other tissues (compartments) such as the fatty tissues. The rate of distribution is determined by a number of factors such as the equilibrium between the affinity (solubility) to one versus the other compartment (blood versus body fat or bone matter) and the blood flow through the tissue, and hence the rate of transport of the compound to the tissue. For these reasons for certain compounds we can see distribution and redistribution over time to several different organs and/or tissues. An example is shown in Fig. 6.5.

9.3 Toxicokinetics – Calculation Models

The one-compartment model

The mathematical approximations made so far relate to the so-called *one-compartment model*. If we analyse this first order equation a little further we find that – for the descending part (the elimination) – the time it takes for the concentration to decrease to half the value is a constant. We call this the plasma half-life, $t_{1/2\ pl}$ (or just the half-life). It can be derived graphically from a blood concentration–time profile drawn based on experimental data. For this purpose a semi-logarithmic presentation is the most convenient.

When we have determined the plasma half-life we can use this to calculate the rate constant k_e for the elimination, as follows.

1. If at time equal to '0' we define the concentration as being $2x$, it will, after one $t_{1/2\ pl}$, be equal to x.
2. Inserting these observations into the equation $\ln C(t) = \ln C(0) - kt$ we get:

$$\ln x = \ln 2x - k_e(t_{1/2\ pl})$$

$$\ln x = \ln 2 + \ln x - k_e(t_{1/2\ pl})$$

$$\ln 2 = k_e(t_{1/2\ pl})$$

$$0.693 = k_e(t_{1/2\ pl})$$

$$k_e = 0.693/t_{1/2\ pl}$$

The two-compartment model

So far we have only looked at how we can mathematically approximate curves that are the result of the two overall processes of absorption and elimination. In this connection we have defined and calculated the rate constant of elimination. There are, however, processes that we have not yet treated in such a numerical way: first of all the process of distribution.

Especially for compounds that distribute to a high degree to compartments other than the circulating blood – be it distribution to one or more of the different fatty tissues or accumulation in the bones (lead, fluorine) – the one-compartment model that we have just discussed does not fully explain the blood concentration–time profile actually observed. Therefore, the so-called *two-compartment model* has been developed (Fig. 9.5).

In the open two-compartment model the 'central compartment' represents the blood and extracellular water, while the 'peripheral compartment' represents the sum of the different possible other compartments.

Presuming that all the processes are of first order, the rate by which a compound will be removed from/conveyed to a compartment will be proportional to the concentration of the compound.

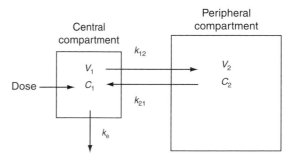

Fig. 9.5. Schematic presentation of the open two-compartment model.

When the absorption is finished, the following will be true for the two-compartment model shown above:

- The *central compartment* – the compound can leave the central compartment both by distribution to the peripheral compartment and by elimination (whether as a result of excretion or metabolism). In addition the compound may return to the central compartment from the peripheral. Hence, we get the following relationship:

$$dC_1/dt = -(k_{12} + k_e)C_1 + k_{21}C_2$$

- The *peripheral compartment* – using the same logic we get the following relationship for the peripheral compartment:

$$dC_2/dt = -k_{21}C_2 + k_{12}C_1$$

If we take an immediate distribution to the whole of the central compartment as the basis of our calculations, for time $t=0$ we get the following relationships:

$$C_1 = D/V_1 \text{ and } C_2 = 0$$

where D is the dose. Using this to find a solution for the two above-shown coupled differential equations, we get:

$$C_1 = Ae^{-\alpha t} + Be^{-\beta t}$$

This equation describes the concentration (C_1) in the plasma (after absorption) as function of time, taking the distribution from the blood and to other compartments into consideration. The result is seen to consist of two elements, namely the first more rapid (re)distribution phase with a rate constant α and the slower elimination phase with a rate constant β (Fig. 9.6).

Depending on the duration of the absorption phase, we get different pictures concerning the overlap of the different phases now described, i.e. the absorption, the distribution and the elimination (Fig. 9.7).

Having access to a blood concentration–time curve we thus already have some information about whether a given xenobiotic compound (toxicant or drug) is distributed to peripheral compartments, and whether this is a quick or slow process (α).

To a certain extent we also can get to know how large a fraction is 'stored':

- If one extrapolates the elimination line back to the y-axis, then one gets to a point called CP0 – a theoretical point representing the concentration that would have existed at the start *if* the dose had been instantly distributed.

- Now we define a theoretical value called the *apparent volume of distribution* (often only the *volume of distribution*; abbreviated V_d). V_d is the ratio of the total amount of compound (the dose) in the body to the actual concentration of the drug in the plasma, or, said in another way, the 'apparent' volume necessary to contain the entire amount of a compound if the compound in the entire body were at the same concentration as in the plasma.

- The numerical value of CP0 is equal to the amount of compound absorbed to the body

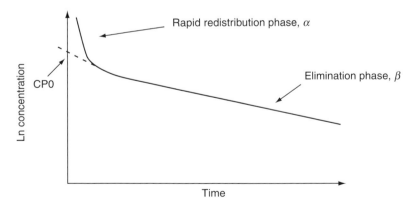

Fig. 9.6. The blood concentration–time curve (ln concentration versus time graph) as approximated by a two-compartment model. Adapted from 4um.com web page.[2]

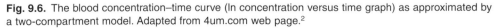

Chapter 9

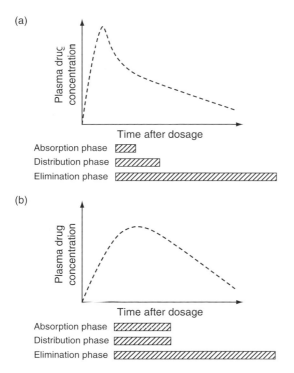

(a)

Plasma drug concentration

Time after dosage

Absorption phase
Distribution phase
Elimination phase

(b)

Plasma drug concentration

Time after dosage

Absorption phase
Distribution phase
Elimination phase

Fig. 9.7. The plasma concentration–time profiles of a chemical following ingestion: (a) oral administration – rapid absorption; (b) oral administration – slow absorption. Adapted from Renwick (2006),[3] reproduced with permission from the Royal Society of Chemistry.

(the dose) divided by the actual concentration in the blood, i.e. D/V_d.

- Now we can calculate V_d as $V_d = D/CP0$.
- Compounds that are highly lipid-soluble, such as digoxin, have a very high V_d (digoxin: 500 litres). Compounds that are lipid-insoluble remain in the blood and have a low V_d.

9.4 Concentration of Parent Compound versus Metabolites

Immediately after the absorption of the first molecules of a xenobiotic its distribution as well as metabolism and excretion start. This means that, at any given time after the start of exposure, we will find a certain mixture of the parent compound together with its metabolite(s) in the blood and maybe also distributed to different organs and tissues, while some of the originally absorbed compound already will have been excreted unchanged and/or as metabolites. This situation is illustrated in Fig. 9.8.

It is important to always be aware of this illustrated situation. First, because metabolites are most often regarded as being physiologically inactive (non-toxic) are not always so; and second, because any chemical analysis to clarify the situation at a given moment must be able to detect and quantify any compound relevant in all the different matrices.

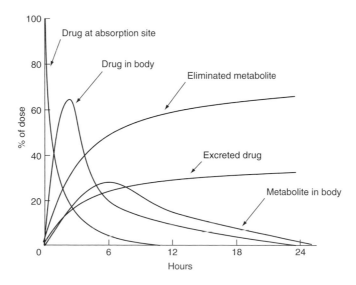

Fig. 9.8. Time course of a toxicant and its metabolites. At any time, the sum of the molar amounts in the compartments equals the dose. Adapted from Tozer and Rowland (2006).[4]

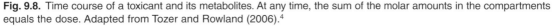

9.5 Conclusion

In the context of chemical food safety and risk assessment associated with chemical food safety, knowledge and understanding of kinetics is important: (i) when planning and carrying out and interpreting results from animal toxicity tests; (ii) when making calculations concerning overall exposure to a given compound coming from different sources and by different routes; and (iii) perhaps especially so, when setting withdrawal periods for veterinary medicinal preparations in different animal species in order to ensure that Maximum Residue Limits (MRLs) are not exceeded.

Notes

[1] Heinrich-Hirsch, B., Madle, S., Oberemm, A. and Gundert-Remy, U. (2001) The use of toxicodynamics in risk assessment. *Toxicology Letters* 120, 131–141.

[2] 4um.com (2002) Basic Pharmacology v1.0, Part 1. Multicompartment Models, Neligan, P. (ed.); available at http://www.4um.com/tutorial/science/pharmak.htm

[3] Renwick, A.G. (2006) Toxicokinetics. In: Duffus, J.H. and Worth, H.G.J. (eds) *Fundamental Toxicology*. RSC Publishing, Cambridge, UK, pp. 24–42.

[4] Tozer, T.N. and Rowland, M. (2006) *Introduction to Pharmacokinetics and Pharmacodynamics – The Quantitative Basis of Drug Therapy*. Lippincott Williams & Wilkins, Philadelphia, Pennsylvania.

Further Reading

Heinrich-Hirsch, B., Madle, S., Oberemm, A. and Gundert-Remy, U. (2001) The use of toxicodynamics in risk assessment. *Toxicology Letters* 120, 131–141.

Klaassen, C.D. (2008) *Casarett & Doull's Toxicology: The Basic Science of Poison*, 7th edn. McGraw-Hill, New York, New York.

Lu, F.C. and Kacew, S. (2009) *Lu's Basic Toxicology: Fundamentals, Target Organs, and Risk Assessment*, 5th edn. Informa Healthcare, New York, New York.

Tozer, T.N. and Rowland, M. (2006) *Introduction to Pharmacokinetics and Pharmacodynamics – The Quantitative Basis of Drug Therapy*. Lippincott Williams & Wilkins, Philadelphia, Pennsylvania.

10   Toxicodynamics

- The concepts of target organs and target cells are defined in this chapter.
- The time aspect and the aspect of reversibility/non-reversibility concerning toxic effects are discussed.
- The general dose–response relationship for one or more effects of a given poison is presented.

10.1   Mechanisms of Toxicity

Target organs and spectrum of toxic effects

A given toxic compound may affect the function of one or more organs. Thus, some compounds show severe adverse effects on several different organs for nearly the same exposure in time and concentration, while others first affect one organ severely, and only at higher concentrations or over a longer time give rise to symptoms due to adverse effects on other organs. All toxic effects are results of biochemical interactions between a compound and/or one or more of its metabolites with structures of the organism. Often we think of specific interactions with a particular subcellular structure or a single type of endogenous molecule; however, the structure may also be non-specific, such as any tissue in direct contact with a corrosive chemical.

A potentially damaging interaction does not always result in an adverse effect with measurable symptoms. This is because the organism possesses a number of defence mechanisms. So overall we can sketch the interaction between a toxicant and the organism as shown in Fig. 10.1.

Organs facing damage/disturbance are called *target organs*; however, these are not always identical to the organs with the greatest concentration of the compound. Thus, cells and organs with special functions that can be inhibited (e.g. enzyme inhibitors such as acetylcholinesterase inhibitors inhibiting the acetylcholinesterase in nerve junctions) or cells with a high energy turnover may be the primary targets while at the same time actual concentrations are higher in other parts of the body.

Toxic effects may be classified in a number of ways. Several such are listed in Table 10.1.

A given toxicity may have a range of secondary effects. This is the case for toxicity to the immune system, which may lead to infections from which the individual may suffer or die. Thus, immunotoxicity is seen for a number of different food toxicants such as trichothecene mycotoxins, a group of structurally similar fungal metabolites capable of producing a range of toxic effects. Among these, deoxynivalenol (DON, vomitoxin), a trichothecene, is prevalent worldwide in crops used for food and feed production. Although DON is one of the least acutely toxic trichothecenes, it should be treated as an important food safety issue since it is a very common contaminant of grain. *In vivo*, DON suppresses a normal immune response to pathogens and simultaneously induces autoimmune-like effects which are similar to human immunoglobulin A (IgA) nephropathy. Besides food-borne exposure, the potential exists for DON to become airborne during the harvest and handling of grains and therefore pose a risk to agricultural workers. Plasma and tissue DON concentrations were shown to be 1.5–3 times higher following intranasal exposure as compared with oral exposure when studied in mice. Immunotoxicity can give rise both to increased susceptibility towards infection and to decreased surveillance against pre-cancer/cancer cells.

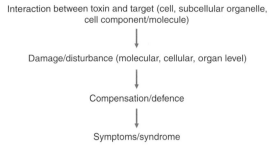

Toxic effects

Interaction between toxin and target (cell, subcellular organelle, cell component/molecule)

↓

Damage/disturbance (molecular, cellular, organ level)

↓

Compensation/defence

↓

Symptoms/syndrome

Fig. 10.1. A sketch of the interaction between a toxic compound and an organism.

Mode of toxic action and molecular targets

The biochemical interaction leading to toxicity may involve a number of basically different molecular targets in the host; these include proteins, lipids (membranes) and nucleic acids.

Proteins

Proteins occur universally in humans and may be divided into a number of groups, each with its important role(s) to play. Here we will look a little further at receptors, enzymes, carriers and structural proteins.

RECEPTORS. The term *receptor* covers a number of different molecular structures located across plasma membranes, or in the cytosol or nucleus, all of which serve to transmit signals to and within the cell. Receptors exert their biological effects upon binding with an appropriate ligand. This may be an endogenous or an exogenous substance. The effect is often not a direct result of the binding of the ligand, rather it is proceeded by a series of biochemical reactions, the signal, which vary according to the structural characteristics of the receptor. Structurally, receptors often are classified into the following four groups:

1. G-protein-coupled receptors

    - G-protein-coupled receptors (GPCRs) are found only in eukaryotes, including yeasts. GPCRs are also known as seven-transmembrane-domain receptors (7TM receptors), heptahelical receptors, serpentine receptors and G-protein-linked receptors (GPLRs). They comprise a large protein family of transmembrane receptors that react to the binding of molecules outside the cell and inside activate signal transduction pathways and, ultimately, cellular responses. Typical ligands for this class of receptors include adrenergic, cholinergic, dopaminergic and muscarinic neurotransmitters.
    - Of non-endogenous compounds one can mention the xenobiotics ephedrine and diphtheria toxin.

2. Ligand-gated ion channels

    - Ligand-gated ion channels (LGICs) are transmembrane proteins that can exist under different conformations. At least one of these conformations forms a pore through the membrane connecting two neighbouring compartments. The equilibrium between the

Table 10.1. Some examples of general classifications of toxic effects.

Site of action	Type
Local effects	Morphological changes (most often irreversible, e.g. necrosis)
• Irritant	Functional changes (often reversible)
• Corrosive	Allergy
Systemic effects	Antibody production
• Organ specific	Inflammatory response (requires previous exposure)
Reversibility	Idiosyncratic
Irreversible	A genetically determined abnormal reactivity to a chemical
Reversible	
Time aspect	
Acute effect	
Delayed effect to time-restricted exposure	
Effect of chronic exposure	

Chapter 10

various conformations is affected by the binding of ligands to the channels. Phenomenologically, the ligands 'open' or 'close' the channel. The LGICs are classified into three different superfamilies, namely:

○ the receptors of the Cys-loop super-family (nicotinic receptors, 5-HT_3 receptors (type 3 serotonin receptors; 5-hydroxytryptamine (5-HT) = serotonin), $GABA_A$ and $GABA_C$ receptors, glycine receptors, and some glutamate-, histamine- and serotonin-activated anionic channels) are made of five homologous subunits, each with four transmembrane segments;
○ the ATP-gated channels (ATP2x receptors) are made of three homologous subunits, each with two transmembrane segments; and
○ the glutamate-activated cationic channels (NMDA (*N*-methyl D-aspartate) receptors, AMPA (α-amino-3-hydroxy-5-methyl-4-isoxazolepropionic acid) receptors, kainate receptors, etc.) are made of four homologous subunits, each with three transmembrane segments.

• Picrotoxin, a bitter crystalline compound derived from the seed of an East Indian woody vine, *Anamirta*, has a strong physiological action. This is because it acts as in a non-competitive way on the $GABA_A$ receptor chloride channels. It is a channel blocker rather than a receptor antagonist. As GABA itself is an inhibitory neurotransmitter, picrotoxin has stimulant and convulsant effects. It has been used in the treatment of barbiturate poisoning.

3. Voltage-gated channels

• We find the voltage-gated channels located across the plasma membrane of excitable cells such as neurons, i.e. on the cell body and on their axons.
• An example of a natural class of toxins – with relevance for chemical food safety – that interact with one such type of channel is the marine biotoxin saxitoxin (together with closely related toxins). Thus, saxitoxin (STX) acts as an hERG channel modifier. This channel, comprising a protein encoded by the human *Ether-à-go-go* Related Gene, is a potassium channel. Potassium (K^+) channels mediate numerous electrical events in excitable cells, including cellular membrane potential repolarization. The hERG K^+ channel plays an important role in myocardial repolarization, and inhibition of these K^+ channels is associated with long QT syndromes that can cause fatal cardiac arrhythmias. In the presence of STX, channels open more slowly during strong depolarizations and close much faster upon repolarization, suggesting that toxin-bound channels can still open but are modified, and that STX does not simply block the ion conduction pore. STX thus decreases hERG K^+ currents by stabilizing closed channel states, visualized as shifts in the voltage dependence of channel opening to more depolarized membrane potentials.

4. Intracellular receptors

• Intracellular receptors are found in either the cytosol or the nucleus. The intracellular receptors are typically hormone receptors with natural ligands including androgens, oestrogens, glucocorticoids and mineralocorticoids.
• An intracellular receptor often mentioned in connection with toxic effects is the so-called aryl hydrocarbon (Ah) receptor. Ah is a cytosolic transcription factor that is normally inactive, bound to several co-chaperones. Upon ligand binding the chaperones dissociate, resulting in Ah translocating into the nucleus and leading to changes in gene transcription. Some chemicals including the very toxic dioxin 2,3,7,8-tetrachlorodibenzo-*p*-dioxin (TCDD) interact with this receptor.

ENZYMES. Many toxic compounds influence the organism by inhibiting enzymes. Such inhibition may be non-specific as is the background for a number of the effects of toxic heavy metals such as lead and mercury. The general mechanism in this case is a high affinity to thiol (–SH) groups present in all enzymes. Even so, some enzymes are more susceptible to inhibition by these metals than others, an example being δ-aminolevulinic acid dehydrase, the activity of which in erythrocytes can be used as an early indicator of lead poisoning.

Inhibition may also be more specific; examples are the following:

• Inhibition of acetylcholinesterase by either organophosphates (which can be insecticides or warfare gases) or carbamate insecticides. In the latter case the inhibition is reversible, which is not always the case for the inhibition caused by organophosphates.

- Dinitrophenols have earlier been used intensively as herbicides. An example is the compound 4,6-dinitro-*o*-cresol (DNOC). Like other dinitrophenols, DNOC increases the oxidative metabolism and heat production by direct cellular reaction. DNOC affects enzyme systems by inhibiting the formation of ATP and by blocking oxidative phosphorylation.

- Inhibition of an enzyme may also happen after several stages of transformation of the original compound absorbed. The key example of this situation, which is also called *lethal synthesis*, is the inhibition of the citric acid cycle enzyme aconitase by fluorocitric acid, a reaction that blocks energy production. The fluorocitric acid is formed if an individual is exposed to either synthetic fluoroacetic acid or to the same compound found as a natural toxic plant constituent in 'gifblaar', a small shrub (*Dichapetalum cymosum*) well known as a livestock poison in South Africa. But we do not stop here. Actually some other species of *Dichapetalum*, such as *D. toxicarium*, contain in its seeds long-chain fluorine fatty acids such as ω-fluoro-oleic acid and ω-fluoro-palmitic acid. After ingestion these fluorine fatty acids are β-oxidized to form the aforementioned fluoroacetic acid. This in turn enters the citric acid cycle where it is metabolized into fluorocitric acid. This cannot be metabolized further since aconitase does not accept this compound instead of its natural substrate citric acid. The cycle is blocked.

CARRIERS. Here we think first of all of haemoglobin, the iron-containing protein capable of transporting oxygen and carbon dioxide in the blood. This pigment of erythrocytes, formed by developing erythrocytes in the bone marrow, has an iron haem moiety and four different polypeptide globin chains that contain between 141 and 146 amino acids. Haemoglobin A is the normal adult haemoglobin and haemoglobin F is fetal haemoglobin. Haemoglobin F is the main oxygen-transport protein in the fetus during the last 7 months of development in the uterus and in the newborn until around 6 months. Functionally, fetal haemoglobin differs most from adult haemoglobin in that it is

able to bind oxygen with greater affinity than the adult form, giving the developing fetus better access to oxygen from the mother's bloodstream.

The iron haem moiety binds reversibly to oxygen to form oxyhaemoglobin and a globin moiety binds reversibly to carbon dioxide to form carbaminohaemoglobin. Under normal conditions around 97% of the oxygen is transported bound to haemoglobin, whereas only 3% is dissolved in the plasma. Only about 20% of the blood carbon dioxide is transported bound to haemoglobin. Oxygen transport can be impaired by interaction with a number of different toxic compounds.

- Carbon monoxide can bind to haemoglobin at the site where oxygen is normally bound.
- Oxygen transport can also be impaired due to the formation of methaemoglobin, i.e. oxidized haemoglobin, with the iron existing in the ferric instead of the ferrous state. Methaemoglobin is incapable of binding reversibly with oxygen. Different toxicants can enhance the formation of methaemoglobin:

  ○ nitrite;
  ○ aromatic amines;
  ○ some aminophenols;
  ○ arylnitro compounds; and
  ○ *N*-hydroxyarylamines.

Infants younger than 4 months of age who are fed formula diluted with water from rural domestic wells are especially prone to developing health effects from nitrite or nitrate exposure. The high pH of the infant gastrointestinal system favours the growth of nitrate-reducing bacteria, particularly in the stomach and especially after ingestion of contaminated water. The stomach of adults is typically too acidic to allow for significant bacterial growth and the resulting conversion of nitrate to nitrite.

A proportion of the haemoglobin in young infants is still in the form of fetal haemoglobin. Fetal haemoglobin is more readily oxidized to methaemoglobin by nitrites than is adult haemoglobin. Therefore, infants, and especially premature infants, are particularly susceptible. In addition, NADH-dependent methaemoglobin reductase, the enzyme responsible for reduction of induced methaemoglobin back to normal haemoglobin, has only about half the activity in infants as in adults.

STRUCTURAL PROTEINS. The replacement of sulfur by selenium upon a chronic intake of high doses of selenium may lead to altered structure and function of cellular components. Especially susceptible are the cells that form keratin (keratinocytes) and the sulfur-containing keratin molecule. Selenium therefore weakens the hooves of animals and hair, which tend to fracture when subjected to mechanical stress.

Selenium in the form of SeMet is easily absorbed by the same mechanism as methionine. Inorganic selenium absorption seems not to be regulated and is quite high (>50%). Bodily storage of inorganic selenium from selenite or selenate occurs as the selenoamino acids SeCys and SeMet. It has been reported that selenium and/or selenoamino acids can be incorporated into sulfur-requiring sites during protein production and thus change the integrity of the protein structure. Cows supplemented with 50 mg of injectable selenium suffered severe claw problems in the postpartum period. It is very likely that the excessive selenium supplement was incorporated into keratin fibres of the maturing keratinocytes with the key Cys and Met sites replaced by SeCys or SeMet. Therefore, critical disulfide bridge formation was reduced or inhibited during the cornification process, creating inferior hoof horn lacking structural rigidity with poor integrity.

Lipids/membranes (permeability/fluidity)

Lipids and lipophilic substances of different types are integrated parts of the cell membrane. Cell membranes are the target of a number of very different toxic agents. These include the phenomenon where anaesthetic ether and halothane as well as other organic solvents accumulate in the cell membrane, thereby altering the membrane characteristics and among others the transport of oxygen and glucose into the cell. Among the metals, lead can increase the fragility of the erythrocyte membrane. The huge group of natural plant glycosides called saponins (see Chapter 6) may also interfere with the structure of cell membranes. A broader definition of the saponins includes the steroidal alkaloid glycosides found in potatoes. Usually, these glycosides have low oral bioavailability and toxicity, but when given intravenously many show strong toxicity and cause haemolysis (rupture of the erythrocyte membrane). The general membrane-disrupting properties of saponins include pore formation by an unknown mechanism.

Nucleic acids

Covalent binding between a toxicant and a base in a DNA string (alkylation) can result in the formation of a point mutation (base substitution or insertion/deletion) upon replication of the DNA. If not repaired such a mutation may further lead to cell death or to the development of cancer. Alkylating (mutagenic) substances in food include two different types, among others, both of which must be activated through metabolism in the liver (and elsewhere) to become the actual mutagens. These are the mycotoxins called aflatoxins and the so-called *frying mutagens* within the group of PAHs, the most potent of the latter being benzo[*a*]pyrene.

10.2 Dose–Response Relationship

Toxic effects may as we have seen be due to interaction with different targets through binding or chemical interaction. Regardless of how an effect occurs, the concentration of the toxicant at the site of action controls the effect. Dose–response data are typically plotted with the dose or dose function (e.g. $\log_{10}$ dose) on the x-axis and the measured effect (response) on the y-axis. Because a toxic effect is a function of dose and time, such a graph depicts the *dose–response relationship* independent of time. Measured effects are most often recorded as maxima at the time of peak effect. Effects may be quantified at the level of molecule, cell, tissue, organ, organ system or organism.

An effect (response) may be *quantal* or *graded*. An example of a quantal response is the percentage of dead animals in an experiment to describe the acute toxicity by determining the so-called LD_{50} value (see Chapter 13), while an example of a graded response could be the increase in blood pressure for a single individual depending on exposure dose or the average increase in blood pressure for different groups of animals depending on the dosing of the group in question. Graded responses can be transformed to quantal responses. Looking at the example with blood pressure this could be done by making a graph of the percentage (the effect/response) of animals that experience at least a 10% increase in blood pressure as a function of the dose. Let us now look at such curves and get to know the possible differences. Two hypothetical dose–response curves are shown in Fig. 10.2.

Both the shape and slope of the dose–response curve are important in predicting the toxicity of a substance at specific dose levels. Huge differences among toxicants may exist not only in the point at which the threshold for the toxic effect is reached, but also in the response increase per unit change in dose (i.e. the *slope*). In the example shown in Fig. 10.2, toxicant A has a higher threshold but a steeper slope than toxicant B.

A given toxicant will normally have different adverse effects, each of which may start at a different threshold. An example could be the different effects of intoxication with methylmercury. Figure 10.3 shows the frequency (% affected) of different symptoms (*y*-axis) seen for adult victims of intoxication with methylmercury in Iraq (1987)

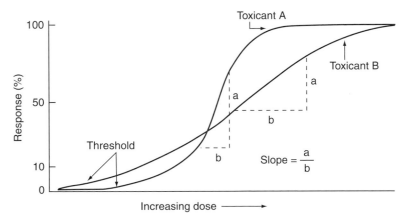

Fig. 10.2. Hypothetical dose–response curves for two different toxicants, A and B. Adapted from The Encyclopedia of Earth web page.[1]

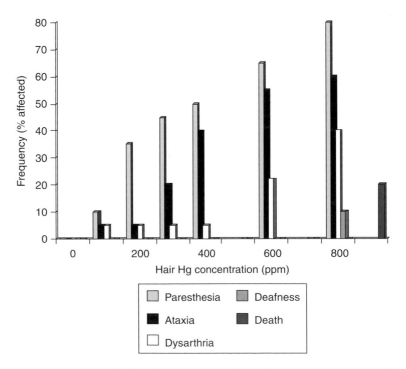

Fig. 10.3. The dose–response relationship for different adverse effects of methylmercury intoxication (frequency of response versus hair concentration).

Chapter 10

due to the use of mercury fungicide-treated cereals for human consumption (bread making). The dose (x-axis) is in ppm of mercury (Hg) as measured in the hair (a biomarker for the exposure).

10.3 Conclusion

Toxic effects are the results of interactions between a toxicant and one or more target molecules in one or more target tissues or organs. Any toxic constituent will normally show a number of different toxic (adverse) effects, each of which will be characterized by a threshold concentration/dose beyond which the effect may be seen. A dose–response relationship will exist, which can be described by a graph. The graphs for different effects of the same compound, as well as for toxic effects of different compounds, may exhibit different slopes, i.e. the response increase per unit change in dose may vary.

Note

[1] The Encyclopedia of Earth (2008) Dose–response relationship. Yuill, T. and Miller, M. (eds). EIC Secretariat, National Council for Science and the Environment, Washington, DC; available at http://www.eoearth.org/article/Dose-response_relationship

Further Reading

Heinrich-Hirsch, B., Madle, S., Oberemm, A. and Gundert-Remy, U. (2001) The use of toxicodynamics in risk assessment. *Toxicology Letters* 120, 131–141.

Klaassen, C.D. (2008) *Casarett & Doull's Toxicology: The Basic Science of Poison*, 7th edn. McGraw-Hill, New York, New York.

Lu, F.C. and Kacew, S. (2009) *Lu's Basic Toxicology: Fundamentals, Target Organs, and Risk Assessment*, 5th edn. Informa Healthcare, New York, New York.

Niesink, R.J.M., de Vries, J. and Hollinger, M.A. (1996) *Toxicology: Principles and Applications*. CRC Press, Boca Raton, Florida.

Omaye, S.T. (2004) *Food and Nutritional Toxicology*. CRC Press, Boca Raton, Florida.

Tozer, T.N. and Rowland, M. (2006) *Introduction to Pharmacokinetics and Pharmacodynamics – The Quantitative Basis of Drug Therapy*. Lippincott Williams & Wilkins, Philadelphia, Pennsylvania.

11 An Introduction to the History of Regulation and Control Worldwide (International Institutions in Risk Assessment and Safety Regulation)

- We look at how legislative regulation started.
- The individual roles of industry versus state authorities.
- The role and influence of international institutions.

11.1 The Beginning – Food Regulations History (the USA with FDA, USDA, etc.)

The modern history of food regulations with respect to chemical substances potentially found in foodstuffs starts in the USA with the 1958 Food Additives Amendment to the Food, Drug and Cosmetic Act of 1938. The amendment regulated the use of food additives such as salt, nitrate, organic acids and other chemical compounds. The Food Additives Amendment requires FDA approval for the use of an additive prior to its inclusion in food. It also requires the manufacturer to prove an additive's safety for the ways it will be used.

In writing this piece of legislation the American Congress felt, however, that a number of substances intentionally added to food would not require a formal scientific premarket review by FDA to assure their safety and hence approve their use. Such trust in a compound could, for example, be based on its safety being 'established' by a long history of use in food. Thus, a two-step definition of a 'food additive' was adopted in the Amendment.

The first step broadly included any substance, the intended use of which results in it becoming a component or otherwise affecting the characteristics of food. The second step, however, excluded from this definition substances that are:

Generally recognized, among experts qualified by scientific training and experience to evaluate their safety ('qualified experts'), as having already been adequately shown through scientific procedures (or, in the case of a substance used in food prior to January 1, 1958, through

either scientific procedures or through *experience based on common use in food*) to be safe under the conditions of their intended use.

Salt, sugar, spices, vitamins and monosodium glutamate were classified as GRAS substances, along with several other substances.

FDA therefore published a list of these generally recognized as safe (GRAS) substances on 9 December 1958. This list came to be called the GRAS list. Following the publication of the GRAS list, FDA made no systematic attempt to evaluate available scientific information on the GRAS substances. By 1969, as a result of a recommendation in the report of the White House Conference on Food, Nutrition, and Health, President Richard M. Nixon directed FDA to make such a critical evaluation of the safety of GRAS food substances. The following GRAS review for years became a major project at FDA's Bureau of Foods.

In 1960, the US Congress passed similar legislation governing colour additives. The Color Additives Amendment requires dyes used in foods, drugs and cosmetics to be approved by FDA prior to their marketing. In contrast to food additives, colours in use before the legislation were allowed continued use only if they underwent further testing to confirm their safety. Of the original 200 provisionally listed colour additives, 90 have been listed as safe. The remainder have been either removed from use by FDA or withdrawn by industry. Both the Food Additives Amendment and the Color Additives Amendment prohibit the approval of an additive if it is found to cause cancer in humans or animals. This clause is often referred to as the Delaney Clause (after Congressman James Joseph Delaney, 1901–1987).

In the USA today, in order to market a new food or colour additive, a manufacturer must first petition FDA for its approval. Approximately 100 new food and colour additive petitions are submitted to FDA annually. A food or colour additive petition must provide convincing evidence that the proposed additive performs as it is intended. Animal studies for long periods are often necessary to show that the substance would not cause harmful effects at expected levels of human consumption. Studies of the additive in humans also may be submitted to FDA.

The Agency considers the composition and properties of the substance, the amount likely to be consumed, its probable long-term effects and various safety factors. If an additive is approved, FDA issues regulations that may include the types of foods in which it can be used, the maximum amounts to be used and how it should be identified on food labels. Additives proposed for use in meat and poultry products also must receive specific authorization by the United States Department of Agriculture (USDA).

Food flavours were not dealt with directly by the governmental agency of FDA in 1958 when setting up the GRAS list. Instead the private sector organization, the Flavor and Extract Manufacturers Association of the United States (FEMA; founded 1909), comprising flavour manufacturers, flavour users and flavour ingredient suppliers, was invited to establish a parallel list of flavours generally recognized as safe in foodstuffs. A FEMA expert panel was appointed in 1960. Substances submitted by manufacturers without sufficient data were taken off the list. FEMA presented its conclusions to FDA prior to publication of the first FEMA GRAS list as *Recent Progress in the Consideration of Flavoring Ingredients under the Food Additives Amendment. III Gras Substances*. This system of authorizing the industrial organization FEMA to perform risk assessments of flavour substances used in foodstuffs has continued in the USA. Thus, FEMA published its first report to include new flavour ingredients in 1970. Today, in determining whether a flavour ingredient is to be considered safe (and thereby allowed to appear on the FEMA GRAS list), the FEMA panel – like FDA for other classes of substances – considers exposure, chemical identity (including purity), metabolic and toxicokinetic characteristics, and animal toxicity. Today this list is available on the Internet as

'GRAS Flavoring Substances'. Edition no. 24 featuring materials nos 4430 through 4666 was launched in December 2008.

11.2 The UN (WHO, FAO, IARC)

The UN is an international organization founded in 1945 after World War II by 51 countries. Today the 192 Member States express their views through the General Assembly, the Security Council, the Economic and Social Council, and other bodies and committees. Soon after being founded a number of very important UN organizations were established. Thus, FAO was established on 16 October 1945 in Quebec City, Canada. In 1951 its headquarters were moved from Washington, DC to Rome. The organization presents itself by a statement saying:

> The Food and Agriculture Organization of the United Nations leads international efforts to defeat hunger. Serving both developed and developing countries, FAO acts as a neutral forum where all nations meet as equals to negotiate agreements and debate policy. FAO is also a source of knowledge and information. We help developing countries and countries in transition modernize and improve agriculture, forestry and fisheries practices and ensure good nutrition for all. Since our founding in 1945, we have focused special attention on developing rural areas, home to 70 percent of the world's poor and hungry people.

The other big and very influential UN organization, i.e. WHO, was founded in 1948 and its headquarters established in Geneva, Switzerland. According to the organization itself:

> WHO is the directing and coordinating authority for health within the United Nations system. It is responsible for providing leadership on global health matters, shaping the health research agenda, setting norms and standards, articulating evidence-based policy options, providing technical support to countries and monitoring and assessing health trends.

In order to ease our discussion about the roles and influences of international organizations on chemical food safety, in addition to FAO and WHO, we also need to present the International Agency for Research on Cancer (IARC). IARC is part of WHO. IARC's mission is to coordinate and conduct research on the causes of human cancer, the mechanisms of carcinogenesis, and to develop scientific strategies for cancer prevention and control. IARC has its headquarters in Lyon, France, and the IARC Monographs Program is a core element of the Agency's portfolio of activities, with international expert working groups evaluating the evidence of the carcinogenicity of specific compounds and exposures.

By the 1960s the two UN organizations FAO and WHO found that they could help to protect the health of people worldwide by developing food standards, guidelines and related texts such as codes of practice. To this end they joined in establishing the Codex Alimentarius Commission (CAC), which was created in 1963. The main purposes of this body, as well as protecting the health of consumers, were to ensure fair trade practices in the food trade and to promote coordination of all food standards work undertaken by international governmental and non-governmental organizations.

CAC establishes its standards (among others for food additives, food contaminants such as mycotoxins and for pesticide residues in food) by getting advice from a number of committees such as the Joint FAO/WHO Expert Committee on Food Additives (JECFA) and the Joint FAO/WHO Meetings on Pesticide Residues (JMPR):

- while not officially part of the CAC structure, JECFA provides independent scientific expert advice to the Commission and its specialist Committees;
- while not officially part of the CAC structure, JMPR provides independent scientific expert advice to the Commission and its specialist Committee on Pesticide Residues.

Let us take a little more detailed look into the work of CAC.

The Commission meets every year alternately in Rome and Geneva and provides a forum for discussion and debate on all major food standards/safety issues of interest and concern to Codex Member States. The task of developing international standards for commodity and general subject areas is spread across specific technical committees.

General Subject Committees are so called because their work has relevance for all Commodity Committees and, since this work applies across the board to all commodity standards, General Subject Committees are sometimes referred to as 'horizontal' committees. There are nine such committees:

- the Committee on General Principles, hosted by France;
- the Committee on Food Labelling, hosted by Canada;

- the Committee on Methods of Analysis and Sampling, hosted by Hungary;
- the Committee on Food Hygiene, hosted by the USA;
- the Committee on Pesticide Residues, hosted by Brazil;
- the Committee on Food Additives and Contaminants, hosted by the Netherlands;
- the Committee on Import and Export Inspection and Certification Systems, hosted by Australia;
- the Committee on Nutrition and Foods for Special Dietary Use, hosted by Germany; and
- the Committee on Residues of Veterinary Drugs in Food, hosted by the USA.

Commodity Committees have responsibility for developing standards for specific foods or classes of food. To distinguish them from the 'horizontal committees' and to recognize their exclusive responsibilities, they are often referred to as 'vertical' committees. There are seven such committees:

- the Committee on Fats and Oils, hosted by the UK;
- the Committee on Fish and Fishery Products, hosted by Norway;
- the Committee on Milk and Milk Products (formerly the Joint FAO/WHO Committee of Government Experts on the Code of Principles Concerning Milk and Milk Products), hosted by New Zealand;
- the Committee on Fresh Fruits and Vegetables, hosted by Mexico;
- the Committee on Cocoa Products and Chocolate, hosted by Switzerland;
- the Committee on Processed Fruits and Vegetables, hosted by the USA; and
- the Committee on Meat and Poultry Hygiene, hosted by New Zealand.

CAC has so far adopted more than 200 *food commodity standards*, more than 40 *hygiene and technological practice codes* and set more than 3200 *maximum residue limits for pesticides and veterinary drugs*. Also within the area of food additives CAC has adopted a high number of *standards*: i.e. (i) specifications for the identity and purity of the individual food additive; and (ii) approved maximum levels for its use in different food categories or individual food items.

Let us look at carnauba wax as an example.

The maximum levels of carnauba wax are established as a result of a calculation based on knowledge of people's food consumption patterns worldwide in order to ensure that its acceptable daily intake (ADI; see chapter 27) is not exceeded. This actually means that a scientific risk assessment has been made prior to the process of establishing the recommended maximum levels in the different commodities. In the case of carnauba wax such a risk assessment was made by JECFA in 1992 at its 39th Assembly. The assessment resulted in an ADI of 0–7 mg kg^{-1} BW for carnauba wax, as reported in the meeting report entitled *Toxicological Evaluation of Certain Food Additives and Naturally Occurring Toxicants* and published in the WHO Food Additives Series no. 30.

The refined wax, obtained from the fronds of the Brazilian tropical palm tree *Copernicia cerifera* (Arruda) Mart. (syn. *C. purnifera* (Muell.)), is a complex mixture of several chemical compounds, predominantly esters; for example:

– aliphatic esters (straight chain acids with even-numbered carbon chains from C_{24} to C_{28} and straight-chain alcohols with even-numbered carbon chains from C_{30} to C_{34}),
– alpha-hydroxy esters (straight-chain hydroxy acids with even-numbered carbon chains from C_{22} to C_{28}, straight-chain acids with even-numbered carbon chains from C_{24} to C_{28}, straight-chain monohydric alcohols with even-numbered carbon chains from C_{24} to C_{34} and dihydric alcohols with even-numbered carbon chains from C_{24} to C_{34}),
– cinnamic aliphatic diesters (*p*-methoxycinnamic acid and dihydric alcohols with even-numbered carbon chains from C_{24} to C_{34}).

This definition is found in the *specification* monograph on carnauba wax as developed by JECFA and approved by CAC. The monograph can be found by searching the online database of JECFA for the specifications of additives. Carnauba wax is described to have a function as an adjuvant, anticaking agent, bulking agent, carrier solvent, glazing agent and/or a release agent. This description of its possible and approved use(s) together with the CAC-approved maximum levels in different food categories and items are given in the *Codex General Standard for Food Additives*, the current pdf version (225 pages) of which can be down loaded from the Codex General Standard for Food Additives online database (http://www.codexalimentarius. net/gsfaonline/index.html?lang=en; the already mentioned JECFA specification report available

online also can be reached from here). The version of the Codex General Standard for Food Additives official while writing this text, i.e. CODEX STAN 192-1995, specifies maximum levels for carnauba wax as follows:

	mg kg^{-1}
Surface-treated fresh fruit	400
Processed fruit	400
Surface-treated fresh vegetables (including mushrooms and fungi, roots and tubers, pulses and legumes, and aloe vera), seaweeds, and nuts and seeds	400
Cocoa and chocolate products	5000
Imitation chocolate, chocolate substitute products	5000
Confectionery including hard and soft candy, nougats, etc., other than food categories 05.1, 05.3 and 05.4	5000
Chewing gum	1200
Decorations (e.g. for fine bakery wares), toppings (non-fruit) and sweet sauces	4000
Bakery wares	Good Manufacturing Practice (GMP)
Food supplements	5000
Water-based flavoured drinks, including 'sport', 'energy' and 'electrolyte' drinks and particulated drinks	200
Coffee, coffee substitutes, tea, herbal infusions, and other hot cereal and grain beverages, excluding cocoa	200
Ready-to-eat savouries	200

Adapting the European E-number system for food additives for international use, CAC has launched the *International Numbering System* (INS) for compound identification. The system indeed largely uses the same numbers (but without the E), i.e. carnauba wax has the INS number 903 and E-number E903. While a lone standing list of INS numbers does not seen to exist, the UK Food Standards Agency (FSA) publishes a listing of E-numbers split into major additive categories (colours, etc.). This can be found on the Agency's website (http://www.food.gov.uk/safereating/ chemsafe/additivesbranch/enumberlist).

While JECFA thus makes the toxicological assessments of food additives and also of food contaminants such as toxic metals, mycotoxins and toxic plant constituents occurring naturally in food plants (e.g. cyanogenic glycosides in manioc or total alkaloids – solanine and chachonine – in potatoes), JMPR makes the corresponding assessments of pesticides. The so-called maximum residue limit (MRL; see Chapter 27), established for a pesticide by CAC on the basis of this work, again is individualized to each major crop for which the pesticide in question is regarded as being relevant. An example could be the insecticide malathion, for which the CAC-recommended MRLs are found by searching the CAC home page facility 'Official Standards – Pesticide MRLs' (presently found at (http://www.codexalimentarius.net/mrls/pestdes/jsp/pest_q-e.jsp). By doing this it is seen that MRLs (in mg kg^{-1}) are given for 27 commodities including apple (MRL 0.5), grapes (MRL 5) and cottonseed oil (edible) (MRL 13). Finally, MRLs are established for residues of veterinary drugs in food; an example could be doramectin. Doramectin (Dectomax®) is a veterinary drug used among other things for the treatment of parasites such as gastrointestinal roundworms, lungworms, eyeworms, grubs, sucking lice and mange mites in cattle. Doramectin is a derivative of ivermectin. If we search the CAC home page facility 'Official Standards – Veterinary Drugs MRLs' for doramectin we get the result shown in Table 11.1.

Before we leave the UN and its organizations it is important to stress that the standards, including the MRLs (for pesticides and veterinary drugs) and

maximum levels for food additives, developed and published by CAC are *recommendations*. The UN and its organizations have no legislative role; however, very often the recommendations are followed/adopted by single national states or by regional political cooperatives such as the EU or others.

11.3 OECD

The Organisation for Economic Co-operation and Development (OECD; in French OCDE) was formed 1961 as a continuation of the Organisation for European Economic Co-operation (OEEC) formed in 1947 to administer American and Canadian aid under the Marshall Plan for the reconstruction of Europe after World War II. The mission of OECD is to help its member countries achieve sustainable economic growth and employment and to raise the standard of living in member countries while maintaining financial stability. The focus of OECD has gradually broadened to include a growing number of other countries in addition to its 30 members, which include the USA, Canada, Mexico, Japan, South Korea, Australia, New Zealand and a number of European countries. Thus, OECD, according to the organization's own web page, now shares its expertise and accumulated experience with more than 70 developing and emerging market economies.

On the basis of this description of OECD it is not immediately evident what the organization

Table 11.1. Maximum residue limit (MRL) values for the veterinary drug doramectin.

Species	Tissue	MRL (µg kg^{-1})	Note
Cattle	Muscle	10	High concentration of residues at the injection site over a 35-day period after subcutaneous or intramuscular administration of the drug at the recommended dose.
	Liver	100	
	Kidney	30	
	Fat	150	High concentration of residues at the injection site over a 35-day period after subcutaneous or intramuscular administration of the drug at the recommended dose.
	Milk	15	Depending on the route and/or time of administration the use of doramectin in dairy cows may result in extended withdrawal periods in milk. This may be addressed in national/regional regulatory programmes.
Pig	Muscle	5	
	Liver	100	
	Kidney	30	
	Fat	150	

has to do with chemical food safety and chemical risk assessment. However, starting its work in the 1970s the Chemicals Group of the Environmental Directorate of OECD gradually launched a number of programmes. In retrospect these today can be recognized as quite outstanding concerning their influence on the world's understanding, as well as handling, of problems with chemicals and their possible adverse effect on the environment and human health.

The development and publication of the *OECD Guidelines for the Testing of Chemicals* is an example of a very practically oriented international activity within this area. The guidelines are a collection of the most relevant internationally agreed test methods used by government, industry and independent laboratories to determine the safety of chemicals and chemical preparations, including pesticides and industrial chemicals. They cover tests for the physico-chemical properties of chemicals, human health effects, environmental effects, and degradation and accumulation in the environment. Since the original publication in 1981, 18 addenda have been published. In 1993, the original publication was revised and Addenda 1–5 were incorporated. The guidelines are divided into five sections as follows:

- Section 1: Physical Chemical Properties.
- Section 2: Effects on Biotic Systems.
- Section 3: Degradation and Accumulation.
- Section 4: Health Effects.
- Section 5: Other Test Guidelines.

Most national and international organizations today will have a stipulation that, as part of the requirements for accepting an application for the approval of a chemical for a certain use, the test results reported originate from tests performed according to the OECD guidelines, or to similar later developed guidelines. Today the guidelines are available electronically (free of charge) from the website of OECD in English and French (http://www.oecd.org/document/40/0,3343,en_2649_34377_37051368_1_1_1_1,00.html).

A second very important achievement of the chemicals programme is the *OECD Principles of Good Laboratory Practice* developed in the early 1980s and revised in 1997. Today, most relevant documents concerning these principles can be downloaded from the OECD web page entitled 'OECD Series on Principles of Good Laboratory Practice and Compliance Monitoring' (http://www.oecd.org/document/63/0,3343,en_2649_34381_2346175_1_1_1_1,00.html).

Chapter 13 ('Safety Assessment Methods in the Laboratory: Toxicity Testing') in this book will to a great extent relate to the OECD Guidelines for the Testing of Chemicals with focus on the assays described in Section 4: Health Effects.

11.4 ECETOC

The European Centre for Ecotoxicology and Toxicology of Chemicals (ECETOC) was established in 1978 by a number of the world's leading companies with interests in the manufacture and use of chemicals. Today it has 50 members including international companies such as Procter & Gamble (toiletries, cosmetics, fragrances, baby care products, household cleaners, etc.), Nestlé (food products), L'Oréal (cosmetics, hair colourants and styling products), Coca Cola (soft drinks), BP (British Petroleum; petrochemical products) and Bayer (pharmaceuticals and products for crop protection). ECETOC assesses and publishes studies on the ecotoxicology and toxicology of chemicals and on existing assays for the testing of chemicals. The spectrum of publications from ECETOC is broad as may be illustrated by quoting just two recent titles: *Toxicity of Possible Impurities and By-products in Fluorocarbon Products* and *Skin Sensitisation Testing for the Purpose of Hazard Identification and Risk Assessment*.

11.5 Conclusion

Above we have discussed both national and international regulations and the scientific backgrounds for regulations concerning food, with special reference to chemical food safety. Laws as well as recommendations change relatively often. To keep up with the latest one can of course go to the primary sources, for example, the Directives within the EU, which can be found using the EUR-Lex online facility (http://eur-lex.europa.eu/). Also concerning the EU one can take advantage of the 'Food Safety – From the Farm to the Fork' portal (at http://ec.europa.eu/food/index_en.htm). However, both when it comes to the EU and when needing a more international view including the latest from the UN organizations etc., it can be an advantage to use some of the existing, indeed very good, privately established net portals such as 'Foodlaw-Reading' established and run by Dr David Jukes, Department of Food Biosciences, University of Reading, UK (found at http://www.rdg.ac.uk/foodlaw/main.htm).

Further Reading

Burdock, G.A. and Carabin, I.G. (2004) Generally recognized as safe (GRAS): history and description. *Toxicology Letters* 150, 3–18.

Hlavacek, R.J. (1981) Codex Alimentarius Commission. *Journal of the American Oil Chemists' Society* 58, 232–234.

Jensen, O.M., Parkin, D.M., MacLennan, R., Muir, C.S. and Skeet, R.G. (1991) History of cancer registration. In: *Cancer Registration: Principles and Methods*. International Agency for Research on Cancer, Lyon, France, pp. 3–6.

The EU with EFSA and EMEA

- We look at the roles of the two EU agencies EFSA and EMEA within chemical food safety.
- We briefly present the food safety control system within the EU.
- We discuss some aspects of novel foods and GMOs as special issues for legislation and control.

12.1 Introduction

The European Economic Community was established in 1957. At that time food safety was not really on the political agenda. This changed slowly during the 1970s and 1980s as the European Commission (EC) gradually took the view that Member State food safety measures constituted illegal barriers to the free movement of foodstuffs within the Community and should be eliminated. During the 1990s a number of food safety scandals (among others the Belgium dioxin scandal and the BSE crisis) reached the headlines, bringing food safety to the top of the European Community's political discussion. An extensive legislative process was initiated. In 1997 the Commission thus published a green paper on the general principles of food law in the EU. This was followed in 2000 by the *White Paper on Food Safety*. On the basis of the ideas in this white paper, in 2002 the foundation of the present legal food safety regime was established in Regulation (EC) No. 178/2002 on the General Principles of Food Law.

Today we can distinguish between the complex food safety control system gradually established by the EU and the EFSA established in Parma, Italy.

The present food safety control system in the EU includes three levels.

1. The primary control is carried out by the individual food businesses.

- Each such business must continuously verify and document that it complies with the food safety rules. If it is discovered that a requirement has not been met it is required to take corrective action. A central instrument here is the HACCP system (see Chapter 28).

2. The secondary control level is the responsibility of the national authorities.

- Each member state is obliged to maintain a system of official controls to monitor and verify that the European Community's around 8 million farms, 300,000 food processers and 600,000 retail outlets carry out the required self-control and take corrective action where necessary.

3. The third control level is by means of the European Communities' own control body known as the Food and Veterinary Office (FVO), a service of the European Commission.

- The FVO control ensures that the Member State food safety authorities fulfil their obligations.

The legal regime on food safety in the EU as established through Regulation (EC) No. 178/2002 on the General Principles of Food Law has a number of characteristics:

- it is coherent, i.e. it covers all types of foodstuffs including imported products;
- it is comprehensive, i.e. it covers the whole food chain from farm to fork;
- its primary purpose is the protection of the consumer;
- transparency is given considerable weight, i.e. public consultation and the right to information have been given prominent roles;

- it is risk-based, i.e. it is based upon independent, scientific advice; and
- the precautionary principle is granted an important role, so that protection of public health is given priority even in situations of scientific uncertainty.

The independent scientific advice is obtained through EFSA as supplemented by the European Medicines Agency (EMEA) in London. EFSA is responsible for doing risk assessments and on the basis of these making recommendations to the European Commission. Recommendations from EFSA may result in new legislation on different levels. Furthermore, EFSA has the responsibility (together with the national food authorities) of producing and conveying the relevant risk communication within the area of food safety in the EU. When it comes to making risk assessments as a basis for proposals concerning acceptable maximum levels for residues of veterinary drugs in food products of animal origin, these are done by EMEA.

12.2 Examples of Risk Assessment-based Regulatory Systems in Place in the EU

The EU has established a number of positive lists. These include the list of food additives (antioxidants, preservatives, colours, sweeteners, etc.), the list of monomers to be legally used in the production of plastics that come into contact with food and the list of food supplements (vitamins, minerals, etc.). These lists set out which compounds may be used in what food products and often they also lay down the maximum level. The lists mentioned are exhaustive: meaning that if an additive, a monomer or a supplement is not on the relevant list, it may not be used. Non-exhaustive lists have also been established, such as a list of additives allowed in the production of plastics that come into contact with food.

In order for a 'new' food additive to be added to the positive list, it must undergo a safety assessment by EFSA whereupon the list must be amended by the Community legislator. In contrast, for a food supplement to be added to the positive list, the addition is made through a so-called *comitology procedure*. This is a simpler procedure, whereby a true safety assessment by EFSA is required only if the use is foreseen to have an effect on public health (Directive 2002/46/EC). In conclusion, if a food business wants to use an additive or supplement not on the positive list, it must apply for authorization.

Also so-called *novel foods* as regulated in the Novel Food Regulation (Regulation (EC) No. 258/97) require prior authorization before being marketed in the EU. Novel foods include the following, among others:

- Foods and food ingredients: (i) with a new or intentionally modified primary molecular structure (e.g. fat substitutes); (ii) consisting of or isolated from microorganisms, fungi or algae (e.g. oil made from microalgae); (iii) consisting of or isolated from plants (e.g. phytosterols); and (iv) isolated from animals (food ingredients).
- Food and food ingredients obtained by traditional propagating or breeding practices with a history of safe food use do not come under the scope of the Regulation.
- Foods and food ingredients to which a production process not currently used has been applied, where that process gives rise to significant changes in the composition or structure of the foods or food ingredients which affect their nutritional value, metabolism or level of undesirable substances (e.g. enzymatic conversion methods).

In case of doubt the European Commission can ask the competent standing committee of the Member States to establish whether a food or a food ingredient is deemed to be novel within the intendment of the Regulation.

The Novel Food Working Group, with experts from the competent authorities and food control bodies, which is regularly convened by the European Commission, examines (among other things) whether foods/food ingredients are to be classified as novel. The results of their discussions are collected in the Novel Food Catalogue. Since June 2008 this catalogue has been published on the website of the European Commission (http://ec. europa.eu/food/food/biotechnology/novelfood/ nfnetweb/index.cfm).

With effect from 7 November 2003, foods and food ingredients containing GMOs (e.g. yoghurt with genetically modified live cultures), which consist of GMOs (e.g. genetically modified vegetable maize) or are produced from but no longer contain GMOs (e.g. purée made from genetically modified tomatoes, oil made from genetically modified rapeseed) no longer come under the scope of the Novel

Foods Regulation but are governed by the following regulations applicable from 18 April 2004:

- Regulation (EC) No. 1829/2003 on genetically modified food and feed; and
- Regulation (EC) No. 1830/2003 concerning the traceability and labelling of genetically modified organisms and the traceability of food and feed products produced from genetically modified organisms and amending Directive 2001/18/EC.

The provisions in the Novel Foods Regulation concerning GMOs were deleted (Article 1 para 2 letters a and b; Article 3 para 2 sub-para 2 and para 3; Article 8 para 1 letter d; Article 9) or revised (Article 3 para 4 sentence 1).

Genetically modified foods and food ingredients placed lawfully on the market in accordance with the Novel Foods Regulation or Directive 90/220/EEC continue to be marketable if the responsible companies informed the European Commission by 18 October 2004 of the date when the product was placed on the market for the first time and submitted information on safety assessment and labelling, as well as a suitable method for detecting the product. Furthermore, additives, flavourings and extraction solutions are not covered by the scope of the Novel Foods Regulation either. Other legal provisions of the EU apply to them to the extent that they comply with the safety level stipulated in the Novel Foods Regulation.

However, 'novel' not only means food products that are the result of technical innovation, but also refers to food products that may have been known and consumed for centuries, but which are new in the European Community. Thus, to market a food product such as noni juice (Box 12.1) from South-East Asia, authorization must first be obtained. The scientific assessment for this juice included laboratory animal studies for toxicity, genotoxicity and allergenicity and took 3 years. An authorization for a novel food product only gives the applicant a right to market the novel food in question. If another food business wants to market the same novel food product, this other food business must submit a new application. However, for such a subsequent application a simplified procedure applies.

12.3 Rules Concerning the Process of Food Production from Farm to Fork

The European Community's food safety regime has to an appreciable extent laid down stringent rules on how to handle the production, processing and distribution of food products. The primary instruments are extensive hygiene obligations and the obligation for food businesses to establish a traceability system. Thus, it is required that all food business operators (with the exception of primary producers) 'put in place, implement and maintain a permanent procedure or procedures based on the HACCP [learn more in Chapter 28] principles' (Regulation (EC) No. 852/2004). For special products even stricter rules exist. Thus, the EU standards for milk and milk products require

---

Box 12.1. The origin of noni juice

Noni, *Morinda citrifolia* L., is a large evergreen shrub or small tree up to 6 m or more in height. The white tubular flowers (Fig. 12.1) are grouped in heads at the leaf axils. The greenish-white to pale-yellow fleshy fruits are ovoid or globose syncarps 5 to 7 cm long. They have an unpleasant odour resembling cheese. They contain a number of seeds about 4 mm long. The plant is commonly known as 'noni', but is also found under the names of 'Indian mulberry', 'great morinda', 'cheeze-fruit', 'morinda', 'mouse's pineapple', 'yellow root', 'jumbie breadfruit', 'hog apple', 'pain killer', 'mengkudu', 'nono', 'feyukke friudem rhubarbe caraïbe', 'bilimbi', 'pomme-macaque' and 'pomme de singe'.

Noni is probably native to the maritime forests of northern Australia as well as those bordering the Western Pacific and Indian Oceans. Beginning 2000 years ago it was spread widely first by people native to the region and more recently by Europeans. Today it is naturalized in most tropical and tropical coastal forests. The fruits of noni are somewhat tasteless and have an unpleasant smell.

Noni juice produced from fruits collected in the wild or grown in plantations is today an economically important botanical remedy and food supplement on the international market. This is based on its reputation as a traditional medicinal plant in the Pacific Ocean region, which has been followed by a limited number of scientific investigations demonstrating for example an analgesic effect.

Continued

Box 12.1. Continued.

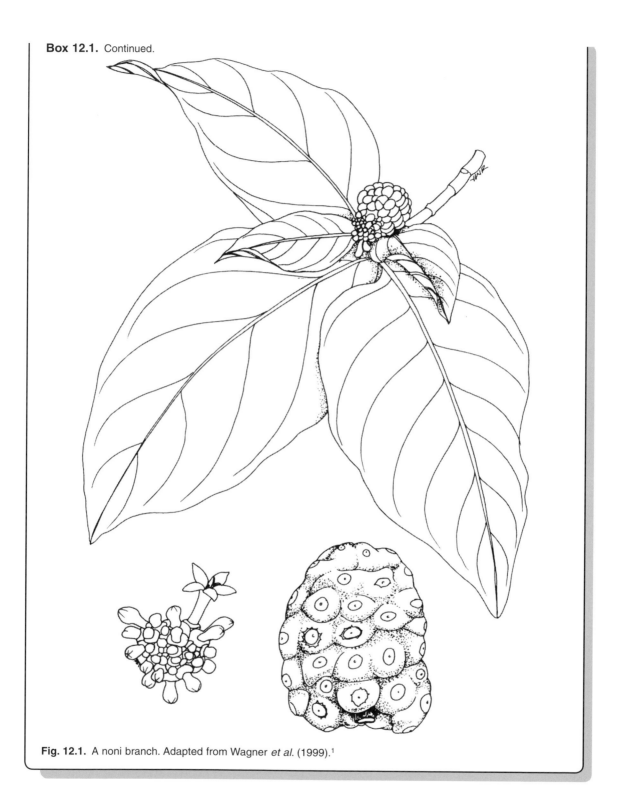

Fig. 12.1. A noni branch. Adapted from Wagner *et al.* (1999).[1]

inspection and monitoring at the level of primary production, i.e. in the stable.

12.4 Import of Food Products to the EU from non-EU Countries

European Community food businesses selling in the European market are not the only businesses that must comply with the EU control requirements including full product traceability. So also must third-country producers. However, to what extent this is the case depends on the type of product produced and exported into the EU. Since products of animal origin are considered to represent the greatest risk, these are subject to stricter controls than are products of non-animal (typical plant) origin.

Third-country food businesses producing or processing food products of animal origin thus must obtain Community approval and registration before export can take place. For food products of non-animal origin there exists no pre-approval requirement. Instead it is incumbent on the EU importer to verify that the third-country food business has met the Community's food safety requirements. Finally it should be noted that products of plant origin may only be exported to the EU if, prior to the export, the national plant protection authority of the export country has inspected (and certified) the products to be free of those pests and diseases that are listed in the Plant Health Directive (Directive 2000/29/EC).

12.5 Influence of the Strict Food Regulations of the EU and Countries in Other Highly Developed Geographical Regions

Obviously strict rules concerning handling in general, traceability and hygiene, together with effective control systems and low maximum levels of acceptance for health-impairing chemical compounds in food, represent an advantage for the consumer. However, it must not be overlooked that such systems and levels also put hard pressures on

developing countries when these want to export food products to, for example, the European market. To obtain a Community approval and registration for export of food products of animal origin thus may simply not be possible, economically speaking. Recently the World Bank in a report also stressed that certain African countries in particular would lose considerable export incomes due to a lowering of the accepted maximum levels for aflatoxins in dried fruits and nuts put in place 1998 by the EU. Intense international negotiations to explore the possibility of establishing slightly higher harmonized levels subsequently made the Commission ask EFSA to make a new risk assessment. The agendum was to look at the effect(s) on health in Europe of increasing the limit value for total aflatoxins from the existing $4\,\mu g\,kg^{-1}$ to 8 or $10\,\mu g\,kg^{-1}$.

Often products intended for export that cannot be exported, however, due to too high a content of an unsafe compound will be sold and consumed at the home market of the producer.

Note

[1] Wagner, L.R., Herbst, D.R. and Sahmer, S.H. (1999) *The Manual of Flowering Plants of Hawaii*, revised edn. Bernice Pauahi Bishop Museum Special Publication. University of Hawaii, Honolulu, Hawaii.

Further Reading

Commission of the European Communities (1999) *White Paper on Food Safety. COM (1999) 719 final, 20.1.2000.* Commission of the European Communities, Brussels.

European Parliament and the Council (2002) *Regulation (EC) No 178/2002 of the European Parliament and of the Council of 28 January 2002 laying down the general principles and requirements of food law, establishing the European Food Safety Authority and laying down procedures in matters of food safety.* Commission of the European Communities, Brussels.

Peterson, J. and Shackleton, M. (eds) (2006) *The Institutions of the European Union*, 2nd edn. Oxford University Press, Oxford, UK.

Safety Assessment Methods in the Laboratory: Toxicity Testing

- The structure of the OECD guidelines for the testing of chemicals is introduced.
- The influence of international approval of toxicity tests is briefly discussed.
- The major overall groups of assay are presented and a few examples, especially *in vivo* assays, are discussed in more detail.
- The concepts of QSAR and *in silico* studies are introduced.
- The concept of required toxicological data set for a risk assessment is introduced.

13.1 Introduction

In order to optimize the results from tests and hence make them as comparable as possible, a process towards standardization has taken place. The international organization OECD started this by their development of the *OECD Guidelines for the Testing of Chemicals*. Later, other national and international organizations developed similar collections of descriptions of standardized tests (assays), examples being the US organizations FDA and EPA, the corresponding agencies in Japan and recently also the corresponding centralized agencies of the EU.

As noted earlier in Chapter 11 the OECD guidelines cover tests for the physico-chemical properties of chemicals, human health effects, environmental effects, and degradation and accumulation in the environment. In the present chapter we look in more detail at the assays found in Section 4: Health Effects of the OECD guidelines.

In Chapter 11 we talked about the role of OECD especially in developing guidelines for the testing of chemicals, i.e. a number of assays specific for toxicity. These guidelines can be reached from the web page 'SourceOECD' (at http://lysander.sourceoecd.org/vl=661567/cl=14/nw=1/rpsv/periodical/p15_about.htm?jnlissn=1607310x), while draft guidelines still open for comment can be downloaded from the page 'Chemicals Testing: Draft OECD Guidelines

for the Testing of Chemicals – Sections 1–5' (http://www.oecd.org/document/22/0,3343,en_2649_34377_1916054_1_1_1_1,00.html).

The OECD guidelines are indeed still very important worldwide, but have been followed by collections of guidelines from other organizations. Thus, the EU today has a number of guidelines for toxicity assay. The EU guidelines were published in Directive 92/69/EEC as Annex V of Directive 67/548/EEC. Over the years since publication, amendments to these methods have been made and new guidelines introduced. Most of the guidelines are, however, transcripts of OECD guidelines (the most notable exceptions being flammability and explosivity guidelines).

Australian guidelines and those of many other countries are based firmly on OECD methods, although the USA and Japan notably have some restrictions on what they require. To overcome national differences, the OECD guidelines are often those indicated to be used – maybe as accompanied by phrases such as 'or similar guidelines'.

The EU guidelines can be downloaded for free from the European Chemicals Bureau website (http://ecb.jrc.it/testing-methods/). Annex V to Directive 67/548/EEC is divided into three parts, which contain Testing Methods for chemicals that address all areas of concern:

- Part A contains methods for the determination of *physico-chemical* properties (e.g. melting and boiling point, density, flash point, flammability, explosivity, oxidizing power, etc.);

- Part B contains methods for the determination of effects on *human health* (e.g. acute or chronic toxicity, skin sensitization, irritancy, corrosivity, carcinogenicity, neurotoxicity, etc., also including *in vitro* or alternative methods); and

- Part C contains methods for *environmental effects*, ecotoxicity and environmental fate (e.g. toxicity to fish, daphnia or algae, bioconcentration, biodegradability, etc.).

Several individual countries as well as organizations with regional and truly worldwide coverage have thus been and are engaged in the development of guidelines (or guides) on how to carry out toxicity assays, but also other different activities in order to ensure and document a specified quality of a process or a product. We have guidelines concerning Good Manufacturing Practice (GMP) and Good Laboratory Practice (GLP), about how to establish and run quality control systems such as a HACCP system, concerning how to perform specific chemical tests and biological assays (validated methods), and recently also about how to more generally validate new methods or how to plan, perform and report a whole sequence of, for example, biological assays such as 'a safety pharmacology package' for a new drug candidate.

Especially within the detailed setup of toxicity assays, small differences between, for example, the guidelines of OECD, the EU, FDA and Japan have led to problems for industries working internationally. Therefore, the International Conference on Harmonization of Technical Requirements for Registration of Pharmaceuticals for Human Use (ICH) was established.

ICH is a unique project that brings together the regulatory authorities of Europe, Japan and the USA and experts from the pharmaceutical industry in the three regions to discuss scientific and technical aspects of product registration.

The purpose is to make recommendations on ways to achieve greater harmonization in the interpretation and application of technical guidelines and the requirements for product registration, with the aim of reducing or obviating the need to duplicate the testing carried out during the research and development of new medicines.

The objective of such harmonization is a more economical use of human, animal and material resources, and the elimination of unnecessary delay in the global development and availability of new medicines, while maintaining safeguards on quality, safety and efficacy, and regulatory obligations to protect public health (http://www.ich.org/cache/compo/276-254-1.html).

The guidelines developed so far by ICH are divided into four major categories, and ICH Topic Codes are assigned according to these categories, as follows:

- Code Q – 'Quality' Topics, i.e. those relating to chemical and pharmaceutical quality assurance (stability testing, impurity testing, etc.);
- Code S – 'Safety' Topics, i.e. those relating to *in vitro* and *in vivo* pre-clinical studies (carcinogenicity testing, genotoxicity testing, etc.);
- Code E – 'Efficacy' Topics, i.e. those relating to clinical studies in human subject (dose-response studies, good clinical practices, etc.); and
- Code M – 'Multidisciplinary' Topics, i.e. cross-cutting topics which do not fit uniquely into one of the above categories.

Looking into the Safety Topics we currently find papers describing the harmonized view on what is needed and how in general it should be performed concerning such topics as immunotoxicity of compounds ('ICH Harmonized Tripartite Guideline; Immunotoxicity Studies for Human Pharmaceuticals – S8'), genotoxicity ('Guidance on Genotoxicity Testing and Data Interpretation for Pharmaceuticals Intended for Human Use – S2(R1)') and 'safety pharmacology'.

Safety pharmacology is defined as 'those studies that investigate the potential undesirable pharmacodynamic effects of a substance on physiological functions in relation to exposure in the therapeutic range and above'. The harmonized guideline within this subject area is the 'ICH Harmonized Tripartite Guideline; Safety Pharmacology Studies for Human Pharmaceuticals – S7A'. This guideline states, among other things, that animal models as well as *ex vivo* and *in vitro* preparations can be used as test systems. *Ex vivo* and *in vitro* systems can include, but are not limited to: isolated organs and tissues, cell cultures, cellular fragments, subcellular organelles, receptors, ion channels, transporters and enzymes. *In vitro* systems can be used in supportive studies (e.g. to obtain a profile of the activity of the substance or to investigate the mechanism of effects observed *in vivo*).

In conclusion it can be said that guidelines have come to stay. They help us a lot but their presence also means that much effort is needed in order to keep up with current guidelines.

13.2 Why Do We Test?

We can test for toxicity in order to obtain knowledge about the effect(s) of a compound or a product (mixture of compounds) on the health (well-being/functional status) of a selected animal species, a plant species or an ecological system.

Very often we do such tests using selected animal species but with the ultimate aim of a subsequent extrapolation of the results to ourselves, i.e. to the most possible effects on man. The reason for testing the compound or product can be different. Perhaps the compound or product: (i) is already in use, e.g. in industry, but is suspected to cause negative health effects; (ii) has been identified as a component of pollution without any knowledge being available about its potential effect on man or animals; or (iii) has been synthesized by a company that wants to market it as a new pesticide, food or feed additive or a human or veterinary medicine, in which case the results of a number of tests for toxicity are required as part of the application for approval by the relevant authorities.

Investigations of the potentially harmful effects of a compound or product (its *toxicity*) may grossly be divided into two main groups. Thus, one can either: (i) test (= assay) for any adverse effect observed when administering the agent to a population (animal/plant) or an ecosystem; or (ii) use a specially developed bioassay optimized to disclose one well-defined effect, such as the ability to cause skin irritation or reproductive failure. We could call these assays *general assays* and *special assays*, respectively.

From around the time after World War II it has been generally agreed, in the international scientific community, that the result of a given test for toxicity depends very much on a number of parameters such as: (i) the genetic identity (strain) of the test organism; (ii) the age and sex as well as the stress level of the test animal; (iii) the physical surroundings including light/darkness cycle; and (iv) a number of details around the administration of the compound or product to be tested. Also the subsequent data handling and presentation may influence the conclusions drawn.

Tests
General assays

The general assays include tests for: (i) acute toxicity; (ii) repeated dose 28-day toxicity in rodents; (iii) repeated dose 90-day toxicity in rodents; (iv) repeated dose 90-day toxicity in non-rodents; and (v) chronic toxicity (the objective of which is to characterize the profile of a substance in a mammalian species (primarily rodents) following prolonged and repeated exposure). Most of these assays are described in detail for oral as well as for dermal exposure and for exposure by inhalation.

Special assays

The special assays today are numerous. In general they can be classified into special *in vivo* assays and special *in vitro* assays. By *in vivo* we mean that the test is performed using a live intact organism with its metabolism and compensations and complex reaction possibilities. *In vitro* (from the Latin: in a glass), on the other hand, refers to biological experiments outside the intact live organism. Within toxicology examples include the '*In vitro* skin corrosion – human skin model test' and the 'Bovine corneal opacity and permeability test method for identifying ocular corrosives and severe irritants'. The latter is an *in vitro* test method that can be used to classify substances as ocular corrosives and severe irritants using isolated corneas from the eyes of cattle slaughtered for commercial purposes, thus avoiding the use of laboratory animals. Further examples are described below.

IN VIVO ASSAYS. The pallet of special *in vivo* assays is indeed broad, from tests using only one or a few animals to tests such as the 'Two-generation reproduction toxicity test' designed to provide general information concerning the effects of a test substance on the integrity and performance of the male and female reproductive systems. The latter uses a lot of animals. A few additional examples of special *in vivo* assays are:

- 'Acute eye irritation/corrosion';
- 'Skin sensitization';
- 'Delayed neurotoxicity of organophosphorus substances following acute exposure';
- 'Neurotoxicity study in rodents'; and
- 'Genetic toxicology: mouse spot test'.

IN VITRO ASSAYS. *In vitro* assays today include a variety of tests using isolated organs, isolated cells, cultured cells or subcellular components. In addition to the already mentioned tests for skin and ocular corrosion, examples include tests as different as:

- '*In vitro* 3T3 NRU phototoxicity test', a method to evaluate photo-cytotoxicity by the relative reduction in viability of cells exposed to the chemical in the presence versus absence of light.
- '*In vitro* mammalian chromosome aberration test', the purpose of which is to identify agents that cause structural chromosome aberrations in cultured mammalian somatic cells. Structural aberrations include any numerical or structural change in the usual chromosome complement (the whole set of chromosomes for the species; in man, the chromosome complement – also called the *karyotype* – consists of 46 chromosomes) of a cell or organism. An example of a structural change includes the gain, loss or rearrangement of chromosome segments after the continuity of the DNA strand in one or more chromosomes is disrupted. Another is the formation of ring chromosomes. When one break occurs in each arm of a chromosome the broken ends of the internal centromeric fragment may join, resulting in the formation of a stable ring chromosome. Each of the two end segments lacks a centromere, and such acentric fragments are lost during cell division.

Special tests using bacteria

Specific concerns about the possibility of a compound or product causing mutations (changes) in the genetic setup have led to the development of a high number of tests for mutagenicity. Here several tests using bacteria have been developed. These have proved to be very useful indeed, especially as both a cheap and a quick instrument for the screening of, for example, a battery of synthesized candidate compounds in the development of a new food additive, pesticide or drug. Positive results (i.e. the compound induces mutations) will most often lead to termination of the further planned programme for the compound in question. In contrast, a negative result will always have to be confirmed in one or more *in vivo* assays using higher animals, typically mammals in the form of a rodent species.

Within the bacterial assays for mutagenesis, the 'Bacterial reverse mutation test' (OECD test no. 471) uses amino acid-requiring strains of *Salmonella typhimurium* (the Ames test) or *Escherichia coli* to detect point mutations by base substitutions or frameshifts. Thus, the test uses amino acid-dependent strains of *S. typhimurium* and *E. coli*. In the absence of, for example, an external histidine source, these cells cannot grow to form colonies. However, colony growth is resumed if a reversion of the mutation occurs, allowing the production of histidine to be resumed. Spontaneous reversions occur with each of the strains, but mutagenic compounds included in the growth medium cause an increase in the number of revertant colonies relative to the background level. Bacterial culture medium is inoculated with the appropriate *S. typhimurium* or *E. coli* strain and incubated overnight. Often a dose range-finding study for the test chemical is carried out using the *S. typhimurium* strain TA100 only, over a wide range of dose.

A special strength of these tests is that to a certain extent they also allow us to test whether a compound is mutagenic after metabolism by cytochome P450 enzymes. Thus, endoplasmic reticulum membranes (in the form of so-called microsomes; also called S9 mix) isolated from rats can be added to the growth medium together with both the tested chemical and the microorganisms. Metabolism often occurs that mimics the true liver metabolism, and hence the effect of the metabolites can be observed.

Combined general and special assays

The objective of OECD test no. 453 'Combined chronic toxicity/carcinogenicity study' is to identify the majority of chronic (i.e. general) and carcinogenic (special) effects and to determine dose–response relationships following prolonged and repeated exposure, within one combined study.

13.3 Quantitative Structure–Activity Relationships and *In Silico* Studies

In 1962 Hansch and co-workers published a study on the relationship between molecular structure and measured activity (potency) of a number of chemicals as plant growth regulators. Although observations concerning systematic rules governing the relationship between molecular structure and a certain biological activity had been published earlier, on the basis of this work Corwin Hansch, Professor of Chemistry at Pomona College in California, is today known as the father of the concept of the *quantitative structure–activity relationship* (QSAR). QSAR soon found its way into the practice of agrochemistry, pharmaceutical chemistry and toxicology.

QSARs are based on the assumption that the structure of a molecule (i.e. its geometric, steric and electronic properties) must contain the features responsible for its physical, chemical and biological properties, and on the ability to represent the chemical by one, or more, numerical descriptor(s). By QSAR models, the biological activity of a new/untested compound can be inferred from the molecular structure of similar compounds whose activity has already been assessed.

Today QSARs are being applied in many disciplines such as risk assessment, toxicity prediction and regulatory decisions, in addition to drug discovery. The development of a good-quality QSAR model depends on a number of factors, such as the quality of the biological data, the choice of descriptors and the statistical methods used. Any QSAR modelling should ultimately lead to statistically robust models capable of making reliable and accurate predictions of biological activities of new compounds.

Gradually *in silico* studies have also gained some popularity. The expression *in silico* means 'performed on computer or via computer simulation'. The phrase was first seen in 1989 as an analogy to the Latin phrases *in vivo* and *in vitro*, which, as already discussed, are commonly used for experiments done in living organisms and outside living organisms, respectively. Thus, the phrase applies to computer simulations that model natural or laboratory processes (in all the natural sciences), such as toxicity testing.

A look into the *OECD Guidelines for the Testing of Chemicals* immediately discloses both the possibility of using *in vitro* assays and that of including knowledge concerning the effects of structurally related compounds, as pointed to in a number of tests. Thus, in the chapter 'Initial considerations', the two test nos 404 ('Acute dermal irritation/corrosion') and 405 ('Acute eye irritation/corrosion') have nearly identical texts, saying (from 405; phrases italicized by the present author):

> In the interest of both sound science and animal welfare, *in vivo* testing should not be considered until all available data relevant to the potential eye corrosivity/irritation of the substance has been evaluated in a

weight-of-the-evidence analysis. Such data will include evidence from existing studies in humans and/or laboratory animals, *evidence of corrosivity/irritation of one or more structurally related substances* or mixtures of such substances, data demonstrating high acidity or alkalinity of the substance, and results from *validated and accepted in vitro or ex vivo tests for skin corrosion and irritation*. The studies may have been conducted prior to, or as a result of, a weight-of-the-evidence analysis.

13.4   Requested Toxicological Data Set

The usual process of approval of a substance or product for use as a food additive, a pesticide or a drug involves a safety evaluation. This requires an extensive toxicological database to be generated for the compound/product in question. If we look at the requirements for a food additive candidate as defined by the EU Scientific Committee for Food in 2001, these include long-term (2-year) chronic toxicity/carcinogenicity studies and reproductive/developmental toxicity studies in addition to short-term toxicity and genotoxicity studies. On this basis an ADI can subsequently be derived using a default uncertainty factor of 100 applied to the No Observed Adverse Effect Level (NOAEL) from the most sensitive of these studies (the pivotal study).

Another example of such a collection of toxicity tests determined by a responsible risk assessment and management body to be required for approval of a compound for a certain type of use could be the very recently published requirements for EFSA to look at an application for approval of a 'Smoke Flavouring Primary Product'. In this case it stated that the dossier of toxicological data must include: (i) a 90-day feeding study in rodents, preferably rats (OECD test no. 408); and (ii) a number of tests for genotoxicity, i.e. a test for induction of gene mutations in bacteria (OECD test no. 471), a test for induction of gene mutations in mammalian cells *in vitro* (preferably the mouse lymphoma *tk* assay) (OECD test no. 476) and a test for induction of chromosomal aberrations in mammalian cells *in vitro* (OECD test no. 473). It is furthermore stated specifically that studies should be conducted using internationally agreed protocols and according to GLP principles as described in Council Directives 87/18/EEC2 and 88/320/EEC3.

With this knowledge in mind we now look a little further into a few tests and the interpretation and use of the results obtained from such tests.

13.5 Acute Toxicity: Determination of/Screening for

Introduction

Knowledge concerning the acute toxicity of a compound or product is of major importance no matter the agent, or its present or planned use. Reasons for this are plenty, including:

- knowledge to allow proper labelling for workers (protection measures, etc.);
- knowledge to allow correct treatment if individuals are poisoned; and
- knowledge to ease the planning of long-term toxicological studies (dose levels to ensure effects as well as survival during the planned period of dosing).

Today all applications to go to authorities in order to obtain approval of a new compound/product – whether for use as a food additive, a pesticide or a drug (human or veterinary) – will have to include solid data for acute (as well as other) toxicity. This includes information concerning the exposure levels to induce toxicity (the potency) as well as the toxic manifestations (target organs and symptoms).

Traditionally, acute toxicity has been determined using rats or mice. The preference for these two species originates in the fact that they are readily available, affordable and easy to handle, especially the rat. Furthermore, there are more toxicological data available on these species than for any other animal species. By generally accepted definition *acute toxicity studies* involve either a single administration of the chemical or several administrations within a 24h period. The route of administration can be oral (through food or by gavage), dermal or by inhalation, or by other parenteral routes.

The *acute* in the test refers to the administration. However, the effect(s) can be acute (the animals drop dead within a few minutes) or can manifest themselves over time (delayed effects including death). Therefore, by general agreement the dosed animals should be observed over a period of usually 7–14 days depending on the test manual used.

During the observation period toxic signs should be observed and written down for later analysis. Such observations may help in characterizing the nature of the toxicant. Table 13.1 lists a number of examples of observable signs of toxicity (toxic manifestations) that may be seen/measured and documented in writing if wanted/needed according to the purpose of the test and/or demands by the protocol used.

At death or at latest at the termination of the test, gross autopsies should be performed on all animals including the animals from the control group(s) (there may be two control groups if a toxicologically not well characterized vehicle is used, i.e. one group with no dosing and one dosed with the vehicle only). Autopsy can provide useful information concerning the target organ(s).

Table 13.1. Relationship between toxic signs and body organs or systems. Adapted from Lu and Kacew (2002).[1]

System	Toxic signs
Autonomic	Relaxed nictitating membrane, exophthalmos, nasal discharge, salivation, diarrhoea, urination, piloerection
Behavioural	Sedation, restlessness, sitting position – head up, staring straight ahead, drooping head, severe depression, excessive preening, gnawing paws, panting, irritability, aggressive and defensive hostility, fear, confusion, bizarre activity
Cardiovascular	Increased or decreased heart rate, cyanosis, vasoconstriction, vasodilation, haemorrhage
Cutaneous	Piloerection, wet dog shakes, erythema, oedema, necrosis, swelling
Gastrointestinal	Salivation, retching, diarrhoea, bloody stools and urine
Gastrourinary	Constipation, rhinorrhoea, emesis, involuntary urination and defecation
Neuromuscular	Decreased or increased activity, fasciculation, tremors, convulsions, ataxia, prostration, straub tail, hind-limb weakness, pain and hind-limb reflexes (absent or diminished), opisthotonus, muscle tone, death
Ocular	Mydriasis, miosis, lacrimation, ptosis, nystagmus, cycloplegia, papillary light reflex
Respiratory	Hypopnoea, dyspnoea, gasping, apnoea
Sensory	Sensitivity to pain, righting, corneal, labyrinth, placing and hind-limb reflex; sensitivity to sound and touch; nystagmus, phonation

13.6 Dose–Response Relationship

The potency of poisonous compounds varies and an assay for acute toxicity will, as already mentioned, ideally give information about symptoms, target organs and potency. Traditionally, assays for acute toxicity as performed using rats or mice have focused on calculating the so-called *median (acute) lethal dose* (abbreviated 'lethal dose, 50%' or LD_{50}). This was introduced as a numeric estimate of the potency of a toxicant by J.W. Trevan in 1927 and is defined as: *the dose, statistically estimated, that, when administered to a population, will result in the death of 50% of the population*. Taking this value as a measure of differences in potency we certainly see a great variation between known toxicants. Thus, the LD_{50} for ferrous sulfate by oral administration to the rat is 1500 mg kg^{-1} BW, while it is 0.00001 mg kg^{-1} BW for botulinum toxin.

When given the same dose as measured in amount of substance per kilogram of body weight, some individuals within a population show an intense response whereas others respond less strongly. For a lethal compound at a particular dose, some animals will succumb to a dose that others will survive. The relationship between dose and response is typically sigmoid in shape.

In practice, determination of the LD_{50} (or 'lethal concentration, 50%' (LC_{50}) for inhaled substances or for toxicity of compounds to water-living organisms) is performed as follows (freely available from the *OECD Guidelines for the Testing of Chemicals* – test no. 401).

- The substance is administered in graduated doses to several groups of animals; one dose per group.
- At least five animals are used at each dose level (of the same sex).
- The doses chosen can be based on the result of a range-finding test.
- The doses administered should be at least three different levels (+ a control group), and spaced appropriately, to produce test groups with a range of toxic effects and mortality rates.
- Subsequent observations of effects and deaths are made.
- The data should be sufficient to produce a dose–response curve.

Figure 13.1 illustrates how an LD_{50} of 20 mg is derived.

Other dose estimates also may be used. LD_0 represents the dose at which no individuals are expected to die. This is just below the threshold for lethality. LD_{10} refers to the dose at which 10% of the individuals will die.

Alternatives to the original LD_{50} determination

For some years now the strict determination of the LD_{50}/LC_{50} value as just described has been gradually phased out in some jurisdictions in favour of tests such as the *Fixed Dose Procedure*, the *Acute Oral Toxicity (AOT) Up-and-Down Procedure* or the *Acute Toxic Class Method*. All of these are alternative acute toxicity tests that provide a way

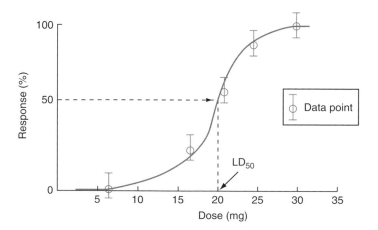

Fig. 13.1. A dose–response curve and derivation of the LD_{50} value. Adapted from The Encyclopedia of Earth web page.[2]

to determine the toxicity of chemicals with fewer test animals by using sequential dosing steps

As an example of this worldwide trend towards using alternatives to the original determination of LD_{50} in rats, one can mention the development in the USA where different offices joined in harmonizing their official methods for the determination of acute oral toxicity. Thus, the Office of Prevention, Pesticides and Toxic Substances (OPPTS) of EPA provides a link on its website (http://www.epa.gov/opptsfrs/publications/Test_Guidelines/series870.htm) to a harmonized test, '870.1100 – Acute Oral Toxicity (December 2002)'. Looking further into this one finds the following introductory presentation:

The Office of Prevention, Pesticides and Toxic Substances (OPPTS) has developed this guideline through a process of harmonization that blended the testing guidance and requirements that existed in the Office of Pollution Prevention and Toxics (OPPT) and appeared in Title 40, Chapter I, Subchapter R of the Code of Federal Regulations (CFR), the Office of Pesticide Programs (OPP) which appeared in publications of the National Technical Information Service (NTIS) and the guidelines published by the Organization for Economic Cooperation and Development (OECD).

And further:

EPA recommends the Up-and-Down Procedure (UDP) as detailed in this guideline and adopted by the Organization for Economic Cooperation and Development (OECD) as test Guideline 425 (see paragraph (n)(1) of this guide-line), to assess acute oral toxicity. This method provides a point estimate of lethality and confidence interval around the LD50. Acute oral toxicity testing may also be performed using the Fixed Dose Method of OECD Guideline 420 (see paragraph (n)(2) of this guideline) or the Acute Toxic Class Method of OECD Guideline 423 (see paragraph (n)(3) of this guide-line). These methods assess lethality within a dose range.

13.7 Repeated Dose 28-Day Oral Toxicity Study in Rodents (OECD test no. 407, adopted 3 October 2008)

A study of repeated dose toxicity such as this or a longer subchronic (90-day) study is most often required as either a stand-alone study of what happens when the exposure is extended in time or as a preparation for a long-term chronic toxicity study. Knowing that a chronic study in rodents runs over a period of 1 year and includes at least four groups of 40 animals each, it is evident that one must have a solid basis for the selection of the dose levels. This is provided by the repeated dose studies, which, in turn, are planned on the basis of knowledge gained from the study of acute toxicity. Thus, the chapter about dosing in test no. 407 says:

Dose levels should be selected taking into account any existing toxicity and (toxico-) kinetic data available for the test compound or related materials. The highest dose level should be chosen with the aim of inducing toxic effects but not death or severe suffering. Thereafter, a descending sequence of dose levels should be selected with a view to demonstrating any dosage-related response and no observed adverse effects at the lowest dose level (NOAEL). Two to four fold intervals are frequently optimal for setting the descending dose levels and addition of a fourth test group is often preferable to using very large intervals (e.g. more than a factor of 10) between dosages.

13.8 Other Tests and Their Interrelationships

We can look at a number of other tests and again find that the design of one as such is dependent on results obtained from another, e.g. the first providing the basis for the selection of the dose levels for the next. Thus, the chapter on the selection of dose levels in the test 'One generation reproduction toxicity study' (OECD test no. 415) states that 'ideally, the intermediate dose(s) should induce minimal toxic effects attributable to the test substance, and the low dose should not induce any observable adverse effects on the parent or offspring'. Clearly, this can only be obtained on the basis of results from a well-designed repeated dose study. Similar recommendations can be found in texts to assays such as 'Prenatal developmental toxicity study' (OECD test no. 414 = teratogenicity) and 'Mammalian erythrocyte micronucleus test' (OECD test no. 474), the latter saying 'the dose being the maximum tolerated dose or that producing some indication of cytotoxicity'.

13.9 Quick and Cheap Screenings for Toxicity of a Compound or Product

In many situations quick information may be wanted on whether a compound or product should be considered toxic or not, including a rough idea of how toxic it is to animals. For such an examination one will rarely use highly developed animals such as mice, out of both ethical and financial considerations. Instead a battery of tests may be used which could also be employed for the elucidation of any environmental consequence of the spreading of the compound, for the screening of a series of compounds extracted and purified from a medical plant, or for the screening of synthetic pesticide candidates, e.g. for insecticidal activity.

One such method uses fruit flies, which may even be wingless mutants to ease the handling. Other test types use larvae of various species of the *Artemia* genus (brine shrimps). The *Artemia* genus is scattered worldwide and the word 'brine' means very salty water. After mating, the 8–10 mm long animals lay their eggs. Under favourable conditions these hatch immediately, while in water which is too saline or with a low oxygen level the eggs develop a thick shell, after which they are called cysts. When hatching, either directly after laying or from the cyst stadium, the larvae are released, called nauplii. These are able to live for about 3 days without food. The nauplii develop into full-grown brine shrimps through 15 different stages.

Cysts such as those of *Artemia salina* can be purchased commercially, since owners of aquariums hatch the cysts and use the larvae as feed for their fish. Some of the cysts on the market derive from large salt lakes in the state of Utah, USA (home of the large town Salt Lake City).

The brine shrimp test

The first to point to *A. salina* as a suitable organism for toxicity tests were A.S. Michael, C.G. Thompson and M. Abramovitz from the Entomology Research Branch, USDA, Beltsville, Maryland. The three scientists developed the test for their work on the identification of new compounds with potential as insecticides. At first different setups of the method were used and so too were both fully developed shrimps and several of the different larval stages. One of the methods included observing the time for the adult animal to sink to the bottom due to paralysis of the swimming movements.

Since the first article on the usage of *Artemia*, many other scientists have developed their own protocols for how to test toxicity using this organism. Meyer *et al.* used nauplii which they fed with yeast during the test. They determined LC_{50} for a long list of plant extracts after 6 and 24 h of exposure and

compared the results with those from two tests for cytotoxicity to cancer cells for the same plant extracts. A long line of other experiments confirm that the brine shrimp test is applicable for many different types of compound. The first to perform the test in a microtitre plate were Pablo *et al.* in 1992. Such tests are today commercially available in kits.

As mentioned above, a large selection of structurally very different compounds has been tested for toxicity using *A. salina*. Hence, when searching on the Internet, it is possible to find a database listing many compounds and their toxic effect(s) on this organism ('Brine shrimp (*Artemia salina*) Chemical Toxicity Studies', available at http://www.pesticideinfo.org/List_AquireAll.jsp?Species=366).

The brine shrimp test for toxicity: how to perform the test

On the first day 25 ml of artificial seawater is measured and placed in a Petri dish. Eggs of the species *A. salina* are used for this test. An appropriate amount of eggs is taken, i.e. about 200 mg, and dispersed on the water surface in the Petri dish and the lid is replaced to protect from pollution, reduce evaporation and ensure a high humidity in the air layer above the water. The Petri dish is then placed under an electric light bulb, ensuring that the temperature is between 25 and 28°C. The eggs are left to hatch overnight.

After 24–48 h the majority of the larvae are hatched and ready for use. A funnel is placed in a large plastic centrifuge tube and the content of the Petri dish is transferred to the tube. If necessary an additional 5 ml of artificial seawater is used to rinse the Petri dish for any remnants of larvae and eggs.

The centrifuge tube is closed and gently turned upside down a few times, then left to rest for a few minutes. This will give the non-hatched eggs an opportunity to gather on the surface. The lid is removed without shaking the tube. The eggs floating on the surface are gently removed using a Pasteur pipette.

Five millilitres of the resulting larvae suspension is transferred to a clean centrifuge tube. The suspension is *taken from the middle of the liquid column to avoid any eggs from the top or the bottom*.

One drop of the suspension with the larvae is placed on a glass slide with a cover slip on top and the larvae can be observed under a microscope.

The centrifuge tube is closed and gently turned upside down to remix the suspension. The tube is opened and 0.1 ml is extracted and placed on a glass slide; this is repeated four times. With a magnifying glass each of the five drops is observed and the number of living larvae is counted and noted. If this is not possible due to a high number of living larvae, a small amount of 0.5 M sulfuric acid is added. When the larvae are lying still (are dead) counting can be done. The average number of larvae per 0.1 ml based on the five drops is calculated. Artificial seawater is added to the examined suspension to dilute this to a resulting concentration of approximately 10 larvae per 0.1 ml.

For the purpose of this discussion we may think of the determination of LC_{50} after 24 h of exposure to potassium dichromate. First, tubes are prepared with the concentrations to be used. A zero concentration is taken directly from the seawater bottle and the highest concentration to be tested (1600 ppm potassium dichromate) is made by preparing a solution at the concentration of 3200 ppm, from which 100 μl will be used. The serial dilution is then started by adding 1 ml from the stock solution to produce a concentration of 1600 ppm. Then 800 ppm is produced by taking 1 ml from the 800 ppm tube and adding 1 ml of seawater. This line of dilution is continued until the lowest concentration has been made.

An eight-channel pipette is prepared with tips for transfer of the larvae suspension to a microtitre plate with 96 wells. The larvae suspension is poured into a 30 ml reservoir called a 'cradle', from where it can easily be sucked up with the eight-channel pipette and distributed in the wells. The suspension should be stirred gently before each round of transfer with the pipette. A volume of 100 μl is added to each well. Then the number of dead larvae is counted with a magnifying glass and noted for each well, as these should be excluded in the final calculation of results. The substance to be tested is then added, in this case the potassium dichromate of which the serial dilution has been prepared. Each concentration is tested in six wells. Starting with the lowest concentration so that the pipette does not need to be changed, 100 μl is added to each well and the final test concentration is thereby half of the dilution concentration.

After the addition of the test compound the microtitre plate is covered/sealed. The plate is then placed in an incubator at 25°C overnight. After incubation for 24 h the microtitre plate is removed from the incubator, placed on a coloured background and the sealing membrane removed. The number of dead larvae in each well is again counted using the magnifying glass and noted on a prepared form. Then from 100 to 150 μl of 0.5 M sulfuric acid is added to each well with the eight-channel pipette. After 15 min all larvae should be immobile (dead) and the total number of larvae in each well is counted and noted. Now the number of live larvae in each well before and after the 24 h of incubation can be calculated. The information needed for determination of the LC_{50} has been obtained.

Analysing the results:
the Reed–Muench method

When using the Reed–Muench method it is assumed that an animal which survives a given dose would also survive any lower dosages of that compound and an animal which dies at any given dose would also die at any higher dosages. The method is demonstrated with the results shown in Table 13.2.

According to Table 13.2, 15 out of 30 larvae survive a concentration of 1000 ppm. At 800 ppm,

Table 13.2. Example of how to calculate LD_{50} from the results of a brine shrimp test using the method of Reed and Muench.

Dose (ppm)	Dosage (log dose)	Dead	Alive	Accumulated dead	Accumulated alive	Accumulated total	Ratio accumulated dead/total	Mortality (%)
1000	3.00	15	15	42	15	57	42/57	73.7
800	2.90	8	22	27	37	64	27/64	42.2
600	2.78	8	22	19	59	78	19/78	24.4
400	2.60	7	25	11	84	95	11/95	11.6
200	2.39	4	26	4	110	114	4/114	3.5

22 of 30 larvae survive. According to the Reed–Muench method the number of surviving larvae at 1000 ppm and 800 ppm are added to one another, meaning that 37 larvae survive at 800 ppm. At 600 ppm a further 22 larvae survive, so the total number of surviving larvae is then 59. The number of dead larvae is calculated by starting with the lowest concentration, i.e. the four dead at 200 ppm are added to the seven dead at 400 ppm and so forth. The total number of dead larvae then equals 42 at 1000 ppm. So, at 1000 ppm, the accumulated number of dead larvae is 42 and the accumulated number of live larvae is 15, i.e. 42 out of 57 are dead, which equals 73.7%. The concentration which statistically will kill 50% of the animals can then be determined on a graph, where the percentage dead (mortality) is plotted as a function of the logarithm of the concentration. According to the literature, the LC_{50} for potassium dichromate towards *A. salina* is somewhere between 500 and 800 ppm at 6 h exposure and between 20 and 40 ppm at 24 h exposure.

The results for screening an unknown compound or extract are regarded as acceptable if a simultaneous determination of LC_{50} for a positive standard (such as potassium dichromate exemplified here) is within the expected – formerly determined – confidence interval for this standard and if the mortality in a negative control is low, i.e. less than 5%. The positive standard is included in the examination to ensure that, among other things, the larvae used are of a suitable quality.

A report would include doing a graphical presentation of the results and the calculations, along with an evaluation of the compound or extract tested in relation to the results.

13.10 Conclusion

Mixtures of compounds (products) as well as pure compounds are today tested in a number of different tests for toxicity using live animals, isolated organs, primary cell cultures or continuous cell cultures. Such testing will in most cases be structured so that simple (short-term, inexpensive) tests come first and are followed by more long-term and expensive tests planned on the basis of the results from the previously performed tests.

Notes

[1] Lu, F.C. and Kacew, S. (2002) Lu's Basic Toxicology: Fundamentals, Target Organs and Risk Assessment. Taylor & Francis, London.

[2] The Encyclopedia of Earth (2008) Dose–response relationship. Yuill, T. and Miller, M. (eds). EIC Secretariat, National Council for Science and the Environment, Washington, DC; available at http://www.eoearth.org/article/Dose-response_relationship

Further Reading

Board on Environmental Studies and Toxicology, Institute for Laboratory Animal Research, Division on Earth and Life Studies, National Research Council (2007) *Toxicity Testing in the 21st Century: A Vision and A Strategy*. National Academies Press, Washington, DC.

Ecobichon, D.J. (ed.) (1997) *The Basis of Toxicity Testing*, 2nd edn. CRC Press, Boca Raton, Florida.

Gad, S.C. (2002) *Drug Safety Evaluation*. John Wiley & Sons, New York, New York.

Hodgson, E. (ed.) (2004) *Modern Toxicology*, 3rd edn. John Wiley & Sons, Hoboken, New Jersey.

Lu, F.C. and Kacew, S. (2009) *Lu's Basic Toxicology: Fundamentals, Target Organs, and Risk Assessment*, 5th edn. Informa Healthcare, New York, New York.

Mongelli, E., Martianez, J., Ananya, J., Grande, C., Grande, M., Torres, P. and Pomillo, A.B. (2003) *Bolax gummifera*: Toxicity against *Artemia* sp. of Bornyl and iso-Bornyl Esters. *Molecular Medicinal Chemistry* 1, 26–29.

In vitro Methods

14

Mette Tingleff Skaanild

Associate Professor of Toxicology, Department of Veterinary Disease Biology, Faculty of Life Sciences, University of Copenhagen, Denmark

- The *in vitro* testing of metabolism is discussed.
- The *in vitro* testing of acute toxicity is presented.
- The *in vitro* testing of genotoxicity is described.
- The *in vitro* testing of developmental toxicity is discussed.

14.1 Introduction

In vitro (Latin: in a glass) refers to biological experiments outside the intact live organism using cultures of isolated organs, primary cells or cell lines and subcellular fractions. The development of *in vitro* methods really took off in 1986 as the Animal Welfare Guidelines were implemented and the EU institutions declared policy was to support the development of alternative methods that can reduce, replace or refine (RRR) the use of animal experiments. The use of *in vitro* methods is therefore increasingly favoured in the EU but similar developments have also been seen in both the USA and Japan. The developments are coordinated by OECD and in 1991 the European Centre of Validation of Alternative Methods (ECVAM; http://ecvam.jrc.it) was founded. Other similar institutions, such as the US Interagency Coordinating Committee on the Validation of Alternative methods (ICCVAM; http://iccvam.niehs. nih.gov/) and the National Toxicology Program Interagency Center for the Evaluation of Alternative Toxicological Methods (NICICEATM; http://iccvam. niehs.nih.gov), also exist. The validation of an alternative method such as an *in vitro* test consists of several stages. First of all the following questions are asked: (i) 'Is the method optimized?' and (ii) 'Can the same results be obtained in another laboratory using the same method?' The next step is to validate its relevance, i.e. how well the *in vitro* test results correlate with the results obtained *in vivo*. If the method is both reliable and relevant, a formal validation is carried out and if the method is scientifically accepted it may be adopted as a regulatory guideline by the EU or OECD.

In this chapter the following *in vitro* methods are described:

- *in vitro* testing of metabolism/toxicokinetics;
- *in vitro* acute toxicity testing;
- *in vitro* genotoxicity testing; and
- *in vitro* testing of developmental toxicity.

14.2 Metabolism/Toxicokinetics Testing

Several metabolizing systems can be used for *in vitro* testing. One of these systems is the so-called *liver S9 fraction*, which is a subcellular fraction of liver cells. This fraction is easily available (Fig. 14.1), but has a much reduced phase II metabolism. It is often used as an 'added phase I metabolism' in order to analyse if compounds are bioactivated or deactivated by the phase I metabolizing enzymes. Another *in vitro* system used for the study of phase I reaction is the *microsomal fraction*, which is also easily available (Fig. 14.1). This fraction is often used to study the cytochrome P450-catalysed reactions as the microsomes are small vehicles of the endoplasmic reticulum and therefore contain high cytochrome activity. The phase I metabolism of new compounds is often studied by incubating microsomes with different concentrations of the compound and detecting and identifying the metabolites formed after incubation using HPLC (high-performance liquid chromatography) and MS (mass spectrometry) or combined LC/ MS. The enzymes catalysing the formation of the different metabolites can be identified by adding different inhibitors (chemical inhibitors or inhibitory

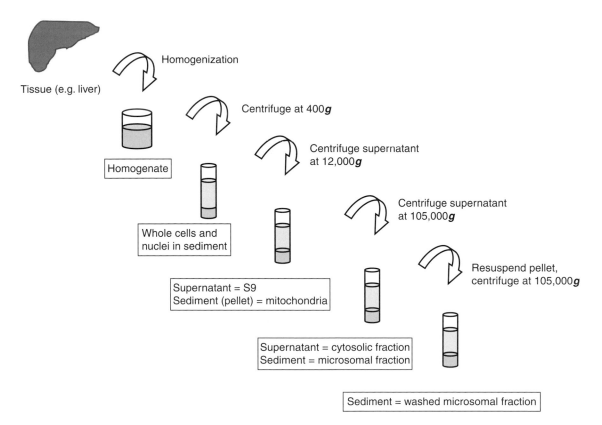

Fig. 14.1. Isolation of subcellular fractions from animal tissue. Adapted from XenoTech web page.[1]

antibodies) to the different isoenzymes; if the metabolism is catalysed by one of the isoenzymes inhibited, the amount of metabolites will be decreased or nil (found by measuring the amount of metabolites after incubation). The microsomes can also be used to test if a compound can inhibit or reduce the activity of the cytochrome P450 enzymes. This is done by incubating the microsomes with the test compound and substrates for the different enzymes. A reduction in metabolism of one of these substrates indicates that the test compound inhibits the enzyme that catalyses that specific reaction.

Metabolism can also be tested by using either primary cultures of hepatocytes or liver slices. This system has the advantage that it contains all phase I and phase II metabolizing enzymes, which makes it possible to measure all the different metabolites. However, the activity of some of the cytochrome P450 enzymes in particular decreases very fast *in vitro* and therefore these systems are applicable only for short incubation periods. Hepatocyte cultures have another advantage

as they can be used to test if compounds induce or reduce the activity of enzymes and this can be estimated at the expression level. A promising new way to test metabolism is under development: genetically engineered cell lines that are capable of both phase I and phase II metabolism. The metabolism should preferably be catalysed by human enzymes.

14.3 Acute Toxicity Testing

General acute *in vitro* cytotoxicity can be estimated using different cell lines or primary cultures and different endpoints to estimate cell death and calculate the LC_{50}, i.e. the concentration of the test compound that kills 50% of the cells. Cells or cell lines are incubated with different concentrations of the test compound, both with and without the S9 fraction, in order to see if the test compound is metabolized into a more or less toxic compound. After incubation the cell death can be measured in several ways. The integrity of the cell membrane can be determined by measuring leakage from the cell (LDH assay, which measures leakage of lactate dehydrogenase into the medium), the exclusion of tryphan blue or the active uptake of neutral red. The cell viability can also be estimated by measuring the mitochondrial metabolism (MTT assay, in which 3-(4,5-dimethylthiazol-2-yl)-2,5-diphenyl-tetrazolium bromide (MTT), a yellow tetrazole salt, is reduced to a purple formazan salt), or the synthesis of DNA and/or of protein. Lately apoptosis assays have been used more extensively. None of these general cytotoxicity tests have been accepted as OECD guidelines but the results found in these tests in different cell lines using different endpoints can be used for screening and ranking compounds as a first approach to selecting and prioritizing them for further studies, i.e. selecting the least toxic candidates for new food additives, pesticides or drugs.

The tests may also give an indication of targets for the toxic effect and help to estimate the first dose in acute *in vivo* toxicity studies, as a certain correlation has been found between the LC_{50} and LD_{50} doses. In this way a reduction in the number of animals used in the first *in vivo* studies has been possible.

In vitro toxicity tests that can replace the 'Draize' acute *in vivo* skin and eye irritation and corrosive test(s) have also been developed, some of which have been accepted as OECD guidelines while others have been accepted only in certain countries, as overviewed in Table 14.1. Examples of these tests include the '*In vitro* skin corrosion – human skin model test', which uses an artificial human skin model, and the 'Membrane barrier test method for corrosion'. The 'Transcutal electrical resistance test (TER)' is also a well-described method measuring the resistance over a cell membrane; a decrease in resistance is a measure for toxicity. The *in vitro* acute eye tests include tests on isolated bovine cornea, isolated chicken eyes and isolated rabbit eyes. These are *in vitro* test methods that can be used to classify substances as ocular corrosives and severe irritants. The use of isolated corneas from the eyes

Table 14.1. Examples of corresponding *in vivo* and *in vitro* methods. Numbers in brackets are the OECD guideline numbers.

Toxicological test	*In vivo* method	*In vitro* method
Skin irritation/corrosion	Acute dermal irritation/corrosion (404)	Transcutal electrical resistance test (TER) (430)
		Skin corrosion: human skin model test (430)
		Membrane barrier test method for skin corrosion (435)
Eye irritation/corrosion	Acute eye irritation/corrosion (405)	Embryonal chicken egg (HET-CAM)[a]
		Isolated bovine cornea (BCOP)[a]
		Isolated chicken eye (CEET)[a]
		Isolated rabbit eye (IRE)[a]
Mutagenicity/genotoxicity	Mammalian erythrocyte micronucleus test (474)	Bacterial reverse mutation test (471)
	Mammalian bone marrow chromosomal aberration (475)	*Saccharomyces cerevisiae* gene mutation assay (480)
	Sex-linked recessive lethal test in *Drosophila melanogaster* (477)	*Saccharomyces cerevisiae* mitotic recombination assay (481)
	Rodent dominant lethal (478)	Mammalian chromosome aberrations assay (473)
	Mouse spot test (484)	Mammalian gene mutation test (476)
	Mouse heritable translocation assay (485)	Micronucleus test (487)
	Unscheduled DNA synthesis (UDS) with mammalian liver cells (486)	Unscheduled DNA synthesis (UDS) in mammalian cell cultures (482)
Teratogenicity	Prenatal developmental study (414)	Whole embryo culture (WEC)[a]
		Micromass test (MM)[a]
		Embryo stem cell test (EST)[a]

[a] These *in vitro* tests have not (yet) obtained regulatory acceptance from OECD.

of cattle slaughtered for commercial purposes thus avoids the use of laboratory animals.

As chemical compounds may be activated by light, the 'In vitro 3T3 NRU phototoxicity test' was developed. This method measures photocytotoxicity by the relative reduction in viability of cells as measured using the uptake of neutral red, a dye that is actively transported into the cells. In order to test the activation of the compound, cells are incubated with the compound in the absence versus presence of a non-toxic dose of UV light.

14.4   Mutagenicity/Genotoxicity Testing

Specific concerns about the possibility of a compound or product causing mutations (changes) in the genetic material have made these tests the most intensively used. The first tests were developed at the beginning of the 1970s by Bruce Ames and they have proved to be very useful indeed, especially as they are both cheap and quick instruments for the screening of, for example, a battery of synthesized candidate compounds in the development of a new food additive, pesticide or drug. Positive results (i.e. the compound induces mutations) will most often lead to termination of the further planned programme for the compound in question. In contrast, a negative result has to be confirmed in other *in vitro* tests using mammalian cell lines and then the compound might be tested in one or more *in vivo* assays using higher animals, typically mammals in the form of a rodent species.

Within the bacterial assays for mutagenesis the 'Bacterial reverse mutation test' uses amino acid-requiring strains of either *Salmonella typhimurium* (the Ames test) or *Escherichia coli* to detect point mutations by base substitutions or frameshifts. Thus, the test uses amino acid-dependent strains of *S. typhimurium* and *E. coli*, which, in the absence of an external amino acid source, cannot grow to form colonies. However, colony growth is resumed if a reversion of the mutation occurs due to exposure to a mutagen, allowing the production of the amino acid. Spontaneous reversions occur within each of the strains, but mutagenic compounds included in the growth medium cause an increase in the number of revertant colonies relative to the background level. Bacterial culture medium is inoculated with the appropriate *S. typhimurium* or *E. coli* strain and incubated overnight. Different concentrations of the test compound are mixed with the bacteria in individual test-tubes and

the S9 fraction is added to half of them. The test-tube contents are spread on agar plates without the amino acid and incubated for 48–72 h. Often a dose range-finding test for the compound under investigation is carried out using the *S. typhimurium* strain TA100 over a wide dose range. The increase in colony numbers as a function of the test compound concentration indicates how mutagenic the compound is.

The addition of the S9 fraction – an external phase I metabolizing system – will give an indication about the metabolites of the compound, i.e. if they are more or less mutagenic than the parent compound. Similar gene mutation assays have been developed using yeast cells (*Saccharomyces cerevisiae*) and mammalian cell lines.

If mutations (microlesions) have been induced by chemicals, UV light or virus infections, the cells will start repairing the mutations. This process has been utilized in two different mutagenicity tests: the UDS ('Unscheduled DNA synthesis test') and the COMET assay. The latter has not yet been accepted by OECD, but is being used increasingly. In the UDS test cells are exposed to different concentrations of the test compound, again with and without the S9 fraction added. Unscheduled DNA synthesis, i.e. DNA synthesis that is not initiated as part of cell proliferation, can be estimated by adding a radioactive nucleotide and by measuring the radioactivity of the cells. The unscheduled DNA synthesis can be estimated and thereby the mutagenicity of the test compound.

In vitro mammalian chromosome aberration test

The purpose of the '*In vitro* chromosome aberration test' is to identify agents that cause structural chromosome aberrations in cultured mammalian somatic cells. Structural aberrations (macrolesions) include any numerical or structural change in the usual chromosome complement (the whole set of chromosomes for the species) in a cell or organism. In humans, the chromosome complement (or karyotype) consists of 46 chromosomes. An example of a structural change includes the gain, loss or rearrangement of chromosomal segments caused by the chemical compound (Fig. 14.2). Another is the formation of ring chromosomes. When one break occurs in each arm of a chromosome, the broken ends of the internal centromeric fragment may join, resulting in the formation of a stable ring chromosome.

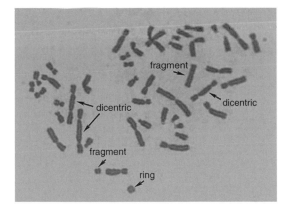

Fig. 14.2. A spread of chromosomes showing aberrations such as dicentric chromosomes and chromosomes without centromeres plus a ring chromosome. With permission from the National Institute of Radiological Sciences, Japan.[2]

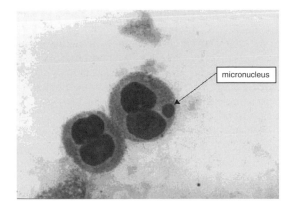

Fig. 14.3. A micronucleus detected by Geimsa staining. With permission from the 'Micronucleus test' web page.[3]

Each of the two end segments lacks a centromere. Such acentric fragments are lost during cell division because the centromeres are essential in the cell division process, being the location for binding of the spindles.

The 'Micronucleus test' is a test that can be used both *in vivo* and *in vitro*. The test detects chemically induced chromosomal damage determined by the increased frequency of micronucleated polychromatic cells. The assay is sensitive to both clastogenic compounds and compounds that interfere with the spindles. Micronuclei are cytospasmic chromatin masses from chromosomes or chromosomal fragments that are not incorporated into daughter cells during mitosis (Fig. 14.3).

14.5 Developmental Toxicity Testing

The effort to find alternative *in vitro* developmental tests has been increasing as the *in vivo* developmental toxicity tests – in particular the two generation test – require by far the largest proportion of animals in safety studies as described by REACH. Three *in vitro* methods, the 'Embryonic stem cell test' (EST), the 'Micromass test' (MM) and the 'Rat post-implantation whole embryo culture test' (WEC), have been validated and are recommended as screening tests for developmental toxicity (Table 14.1). However, no OECD guidelines have yet been made. These tests cover only certain aspects of developmental toxicity and mainly measure embryotoxicity as an endpoint.

In the EST assay embryonic stem cells that can be maintained in the undifferentiated stage are exposed to the test compound. The inhibition of cellular differentiation mainly into cardia myoblasts is measured to estimate the embryotoxicity of the compound. In the MM assay cultured chick embryo limb cells are exposed to the test compound and toxicity is measured with a focus on the differentiation of limb bud cells into cartilage-producing chondrocytes. The WEC utilizes rat embryo cultures on day 9.5 of gestation. During 48 h of culture major aspects of organogenesis occur, such as heart development, closure of the neural tube and development of ear, eye, limb buds and brachial bars. Exposure to chemicals at this time can lead to retardation of growth and malformation of one or several of the organs under development. These malformations are evaluated using a morphological scoring system. This test and the EST have shown excellent predictivity and precision for strongly embryotoxic compounds (100%), and for non-embryotoxic compounds the precision was 65 and 72%, respectively. However, these tests have only been used to test compounds with a limited number of toxicological mechanisms, and an external metabolizing system such as the S9 fraction has not been applied.

14.6 Toxicogenomics – Proteomics

In recent years toxicogenomics and proteomics have increasingly been used to study the mechanisms of toxic effects caused by exposure to chemical compounds. In *toxicogenomics* the expression or change in expression of genes is analysed by use of cDNA microarrays or by quantitative PCR (qPCR). Such changes in gene expression will cause a change in protein level in the cell. These changes can be analysed by using *proteomics* to isolate the proteins and running a two-dimensional polyacrylamide gel electrophoresis. By doing this it is possible to distinguish all the proteins and find the changes. These methods are often used to identify biomarkers for the toxic effect. Such biomarkers found *in vitro* using different cell lines can afterwards be used *in vivo*.

14.7 Conclusion

Over the last three decades the area of *in vitro* toxicological methods has progressed tremendously, owing to the development in knowledge of cell biology and cell and tissue culture methodologies. Nevertheless there are still some drawbacks including the loss of tissue-specific functions in many *in vitro* systems, such as the loss of metabolic activity in hepatocyte cultures. Also the tissue–tissue interaction is lacking in the *in vitro* assays. Furthermore, the *in vivo* bio-availability of the test compound has to be considered because, if its intake is oral, then the compound first of all has to be absorbed in the gastrointestinal tract and then distributed to the different organs. In addition the compound may be accumulated in certain tissues *in vivo*, e.g. adipose tissue. On the other hand, the use of *in vitro* methods reduces the number of animals used in the initial phase of toxicity testing, and elucidation especially of the toxicological mechanisms and the kinetic studies permitted by *in vitro* systems will have regulatory impact.

Notes

[1] XenoTech (not dated) Subcellular Fractions. XenoTech LLC, Lenexa, Kansas; available at http://www.xenotechllc.com/Products/Subcellular-Fractions

[2] NIRS (2007) Inevitable aspect to radiation emergency medicine. National Institute of Radiological Sciences, Chiba, Japan; available at http://www.nirs.go.jp/ENG/research/radiation_emergency/04.shtml

[3] Vrije Universiteit Brussels (not dated) Micronucleus test. Laboratory Cell Genetics, Vrije Universiteit Brussels, Belgium; available at http://we.vub.ac.be/~cege/volders/ENG/tests/MN.htm

Further Reading

Attenwill, C.K., Goldfarb, P. and Purcell, W. (eds) (2000) *Approaches to High Throughput Toxicity Screening*. Taylor & Francis, London.

Eisenbrand, G., Pool-Zobel, B., Baker, V., Balls, M., Blaauboer, B.J., Boobis, A., Carere, A., Kevekordes, S., Lhuguenot, J.C., Pieters, R. and Kleiner, J. (2002) Methods of *in vitro* toxicology. *Food and Chemical Toxicology* 40, 193–236.

Gad, S.C. (2000) *In Vitro* Toxicology. Taylor & Francis, London.

Gad, S.C. (2002) *Drug Safety Evaluation*. John Wiley & Sons, New York, New York.

O'Hare, S. and Atterwill, C.K. (eds) (1995) *In Vitro Toxicity Testing Protocols. Methods in Molecular Biology*, vol. 43. Humana Press, Totowa, New Jersey.

Stacey, G.N., Doyle, A. and Ferro, M. (eds) (2001) *Cell Culture Methods for In Vitro Toxicology*. Kluwer Academic Publishers, Norwell, Massachusetts.

Tiffany-Castiglioni, E. (ed.) (2004) *In Vitro Neurotoxicology: Principles and Challenges. Methods in Pharmacology and Toxicology*. Humana Press, Totowa, New Jersey.

15 Naturally Inherent Plant Toxicants: Introduction and Non-glycosidic Compounds

- We define secondary metabolites and relate them to poisonous effects.
- We look at their distribution.
- A number of classes of non-glycosidic plant toxins are discussed separately.

15.1 Primary and Secondary Metabolites as Toxicants

The plant kingdom (*Plantae*) comprises a number of groups with an amazing range of diverse forms. This kingdom is second in size only to the arthropods. *Plantae* include the water-living algae, which range from single-cell organisms to seaweeds more than 10 m long, and a number of terrestrial groups of so-called *spore plants*, i.e. the mosses, plants belonging to the families *Lycopodiaceae* (e.g. club moss or stag's horn) and *Equisetaceae* (e.g. horsetail), respectively, and the ferns. In addition the plant kingdom includes the *seed plants* (*Spermatophyta*) made up of the gymnosperms (the cycads, *Ginkgo biloba* (the maidenhair tree) and the conifers) and the angiosperms (the flowering plants), which are subdivided into the monocotyledonous (monocots) and the dicotyledonous (dicots) plants. The first of these two groups includes all of the grasses – and hence the cereals – together with palms, lilies (including onions) and tulips, just to give some examples. Of food-relevant plants the dicots include the fruit trees, all of the cabbages, etc. An overview of the plant kingdom (*Plantae*) according to the scientific understanding used here (other systems exist) is given in Table 15.1.

Plants were shown early in the 20th century to contain a high number of so-called *secondary metabolites*, i.e. low-molecular-weight organic compounds biosynthesized by the plant but not essential to its growth and survival if isolated from interactions with other organisms. Such compounds typically are thought to be protective to the plant by deterring herbivorous organisms from eating it by being bad tasting or toxic, or both.

From the point of view of the mechanisms of deterring animals from eating the plant, we often divide the secondary compounds into anti-nutritional and toxic compounds:

- toxic (poisonous) compounds destroy life or impair health by their own action or by the action of their metabolites formed (in the body) after uptake; and
- anti-nutritional compounds impair health by destroying nutrients/vitamins or by reducing the uptake of such essential compounds (by different mechanisms).

Macromolecular compounds such as polynucleic acids (DNA, RNA), proteins and polysaccharides are seldom toxic, and especially not upon ingestion. In saying this maybe we should just mention that we thereby exclude the elicitation of an allergenic response by an ingested protein as a toxic effect. Also it should be remembered that the harmful effects potentially caused by DNA/RNA in the form of viruses and proteins in the form of prions are not toxic effects.

In spite of what has just been stated, a few individual proteins and classes of protein still have the ability to cause toxic or anti-nutritional effects in higher animals including man. Thus, the plant proteins ricin and abrin are highly toxic, while the two groups of proteins called lectins and proteinase inhibitors possess anti-nutritional effects. The enzyme thiaminase, which degrades the B vitamin thiamine, can act as an anti-nutritional factor in

Table 15.1. The plant kingdom *Plantae* and its subdivision. Adapted from ITIS Report (2009).[1]

Kingdom *Plantae*
   Division *Anthocerotophyta*
   Division *Bryophyta* – hornworts, mosses
   Division *Charophyta* – stoneworts
   Division *Chlorophyta* – green algae
   Division *Chrysophyta* – golden-brown algae
   Division *Craspedophyta*
   Division *Cryptophycophyta*
   Division *Euglenophycota* – euglenoids
   Division *Haptophyta*
   Division *Hepatophyta* – liverworts
   Division *Phaeophyta* – brown algae
   Division *Prasinophyta* – green flagellates
   Division *Pyrrophycophyta* – dinoflagellates
   Division *Rhodophyta* – red algae
   Division *Xanthophyta* – yellow-green algae
   Subkingdom *Chromista*
   Subkingdom *Tracheobionta* – vascular plants

this way, although primarily in ruminants that ingest it via plants such as horsetail.

The secondary plant metabolites include compounds from many different structural classes. Toxic and anti-nutritional agents are found within the following, among others:

- macromolecular polyphenolic substances (hydrolysable and condensed tannins);
- toxic fatty acids/lipids;
- non-protein amino acids;
- alkaloids;
- furanocoumarins;
- polyacetylenes;
- mono-, sesqui- and diterpenes; and
- toxic glycosides of various types (glucosinolates, cyanogenic glycosides, saponins).

A number of these compounds are dealt with further in this chapter, along with phytic acid, gossypol, fluoroacetic acid and certain oligosaccharides present especially in legume seeds.

Before the 1960s, general anatomic traits and in particular those of the sexual organs (flower anatomy) were the most important when botanists within plant systematics grouped the different species into genera, families, orders, etc. However, gradually the content of secondary metabolites was also taken into account. Thus, Professor Dahlgren from the Botanical Museum of the University of Copenhagen constructed the so-called 'Dahlgrenogram' showing the evolution of the mono- and dicots into overorders

and orders of plants by including both anatomic and chemical characteristics. Figure 15.1a and b shows two-dimensional Dahlgrenograms on the level of plant orders (groups of plant families).

Figure 15.1 clearly demonstrates that both groups of secondary constituents mapped, i.e. the glucosinolates (the flavouring compounds in cabbage and mustard and the toxic constituents in rapeseed; Fig. 15.1a) and the benzylisoquinoline alkaloids (the opium alkaloids such as morphine and codeine used in medicine; Fig. 15.1b), occur in only a very restricted number of plant species within the angiosperms (monocots + dicots). However, if we had been looking at the group of cyanogenic glycosides, toxic constituents which are closely related to the glucosinolates with regard to their biosynthesis, we would have found that they are more widespread in occurrence.

In conclusion we can say that certain toxic and anti-nutritional secondary plant constituents are relatively widely distributed throughout the plant kingdom, while others have been found in only a few genera or families. The remainder of this chapter is organized by compound class with the emphasis being on natural plant constituents and chemical food safety, although other topics are dealt with.

15.2 Plant Toxicants and Anti-nutritional Substances

Proteins

Proteinase inhibitors are known from bacteria, animals and plants. When our interest is on food, the plant proteinase inhibitors are those to discuss. Legumes are particularly rich in these constituents. Proteinase inhibitors are proteins themselves and are classified according to the type of proteinase they inhibit, i.e. into serine-, sulfhydryl-, acid- and metallo-proteinase inhibitors.

It was observed quite early that certain monogastric animals such as rats faced growth depression, hypersecretion of pancreatic enzymes and, as a result of this, enlargement of the pancreas over time when fed, for example, raw soybeans. The reason for this is that the soy plant, which belongs to the *Leguminosae* (= *Fabaceae*), and in particular the seeds (the soybeans) contain relatively high concentrations of the so-called Bowman–Birk serine proteinase inhibitors, inhibiting the digestive proteinases trypsin and chymotrypsin.

The content of such inhibitors in a number of mature legume seeds is one of the reasons why these in general are (have to be) cooked before consumption. The cooking not only improves the palatability and general acceptability of the seeds, but at the same time also denatures and thereby inactivates the proteinase inhibitors (these being proteins themselves).

Macromolecular polyphenolic substances (hydrolysable and condensed tannins)

Tannins also interfere with protein digestion as do the proteinase inhibitors. However, the mechanism is very different. As macromolecular polyphenolic substances they can bind to proteins through a high number of hydrogen bonds. Thereby they may either inhibit the action of such proteins as the digestive proteinases or make the proteins from food less susceptible as substrates for these proteinases.

Tannins have molecular weights ranging from about 500 to over 3000. Chemically they are usually classified into two major structural groups: the hydrolysable tannins and the condensed tannins (proanthocyanidins). On heating with acid the hydrolysable tannins yield gallic acid or ellagic acid. The centre of a hydrolysable tannin molecule comprises a carbohydrate (usually D-glucose). The hydroxyl groups of the carbohydrate are partially or totally esterified with phenolic compounds such as gallic acid in gallotannins or ellagic acid in ellagitannins. Condensed tannins, also known as proanthocyanidins, are polymers of two to 50 (or more) flavonoid units that are joined by carbon–carbon bonds, which are not susceptible to being cleaved by hydrolysis.

Tannins are found in many different plant organs and are commercially produced by extracting them from tree barks such as the bark of oaks and certain acacias. These tannins are used to transform skin to leather: the tanning process. Furthermore, certain tannins are also used in cosmetic/toiletry products such as skin tonics; this is the case, for example, for tannins from certain *Hamamelis* spp. (e.g. *Hamamelis virginiana* = witch hazel).

When fed to animals, tannins (like proteinase inhibitors) result in growth impairment and/or reduced feed efficiency. The dose needed for growth depression has been observed to vary from species to species, but was found to be in the range of 0.5 to 5.0% by weight of the diet. Similar figures are not available for man.

In a food context we find tannins in a lot of raw materials and processed products. While some leafy green vegetables do contain tannins in detectable amounts, the most important sources again include seeds such as a number of beans and a number of cereals. For the beans rather a great variation is seen; thus, light and dark red kidney beans have been reported to contain 100–150 mg tannins per 100 g, while faba beans may reach tannin levels up to 200 mg $100 g^{-1}$. Among the cereals one must first of all point to grain sorghum as a commodity which may contain high concentrations of tannins depending on the cultivar in question. An investigation of 30 sorghum varieties grown in Burkina Faso showed that 20 of these had a total content lower than 0.2% of dry weight; these were preferably used for cooking (to produce a kind of porridge named 'to'). The second group of sorghum (high-tannin varieties), which included ten varieties, was used for the preparation of a local alcoholic drink (a kind of beer named 'dolo'). The tannin content in these varieties was found to be in the range from 0.5 to 1.3% of dry weight.

Since tannins most often are present in the outer layers of, for example, a fruit/seed, processing such as de-shelling and de-hulling reduces the overall content. The same is true for germination.

Processed products such as tea, coffee and wine also contain tannins. The reaction of these tannins with the surface proteins of the mouth mucous membrane is part of what we observe as the total olfactory impression the products give us upon consumption – namely astringency. Especially for wine and tea, differences in tannin content are regarded as very important.

Phytic acid

Phytic acid (inositol hexakisphosphate, IP_6; or phytate when in salt form) is the principal storage form of phosphorus in many plant tissues, especially in different seeds. Phytic acid is a strong chelator of important minerals such as calcium, magnesium, iron and zinc, and can therefore contribute to mineral deficiencies in people whose diets rely on foods with a high phytic acid content while having a low mineral intake from other sources at the same time.

Fluoroacetic acid and toxic fatty acids

As already described in Chapter 10 on toxicodynamics, inhibition of an enzyme crucial to the

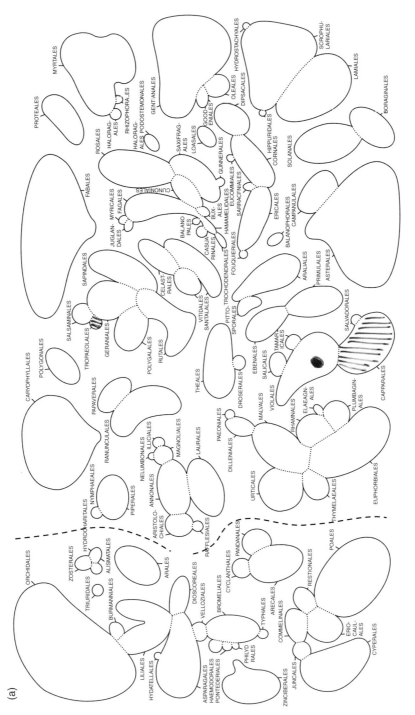

Fig. 15.1. The distribution in the angiosperms of the glucosinolates (a) and the benzylisoquinoline alkaloids (b).

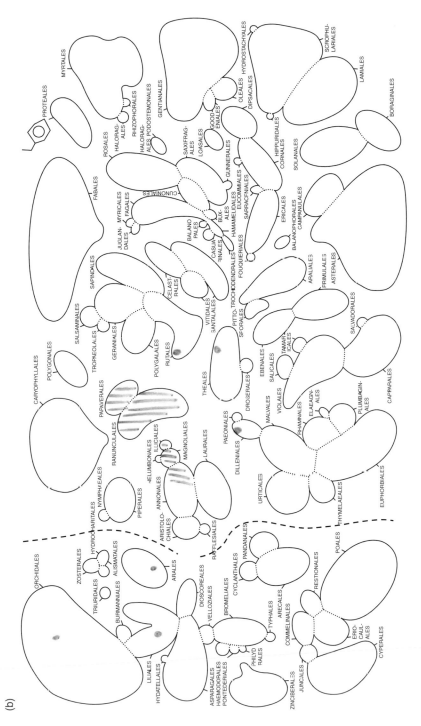

Fig. 15.1. Continued.

normal function of the cell may be caused by a xeno-biotic metabolite formed by several steps of metabolism. This is what we see with the so-called lethal synthesis of fluorocitric acid from, for example, ω-fluoro-oleic acid or ω-fluoro-palmitic acid present in the seeds of the South African plant *Dichapetalum toxicarium*. After ingestion these fluorine fatty acids are β-oxidized to fluoroacetic acid, which in turn enters the citric acid cycle where it is metabolized into fluorocitric acid. The citric acid cycle enzyme aconitase is inhibited by fluorocitric acid; thus, the fluorocitric acid cannot be further metabolized since aconitase does not accept this compound instead of its natural substrate citric acid. The cycle is blocked and the cell dies.

Non-protein amino acids

Plants synthesize and store a number of so-called non-protein amino acids. The legumes especially are well known to accumulate such compounds in their seeds. Many of the more than 200 or so non-protein amino acids synthesized by higher plants are structurally very closely related to the amino acid constituents of common proteins.

Several non-protein amino acids are among the more often described toxicants affecting animals and husbandry in particular. In a food context this group of secondary plant constituents is less important, which is why we restrict ourselves here to describing three examples of non-protein amino acids and their mechanism of toxicity.

L-*Canavanine*

The first example is L-canavanine, a toxic arginine anti-metabolite, which is a principal non-protein amino acid of many leguminous plants. The compound was given its name after *Canavalia ensiformis* (L.) DC. (Family: *Leguminosae*), also called 'jack bean'.

Owing to its structural similarity to L-arginine, L-canavanine, the β-oxa analogue of L-arginine (Fig. 15.2), thus is a substrate for arginyl tRNA synthetase and is incorporated into nascent proteins in place of L-arginine. Although L-arginine and L-canavanine are structurally similar, the oxyguanidino group of L-canavanine is significantly less basic than the guanidino group of L-arginine. Consequently, L-canavanyl proteins lack the capacity to form crucial ionic interactions, resulting in altered protein structure and function, which leads to cellular death.

The compound is not very acutely toxic when tested in rodents such as rats. However, repeated administration of canavanine results in more severe toxicity. Weight loss and alopecia were observed in rats given daily subcutaneous canavanine injections for 7 days. Food intake was decreased by 80% in adult rats subjected to this dosing regimen, but returned to normal after canavanine injections were terminated. Histological studies of tissues from adult rats treated with 3.0 g canavanine kg^{-1} BW day^{-1} for 6 days revealed pancreatic acinar cell atrophy and fibrosis. Further adverse effects that may occur according to some references include a syndrome that closely resembles the autoimmune systemic lupus erythematosus-like syndrome.

Hypoglycin A and B

The second example concerns the two compounds hypoglycin A and B. Hypoglycin A is β-(methylenecyclopropyl)alanine, also called 2-amino-3-(methylenecyclopropane)propanoic acid, a non-protein α-amino acid identified as the hypoglycaemic and toxic principle of the unripe fruit of 'ackee' (*Blighia sapida*; Family: *Sapindaceae*), the national fruit of Jamaica. In the unripe fruit it is present in high amounts in both the fleshy aril (an extra seed covering) and the seeds. The compound was linked to the well-known illness called 'Jamaican vomiting sickness' in 1976. In the seed it also occurs as the N-L-glutamyl derivative, hypoglycin B.

The compounds are degraded in animals to methylenecyclopropylacetate, either free or conjugated to glycine or coenzyme A. Methylenecyclopropylacetyl-CoA interferes with fatty acid metabolism and gluconeogenesis. A number of biochemical reactions are affected, which eventually results in mitochondrial β-oxidation being impaired and long-chain fatty acids seeming to undergo ω-oxidation in the liver, resulting in accumulation of short- and medium-chain dicarboxylic acids such as glutaric acid and a metabolic acidosis.

The plant was introduced to the Americas from West Africa in 1778. 'Ackee' was banned by the

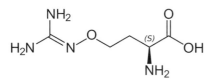

Fig. 15.2. L-Canavanine.

FDA in 1973, a ban that remained effective until several companies demonstrated that their canned products were safe for consumption. In the fresh state the fruit should not be eaten before the hill has split open of its own accord as a sign of being ripe.

β-ODAP

The third example is the non-protein amino acid β-N-oxalyl-α,β-diaminopropionic acid (β-ODAP). This compound is present in the seeds of *Lathyrus sativus* (grass pea or chickling pea), a drought-tolerant legume grown among other places in India, Bangladesh and Ethiopia. Grass pea has extraordinary environmental tolerance in that it also withstands flooding, while it also fixes nitrogen, as do many other legumes, and hence needs no or little fertilizer.

Decades of study have made it fairly clear that the disease neurolathyrism is the result of excessive consumption of *L. sativus* for prolonged periods. Vast populations are known to traditionally consume this pulse over many years as part of their diet without any adverse effects; however, when neurolathyrism strikes (mostly men) it is indeed a serious disease. It was reported very early in history by Hippocrates (460 BC) among others and in 1977 crippled over 2500 individuals in Ethiopia.

The disease causes paralysis, characterized by lack of strength in or inability to move the lower limbs, i.e. a walking disability. A unique symptom of lathyrism is emaciation of the gluteal muscles (buttocks). Today most scientists agree that exposure to β-ODAP is the causative factor, the amino acid being a glutamate analogue at AMPA/kainate receptors in motor neurons and therefore an excitotoxic substance. However, most also believe that other factors such as depletion of the sulfur pool is essential to trigger the disease. Clearly the last word has not yet been said concerning the mechanism behind neurolathyrism.

Alkaloids

The name alkaloid was first used by W. Meisner at the beginning of the 19th century. According to this original use, *alkaloid* is a collective designation for natural substances reacting like bases, in other words like alkalis (from the Arabic *alkaly* = soda and the Greek *eidos* = appearance). We still use the term alkaloids today, and the group of compounds

falling under presently accepted definitions is indeed very broad in structural diversity as well as in numbers of characterized compounds, so the definition varies a little, one being: *any of various naturally occurring organic compounds normally with basic chemical properties and usually containing at least one nitrogen atom in a heterocyclic ring.*

Often it is added to the definition that compounds should have a *marked physiological effect on animal physiology*. This is in accordance with the fact that many of our medicinally used natural compounds such as atropine, morphine, codeine, cocaine, colchicine, ephedrine, vinblastine and quinine are plant alkaloids, as are several stimulants in beverages such as caffeine (Fig. 15.3) and nicotine inhaled from tobacco. Today the term is also applied to synthetic substances which have structures similar to plant alkaloids, such as the medicinally used procaine.

The classification of the alkaloids is based on the general structure that reflects the biosynthetic origin, which in most cases includes a contribution from one (very occasionally more) amino acids. Examples of classes (with compound examples) are: the pyrrolidine group (nicotine); the tropane group (atropine, cocaine, scopolamine); the indolizidine group (senecionine); the quinoline group (quinine, quinidine); the phenanthrene group (morphine, codeine); the phenethylamine group (mescaline, ephedrine); the purine group (caffeine, theobromine); and the indole group, subgroup ergolines (the ergot alkaloids including ergotamine). Some alkaloids like α-solanine and α-chaconine in Irish potatoes are glycosylated. In the present text these are discussed under glycosides.

Alkaloids are very common plant metabolites. The number of known structures is high and steadily growing. Thus, the second edition of the *Dictionary of Alkaloids* edited by John Buckingham and colleagues and published January 2010, in its ambition to categorize and describe (give concise chemical, structural and physical data) all known alkaloids, includes more than 20,000 compounds. Some plants and fungi (e.g. opium poppy, ergot

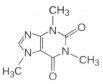

Fig. 15.3. Caffeine – a purine alkaloid.

fungus) produce many different alkaloids, but most produce only one or a few. Certain plant families, including the poppy family (*Papaveraceae*) and the nightshade family (*Solanaceae*), are particularly rich in alkaloids.

Alkaloids in food

Alkaloids may be present in food and food-like products for a number of different reasons. They can be naturally occurring in one of the major food ingredients or in an ingredient added to give flavour (spices); they can be added as pure compounds to soft drinks to give taste (bitterness as with quinine) or to market the beverage as a stimulating soft drink (caffeine in soft drinks); or they can be present in herbal products sold as food supplements or green medicines (seen for pyrrolizidine alkaloids). Also alkaloids may be present in food as a mycotoxin contamination since, as already mentioned, the so-called ergot alkaloids can be formed by the fungus *Claviceps purpurea* when it grows on rye or other cereals. Ergot alkaloids are treated in Chapter 19 under mycotoxins.

Opium alkaloids

Many different alkaloids are present in the latex of (opium) poppy (*Papaver somniferum* L.), with morphine as the major constituent. The plant originates in Asia Minor but is grown for different purposes around the world. Thus, the poppy is grown for production of opium (the dried latex) from which the alkaloids are purified, for production of poppy seeds commonly used in dishes and pastries in Europe, and as ornamental plants.

The alkaloids, in addition to morphine, include codeine, thebaine, noscapine and papaverine, several of which are used medicinally. Morphine is a potent analgesic which is used for short-term treatment of post-surgical and traumatic pain as well as for long-term treatment of severe pain in cancer patients. Besides these clinical applications, morphine is a common drug of abuse.

From about 2000 onwards, concerns were raised, for example, in the press, as to whether the intake of poppy seeds could lead to an unacceptable opiate alkaloid exposure. For this reason a risk assessment was made for the use of EFSA by an external expert group.

Poppy seeds for food use are produced in several countries, of which Turkey by far is the most important. The annual production of poppy seeds exceeds 32,000 t in Turkey with 18,000 t of this amount being produced in Afyon alone, a province in the central west of Turkey.

Before this risk assessment was made some countries already had tried to minimize the risk of alkaloid exposure, and probably also of the risk of misuse in a broader perspective. Thus, only the low-morphine variety Mieszko is certified for cultivation in Germany. However, Germany's annual poppy seed requirement for baking and food use of up to 10000 t is still almost exclusively covered by imported goods. Important producer countries are Turkey, the Czech Republic, Hungary and Austria.

For seeds with high alkaloid content there are already some procedures that have been implemented by a number of producers to reduce the content before marketing, such as different washing procedures, which do reduce the alkaloid level. Indeed, there is scientific evidence that poppy seeds contain low levels of these alkaloids including morphine. The content differs with botanical variety, harvesting time and whether the poppy plant has been subject to stress, which tends to increase the alkaloid content. A recent review of published data on the content of morphine and codeine in poppy seeds found that the concentrations of these alkaloids are within the ranges of 1.5–294 mg kg^{-1} seed and 2.1–294 mg kg^{-1} seed, respectively. In agreement with this, various toxicological studies report that consumption of large amounts of commercially available poppy seeds can lead to light-headedness and enteroparesis in sensitive individuals. The symptoms described are in agreement with the range of toxicological actions of morphine.

The above-mentioned risk assessment came to the following conclusions, among others:

- The fear mongering by the tabloid press, stating that all foods containing poppy seeds are 'toxic' and have to be banned from the market, should be disregarded.
- If the poppy seed is used for baking purposes or for decoration of bakery products, it is recommended that the baking should be done at the highest possible temperature. This has been demonstrated to reduce the level by degrading the alkaloids.
- The use of seed with morphine contents below 4 mg kg^{-1} from controlled producers should be enforced, so that morphine reduction can become superfluous in future.

- The preparation of guidelines for pre- and post-harvest management of poppy and its seeds to minimize morphine content was suggested.

No maximum limits for morphine in poppy seeds have as yet been established in the EU.

Caffeine (and other methylxanthines)

The methylxanthine alkaloids caffeine, theobromine and theophylline are, in different relative concentrations, naturally present in a number of plants from which we produce foods and beverages. Thus, methylxanthines occur naturally in as many as 60 different plant species and include caffeine (the primary methylxanthine in coffee) and theophylline (the primary methylxanthine in tea). Theobromine is the primary methylxanthine found in products of the cacao tree (*Theobroma cacao*), beans and shells (Table 15.2 and Fig. 15.4).

Caffeine is used as a psychostimulant and increases physiological arousal, wakefulness and alertness. Years of discussion concerning a possible carcinogenic effect of caffeine now have been concluded with a 'no concern' consensus. However, the chemical structure of caffeine resembles that of adenosine, and the compound (together with other xanthines) has been found to act as a competitive inhibitor at the adenosine receptor sites on inhibitory neurons in the CNS.

In man four adenosine receptors (A_1, A_{2A}, A_{2B} and A_3) have been characterized, each of which is encoded by a separate gene. The receptors have different functions, although with some overlap. Both the A_1 and A_{2A} receptors play roles in the heart, regulating myocardial oxygen consumption and coronary blood flow, while the A_{2A} receptor also has broader anti-inflammatory effects throughout

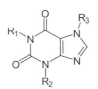

Fig. 15.4. The general structure of methylxanthine alkaloids.

the body. Both of these receptors also have important roles in the brain, regulating the release of other neurotransmitters such as dopamine and glutamate. In contrast the A_{2B} and A_3 receptors are located mainly peripherally and are involved in processes such as inflammation and immune responses. The methylxanthine derivatives such as caffeine and theophylline act as non-selective antagonists at A_1 and A_{2A} receptors in the heart as well as the brain and so have the opposite effect to adenosine, producing a stimulant effect and rapid heart rate.

In the EU the Scientific Committee on Food concluded in 1999 that caffeine used as an ingredient in 'energy drinks' does not appear as a cause for concern when looking at adults and assuming that 'energy drinks' replace other sources of caffeine. For children, however, an increase in the daily intake of caffeine to a certain level of consumption per day may bring about temporary changes in behaviour, such as increased excitability, irritability, nervousness or anxiety, according to the Committee. In addition, for pregnant women, the Committee's view is that moderation of caffeine intake is advisable.

Therefore the EU Directive 2002/67/EC of 18 July 2002 on the labelling of foodstuffs containing quinine, and of foodstuffs containing caffeine

Table 15.2. Methylxanthines occurring in food and beverages[a].

Common name	R_1	R_2	R_3	IUPAC name	Isolated from (examples)
Caffeine	CH_3	CH_3	CH_3	1,3,7-Trimethyl-1*H*-purine-2,6-(3*H*,7*H*)-dione	Coffee, guarana, Yerba mate, tea
Theobromine	H	CH_3	CH_3	3,7-Dihydro-3,7-dimethyl-1*H*-purine-2,6-dione	Cacao, Yerba mate
Theophylline	CH_3	CH_3	H	1,3-Dimethyl-7*H*-purine-2,6-dione	Tea

Cacao = *Theobroma cacao*; coffee = *Coffea arabica* and *Coffea canephora*; guarana = *Paullinia cupana*; Yerba mate = *Ilex paraguariensis*; tea = *Camellia sinensis*.
[a] R_1, R_2 and R_3 refer to the general structure shown in Fig. 15.4.

states that quinine and/or caffeine used as flavouring in the production or preparation of a foodstuff must be mentioned by name in the list of ingredients immediately after the term 'flavouring'. Furthermore, for beverages intended for consumption without modification which contain caffeine in excess of 150 mg l^{-1}, the following message must appear on the label in the same field of vision as the name under which the product is sold: 'High caffeine content'.

Quinine

Quinine salts such as quinine sulfate, quinine hydrochloride and quinine monohydrochloride dihydrate are added to soft drinks as bitter compounds. For this reason JECFA evaluated the compounds in 1993 and expressed no concerns up to a concentration of 100 mg per litre of soft drink. However, the compounds are on the list of flavouring compounds given special priority in the evaluation process of flavourings in EFSA (see also Chapter 24). For this reason we will take a closer look at quinine.

Quinine occurs together with related alkaloids in the bark of the stem and the roots of the evergreen tree *Cinchona succirubra* Pavon et Klotzsch (Family: *Rubiaceae*), known in commerce as 'red cinchona'; in the barks of the related species *Cinchona ledgeriana* (Howard) Moens et Trimen and *Cinchona calisaya* Weddell; and hybrids of these with other species of *Cinchona*, known in commerce as 'calisaya' or 'yellow cinchona'. *Cinchona* was named in honour of the Countess of Chinchon, wife of the Viceroy of Peru; *succirubra* is Latin for 'red juice'. The trees are indigenous to the Andes of Ecuador and Peru (from which the more generally used name of 'Peruvian bark' stems) at an elevation of 1000–3000 m. *Chincona* species contain some 25 closely related alkaloids, of which the most important are quinine, quinidine, cinchonine and cinchonidine. The average yield of alkaloid extraction is about 6–7%, of which quinine makes up the major fraction in the yellow barks, whereas cinchonidine is relatively more abundant in the red bark.

Peruvian bark was introduced to Europe from South America in 1640, but the plant producing it was not known to botanists until 1737. It was the first effective treatment for malaria caused by *Plasmodium falciparum*. It was known and used by the Jesuits very early in history, but was first adver-tised for sale in England by James Thompson in 1658 and was made official in the *London Pharmacopoeia* of 1677, appearing in general therapeutics in the 17th century. In 1854 the Dutch began its introduction into Java (Indonesia) and in 1860 the English introduced it into India. So, cultivated commercially, the bark and later the alkaloid quinine remained the antimalarial drug of choice until the 1940s, when other drugs started to replace it. In addition to its use in the treatment of the protozoan diseases of malaria (different *Plasmodium* spp.), it was also gradually introduced in the treatment of nocturnal leg cramps. Since the end of World War II many effective antimalarials have been introduced; however, quinine is still used to treat the disease in certain situations.

The bark is spongy with a very slight odour, an astringent taste and a strongly bitter flavour. Due to its bitter taste quinine, as quinine salts or extracts from cinchona bark, is used as a bittering agent in tonic-type drinks, usually at a concentration of approximately 80 mg quinine hydrochloride per litre. Quinine is also used in some bitter alcoholic beverages and to a small extent in flour confectionery. Tonic water is a carbonated soft drink flavoured with quinine, which gives it a distinctively bitter taste. The tonic drink (originally called 'Indian tonic') was actually developed by the English as a drink prophylactic against malaria, since it was originally intended for consumption in tropical areas of South Asia and Africa. However, the original Indian tonic was bitterer than what we know now, which is why the mixed drink gin and tonic was developed in British colonial India when the British population would mix their medicinal quinine tonic with gin to make it more palatable.

Quinine has local anaesthetic action but also is an irritant. The irritant effects may be responsible in part for the nausea associated with its clinical use. Several features are common to both an acute single overdose in self-poisoning and accumulation of quinine during therapy for malaria: together they are termed cinchonism. Auditory symptoms, gastrointestinal disturbances, vasodilation, sweating and headache occur with a moderately elevated plasma quinine concentration. As plasma concentrations rise, increasingly severe visual disturbances and then cardiac and neurological features occur. Visual symptoms usually are delayed, and blindness may not be discovered for a day or more. Aspirin-sensitive patients, and others, may develop angio-oedema by non-immunological mechanisms in response to drugs, and quinine has been reported to produce pseudo-allergic reactions in aspirin sensitive patients. With this knowledge about the observed toxic effects of quinine we can understand the conclusion of JECFA (1993), that data evaluated demonstrated a clear NOAEL with respect to the ocular effects of 80 mg of anhydrous quinine hydrochloride per day, equivalent to 72 mg of quinine free base, and that no treatment-related effects on audition or clinical biochemical abnormalities were observed at doses up to 160 mg of anhydrous quinine hydrochloride per day.

JECFA further concluded that current use levels in soft drinks of up to 75 mg l^{-1} (as quinine base) were not of toxicological concern, but also noted that a small group of consumers showed an idiosyncratic hyper-reactivity to quinine (see also above) and recommended that the consumer should be informed by appropriate means of the presence of quinine in foods and beverages in which it is used.

The EU Directive 2002/67/EC of 18 July 2002 on the labelling of foodstuffs containing quinine, and of foodstuffs containing caffeine, states that quinine used as flavouring in the production or preparation of a foodstuff must be mentioned by name in the list of ingredients immediately after the term 'flavouring'. At present FDA in USA limits the quinine content in tonic water to 83 ppm.

Pyrrolizidine alkaloids

Pyrrolizidine alkaloids (PAs), formerly also called senecio alkaloids, are widely distributed among plant species. Thus, it is assumed that more than 6000 plant species belonging to the families of *Boraginaceae*, *Compositae* (*Asteraceae*) and *Leguminosae* (*Fabaceae*) alone contain PAs at different levels and in different patterns. In turn it has been estimated that about 3% of all flowering plants contain one or more of the more than 350 toxic PAs, including a number of economically important species. The pattern of PAs in plants varies not only depending on species but also on the plant variety, the climatic growth conditions, the period of sampling and the plant organ/tissue. Basic alkaloids accumulate mostly in the seeds, whereas the respective N-oxides dominate in the green parts of a plant.

The term *pyrrolizidine alkaloid* describes individual compounds that share as a basic structure one of the four necine bases: platynecine, retronecine, heliotridine or orotonecine. PAs in plants

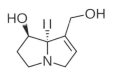

Fig. 15.5. Retronecine.

are esterified and the esters can be divided into monoesters, non-macrocyclic diesters and macrocyclic diesters of a necine base (Fig. 15.5).

Monoesters are the least toxic group and non-macrocyclic diesters posses intermediate toxicity, while macrocyclic diesters are the most toxic compounds within the PAs. The degree of toxicity is to a large extent associated with the hepatic metabolism of individual compounds. PAs are metabolized in the liver and the critical step is the formation of the reactive bifunctional pyrrolic derivative, 6,7-dihydro-7-hydroxy-1-hydroxy-methyl-5H-pyrrolizidine (DHP). DHP reacts with cellular macromolecules including proteins and DNA and accounts for the organ- and cell-specific toxicity, as well as for the genotoxiciy and mutagenicity, as it is able to form DNA adducts.

Newer results indicate that three classes of PAs – the retronecines, the heliotridines and the orotonecines – are genotoxic, whereas the platynecine type, which does not contain a double bond in the base, is not. The pyrrolic metabolites formed by the three first mentioned classes form DNA adducts, DNA cross-links and DNA–protein cross-links, which form the basis for the observed mutagenicity and carcinogenicity. As already mentioned, the pyrrolic metabolites also play a key role in liver toxicity, which is characterized by megalocytosis of parenchymal cells, followed by necrosis and finally liver cirrhosis.

Examples of acute toxicity of some PAs to the rat (intraperitoneal injection, mg kg^{-1} BW) are: retrorsine, 34; senecionine, 50; seneciphylline, 77.

Today human exposure is due to PA-containing herbs, teas and dietary supplements. A number of herbal medicines and dietary supplements containing comfrey (*Symphytum officinale*) have been widely used for more than 200 years in traditional/green medicine, and it was only in 2001 that FDA requested all manufacturers to withdraw these products from the market (with the exception of products intended for external use).

Colchicine

Colchicine-containing plant material is by no means included in a human diet intentionally.

However, during spring in the Alps, people go and pick leaves of wild garlic (*Allium ursinum*) for use in the preparation of meals. Young leaves of *Colchicum autumnale* (autumn crocus) are sometimes collected instead. During the period from 1999 to 2009, both years inclusive, at least seven reports on serious or fatal poisonings due to such incidents can be found, some including more than one person. Death actually occurred in six cases. The symptoms can range from nausea, vomiting and diarrhoea to liver injuries and multiple organ failure.

Colchicine is an antimitotic compound that interferes with a main group among the protein filaments responsible for the cytoskeleton, i.e. the microtubules. Colchicine binds to tubulin, which then cannot form polymers. The normal elongation of the microtubules prior to cell division is inhibited and the mitotic spindle is disrupted, which means that cell division is no longer possible. The first and most affected tissues are naturally those with the highest mitotic activity, like gastrointestinal epithelia cells, hair follicles and haematological stem cells, together with cells with a high number of microtubules such as sperm cells.

As a result of the described toxic mechanism, colchicine is genotoxic *in vitro* and *in vivo* in low concentrations, can cause malformations in offspring and can affect fertility. Nevertheless, the compound also can be used in therapy and as such was approved by FDA in 2009 for the treatment of acute gout and familial Mediterranean fever.

Furanocoumarins (psoralens)

The existence of furanocoumarins in many species of the *Rutaceae* and *Umbelliferae* (= the carrot family) is well documented. The *Rutaceae* include the citrus fruit trees, while a large number of vegetables such as parsnip, skirret, carrot, celery, parsley and Florence fennel belong to the umbelliferous plants. The chemical structure of furanocoumarins consists of a furan ring fused with coumarin. The furan may be fused in two different ways producing linear or angular compounds with the basic ring structure, e.g. bergapten and angelicin, respectively (Fig. 15.6).

The linear furanocoumarins in particular cause photodermatitis and are photo-activated carcinogens. After application to the skin and irradiation of the exposed surface with long-wave UV light (occurring as a component of sunlight), eczema

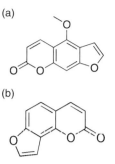

(a)

(b)

Fig. 15.6. (a) A linear furanocoumarin (bergapten); (b) an angular furanocoumarin (angelicin).

with skin erythema and oedema followed by hyperpigmentation is seen. In the skin cells the furanocoumarins yield products that are able to interact with DNA, forming mono- and di-adducts. These acute toxic as well as mutagenic and carcinogenic effects have been demonstrated in animal studies. From the use of certain of these compounds in the treatment of the diseases vitiligo and psoriasis, it is further known that after oral administration the compounds also distribute under the skin, to render this sensitive to the combined effect of the compounds and external UV light. Thus, not only handling plants with high content of furanocoumarins but also consumption theoretically may pose a risk. However, the current toxicological database concerning these compounds is far from complete.

A quite detailed study published in 2007 including a number of commodities showed that the levels of furanocoumarins in celery, celeriac, parsnip, carrot, lemon and other foods purchased from a Czech retail market in the years 2003–2004 varied over a wide range; the highest contents were determined in parsnip (*Pastinaca sativa*), while the levels of these toxins in carrots and citrus pulps were relatively low. The total content of furanocoumarins found in parsnip ranged from 5 to 89 $\mu g\ g^{-1}$ ($n=50$). In good agreement with these results, this class of phytochemical is known to be responsible for the phytophotodermatitis seen after exposure to the juice of the wild parsnip.

Furanocoumarins have other biological effects. Thus, in humans, bergamottin and dihydroxybergamottin are responsible for the 'grapefruit juice effect', in which these furanocoumarins affect the metabolism of certain drugs.

Simple mono-, sesqui- and diterpenes

A large number of mono- and sesquiterpenes are components in natural flavours and as such are discussed in Chapter 24 on food additives and flavourings. Here we take a look at diterpenes that make up the group of toxins called *grayanotoxins* (GTXs; previously called andromedotoxins or rhodotoxins). GTXs are believed to be the causative agent behind the earliest case of food poisoning described, namely a mass intoxication of soldiers of the Cyrus army around 400 BC. The author 'Xenophon' tells us that the soldiers had consumed honey harvested along the way. In the evening they lost their senses, vomited and were not able to stand upright. Today we know that plants belonging to the family *Ericaceae* including *Rhododendron* spp. contain GTXs in their honey, and actually this poisoning is known as 'mad honey poisoning' in the Black Sea region of the present-day Turkey where the old incident took place. A number of such poisonings have been described in the recent literature (from the 1980s to date) from the very same region, probably as a result of bees feeding on, for example, *Rhododendron ponticum*.

Of the over 30 GTXs that have been structurally elucidated, the compounds GTX1, -2 and -3 seem to be the most toxic (Fig. 15.7).

GTX was found to bind to closed sodium ion channels in cell membranes, resulting in a modified continuously open channel. Initial symptoms on poisoning are salivation, perspiration, vomiting, dizziness, and paraesthesia in the extremities and around the mouth. Furthermore, low blood pressure and bradycardia are seen. In higher doses loss of coordination and severe and progressive muscular weakness, still followed by bradycardia, occur. Despite the cardiac problems the condition is rarely fatal and generally lasts less than a day.

Gossypol

In 1957 it was reported that in a village in Jiangsu Province in China, no children had been born between the 1930s and 1940s, although the villagers were fecund before and after that period. Investigations showed that the infertility was due to gossypol in the food oil used. Later, in the 1960s, farmers from Hubei and Hebei Provinces in China who ingested home-made unheated cottonseed oil developed fatigue and a burning sensation on the face and other exposed parts of the body.

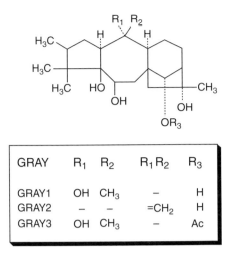

GRAY	R_1	R_2	$R_1 R_2$	R_3
GRAY1	OH	CH_3	–	H
GRAY2	–	–	$=CH_2$	H
GRAY3	OH	CH_3	–	Ac

Fig. 15.7. The structures of the three toxins GTX1, -2 and -3 (equal to GRAY1, -2 and -3). Ac, acetyl.

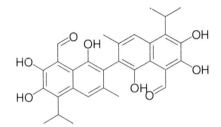

Fig. 15.8. Gossypol.

The syndrome was named 'Hanchuan fever or burning fever'. Soon gossypol (Fig. 15.8) attracted attention as a possible male anti-fertility agent or a therapeutic agent for some gynaecological diseases, but the research in this area was discontinued due to the irreversibility of its anti-spermatogenic effect at low doses.

Gossypol occurs in cotton plants, mostly in the seeds, which are grown for the production of fibre and oil. The oil must be rectified before use as a food oil in order to avoid its toxicity, including the influence on male fertility described above.

15.3 Conclusion

Plants defend themselves against herbivores, whether mammals or insects, and from attacks by fungi, etc. For this defence they biosynthesize a large pallet of organic compounds, many of which are also toxic to man. Throughout history we have learned to avoid the most poisonous and we have used breeding to lower the content of non-desired compounds. At the same time we have found certain potentially toxic compounds to be of value, e.g. as food additives, a development that has called for risk assessments to set limits for their use.

Note

[1] ITIS Report (2009) Plantae, Taxonomic Serial No. 202422. International Taxonomic Information System, Washington, DC; available at http://www.itis.gov/servlet/SingleRpt/SingleRpt?search_topic=TSN&search_value=202422

Further Reading

Backshall, S. (2007) *Venomous Animals of the World.* Johns Hopkins University Press, Baltimore, Maryland.

Bevan-Jones, R. (2009) *Poisonous Plants: A Cultural and Social History.* Windgather Press/Oxbow Books, Oxford, UK.

Cheeke, P.R. (1997) *Natural Toxicants in Feeds, Forages, and Poisonous Plants*, 2nd edn. Prentice Hall, Upper Saddle River, New Jersey.

Dauncey, E.A. (2010) *Poisonous Plants. A Guide for Parents and Childcare Providers.* Kew Publishing, London.

EFSA (2009) Marine biotoxins in shellfish – Summary on regulated marine biotoxins. Scientific Opinion of the Panel on Contaminants in the Food Chain. *EFSA Journal* 1306, 1–23.

EFSA (2009) Scientific Opinion. Influence of processing on the levels of lipophilic marine biotoxins in bivalve molluscs. Statement of the Panel on Contaminants in the Food Chain (Question No. EFSA-Q-2009-00203). Adopted on 25 March 2009. *EFSA Journal* 1016, 1–10.

Juneja, V.K. and Sofos, J.N. (eds) (2010) *Pathogens and Toxins in Foods; Challenges and Interventions.* ASM Press, Washington, DC.

Wagstaff, D.J. (2008) *International Poisonous Plants Checklist: An Evidence-Based Reference.* CRC Press, Boca Raton, Florida.

16 Naturally Inherent Plant Toxicants: Glycosides

- Potatoes contain alkaloidal glycosides and more so if sprouted.
- Cassava root contains toxic cyanogenic glycosides – in toxic amounts in the so-called bitter varieties.
- Many other food plants are restricted in their use due to the presence of different glycosides.
- The problems and their solutions are discussed.

16.1 Introduction

A great number of different glycosides and oligosaccharides, causing physiological effects (toxins) or reduced uptake or use of nutrients (anti-nutritional compounds) after ingestion, are known in the plant kingdom, as are a number of especially bitter-tasting glycosides which reduce the palatability of the plant organ whether used for food or as feedstuff (Table 16.1). The human palate is very sensitive to the bitter taste, which, although often regarded as disagreeable in itself, in conjunction with other tastes may contribute significantly to product acceptance. Three classes of naturally occurring organic constituents encountered in food materials are particularly associated with bitterness: alkaloids, glycosides and peptides. Thus, there is no obvious chemical relationship between the main groups of compounds having a bitter taste, a pattern that in general seems to hold even when looking into each of the three groups, although some very rough structural relationships may be found. While a few of the glycosides listed in Table 16.1 actually have been demonstrated to be protective to the plant in reducing natural herbivory or infection by bacteria, fungi or viruses, most have been identified as possessing one or more of the above-mentioned properties when looking at domestic animals or humans as consumers. That is, a number of these compounds are found in plants of known nutritional value to humans, and others in vegetable resources regarded as promising for food or feed as discussed below.

In this chapter, only glycosides with a known history as poisons in food, as sources of described human intoxications or as compounds found in plants from which food ingredients are produced are discussed further.

Bitter versus sweet varieties, forms or cultivars

Several toxic glycosides (including various saponins and cyanogenic glycosides, etc.; see below) are known to be bitter tasting (as pure compounds) in addition to their toxicity. Hence, the term 'bitter', as opposed to 'sweet', has traditionally been used to designate naturally occurring or selected groups within a plant species that contain high amounts of the toxic (and bitter) substance. Depending on the view of the botanical author the groups in question may be divided on the level of variety, form or cultivar. Examples of species for which such a division into 'bitter' and 'sweet' has been used are *Prunus dulcis* and other *Prunus* spp., as well as *Manihot esculenta* (cassava). In most such cases a certain correlation between the toxicity (content of glycoside) and the degree of bitterness of the plant part has been established. However, it is only seldom that a proper investigation has been performed concerning the degree to which this correlation holds.

16.2 Single Classes of Toxic or Anti-nutritional Glycosides

The broad range of compounds listed in Table 16.1 illustrates the diversity of chemical structures found

Table 16.1. Toxic, anti-nutritional and bitter-tasting glycosides and oligosaccharides.

Compound group or compound	Example(s)	Toxicity, taste, etc.
A. *O*-Glycosides, sugar esters and oligosaccharides		
In sources of food and feed		
Cyanogenic glycosides	Linamarin in *Manihot esculenta*, *Euphorbiaceae*, in general widespread in the plant kingdom (*Tracheophyta* and *Spermatophyta*)	Acute and chronic toxicity due to release of HCN. Neurotoxicity of intact glycosides discussed. Bitter taste
Glycoalkaloids	Chachonin and solanin in *Solanum tuberosum*, *Solanaceae* (*Angiospermae*)	Corrosive to the gastrointestinal tract, acutely toxic upon absorption due to several mechanisms. Bitter taste
Glycosides of organic nitriles	Simmondsin in *Simmondsia californica* (jojoba), *Buxaceae* (*Angiospermae*)	Causes chronic toxicity by unknown mechanism
Glycosides and sugar esters of aliphatic nitrocompounds	Miserotoxin in *Astragalus* spp., *Fabaceae* (= *Leguminosae*; *Angiospermae*)	Acutely toxic to ruminants; inhibits the citric acid cycle of cells
Methylazoxymethanol (MAM) glycosides	Cycasin in *Cycas* spp., *Cycadaceae* (*Gymnospermae*)	Carcinogenic
Naringin	In *Citrus* spp., especially *Citrus paradisi* (grapefruit), *Rutaceae* (*Angiospermae*)	Bitter taste
Oligosaccharides	In seeds of several legume spp., *Fabaceae* (= *Leguminosae*; *Angiospermae*)	Flatulence-producing
Platyphylloside	In *Betula pendula*, *Betulaceae* (*Angiospermae*)	Anti-nutritional (deterrent) to several animal species
Polyphenols	2-Hydroxyarctiin in *Carthamus tinctorius* (safflower), *Asteraceae* (= *Compositae*; *Angiospermae*)	Cathartic (laxative). Bitter taste
Ptaquiloside	In *Pteridium aquilinum*, *Polypodiaceae* (*Tracheophyta*)	Acutely toxic and carcinogenic
Saponins	Triterpene or steroid saponins in *Quinoa* spp., *Borassus flabellifer*, *Glycyrrhizae glabra* and *Balanites* spp. (*Angiospermae*)	Some acutely toxic, others mildly to strongly toxic. Several are bitter tasting
Vicine and convicine	In *Vicia faba* (faba bean), *Fabaceae* (= *Leguminosae*; *Angiospermae*)	Acutely toxic to G6PD-deficient individuals
In medicinal and toxic plants		
Carboxyatractyloside (CAT) and related compounds	CAT in *Atractylis gummifera*, *Asteraceae* (= *Compositae*; *Angiospermae*)	Acutely toxic, inhibit mitochondrial oxidative phosphorylation
Cardeno- and bufodienolides	'Digitalis glycosides' in *Digitalis* spp. (cardiac glycosides), *Scrophulariaceae* (*Angiospermae*)	Acutely toxic to the heart
Cucurbitacins	Cucurbitacin L in *Citrullus colocynthis*, *Cucurbitaceae* (*Angiospermae*); some cucurbitacins also present in food plants	Intensely bitter substances, some of which are acutely toxic
Glycosides of vitamin D$_3$	Glycosides of 1α,25-(OH)$_2$D$_3$ in *Solanum glaucophyllum*, *Solanaceae* (*Angiospermae*)	Chronic toxicity (vitamin D intoxication – calcinosis)
Ranunculin	In *Ranunculus* and *Caratocephalus* spp., *Ranunculaceae* (*Angiospermae*)	Acutely toxic. Irritant to mucous membranes. Upon absorption affects several organs such as heart, lungs, etc.
B. *C*-Glycosides (some also occurring as *O*-glycosides)		
In medicinal plants		
Anthraquinone, anthrone and dianthrone glycosides	Sennosides in *Cassia angustifolia*, *Fabaceae* (= *Leguminosae*; *Angiospermae*)	Laxative effect; some compounds are *drastica*
C. *S*-Glycosides (thioglycosides)		
In food and feed resources		
Glucosinolates	In many species within the family of *Capparales* (*Angiospermae*)	Chronic toxicity due to release of thiocyanate and other compounds. Sharp (burning) taste

even within the restricted field of toxic and anti-nutritional glycosides and oligosaccharides. Since this diversity means a broad range of different mechanisms of action, each group from Table 16.1 is commented upon below (in alphabetic order). Structure examples are also presented in a number of figures.

Anthraquinone, anthrone and dianthrone glycosides (cathartic)

The chemical class of naturally occurring anthranoids comprises some hundreds of structurally related compounds present in many plant families within both the mono- and dicots. Laxative and/or cathartic compounds are found mainly within the genera *Aloe*, *Cassia*, *Rhamnus*, *Rheum* and *Rumex*. The anthranoids are oxo-, hydroxy- and hydroxy-oxo-derivatives of anthracene. Most compounds found in nature are derivatives of 9,10-anthraquinone (AQ). They occur in plants both as free anthranoids and as glycosides (Fig. 16.1). The glycosides may be hydrolysed to a limited extent in the small intestine. However, the main part is transported to the colon, where microbial hydrolysis releases the aglycone. If the genuine compound contains a 1,8-dihydroxy structure, highly reactive anthrones will be formed, directly or by reduction, which are responsible for the laxative action. The laxative effect is used in medicine; however, certain plant organs are so strong in their action that we talk about a *drasticum*. During the 1990s discussions were intense as to whether anthranoid laxatives present a risk of human colon cancer, but it was concluded in 2000 that several cohort studies failed to find any association between anthranoid laxative use and colorectal cancer.

A special problem to be faced in a food context is the production of cassia gum with a low content of anthraquinones and anthrones. Cassia gum is used as a food additive (in Europe designated E499), i.e. as a thickener, emulsifier, foam stabilizer, moisture retention agent and/or texturizing agent in cheese, frozen dairy desserts and mixes, meat products and poultry products. Cassia gum is primarily the ground purified endosperm of the seeds of *Cassia tora* and *Cassia obtusifolia* (Family: *Leguminosae*). The seeds are de-husked and de-germed by thermal mechanical treatment followed by milling and screening of the endosperm. Cassia gum consists mainly of high-molecular-weight (approximately 200,000–300,000) polysaccharides composed of galactomannans; the

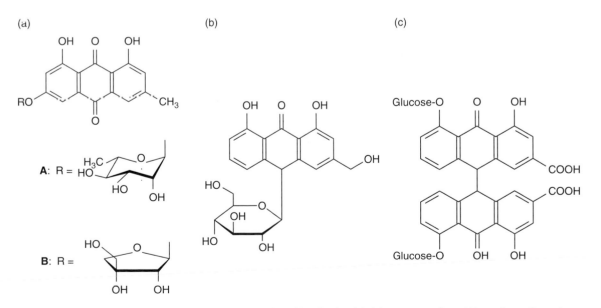

Fig. 16.1. Anthraquinone, anthrone and dianthrone glycosides (cathartic): (a) structures **A** and **B** are the anthraquinone glycosides frangulin A and B, respectively; (b) the anthrone glucoside (a *C*-glucoside) aloin; (c) a structure representing the two compounds sennoside A and B. The two latter are diastereoisomers (*R,R'* and *R,S'*) respectively around the C9–C9' bond which connects the two parts of the molecule.

mannose:galactose ratio is about 5:1. Other galactomannans used in food production include carob bean gum, guar gum and tara gum.

C. tora and C. obtusifolia seeds naturally contain anthraquinones, the content of which is reduced from around 10,000 ppm to 250 ppm during the mechanical processing. This level is still not low enough though, which is why the ground endosperm is further purified by extraction with isopropanol to remove all anthraquinones.

The international quality standards for cassia gum all also require that the production starts with a material that contains less than 0.1 or 0.05% of seeds of Cassia occidentalis. C. occidentalis generally does not grow in conjunction with C. tora or C. obtusifolia, but still is an occasional impurity for which the collected seeds need to be inspected. C. occidentalis seeds are noticeably smaller and differently shaped (flat discs instead of the longish seeds of C. tora and C. obtusifolia) and can be recognized, both as seeds and later on as splits.

The reason for this restriction is that C. occidentalis is associated with muscle toxicity. Signs of C. occidentalis poisoning in general include, independent of species affected: ataxia, muscle weakness, stubbing, and body weight loss eventually leading to death. Skeletal muscle degeneration is the predominant lesion found in the majority of animal species intoxicated with C. occidentalis; other lesions such as degenerative myopathy of myocardial muscle, congestion and pulmonary oedema, hepatic cell hypertrophy and vacuolization have also been reported.

Although many studies have been carried out to identify the toxic principles of C. occidentalis, we had to wait until 1996 when a dianthrone – an anthraquinone-derived compound – was isolated and shown to cause the characteristic mitochondrial myopathy produced by the plant.

Semi-refined cassia gum normally containing detectable amounts of anthraquinones has been accepted for use in pet food by several countries.

Carboxyatractyloside and related compounds

Carboxyatractyloside/atractyloside was shown in 1972 to be the toxic principle in *Atractylis gummifera*. This plant was known both as a toxic and a medicinal plant as far back in history as about 300 BC. In about 1982, the work of a number of research groups revealed that a veterinary toxicosis resulting from the eating of young sprouts of *Xanthium strumarium* is due to contents of carboxyatractyloside (CAT). Fatal intoxications due to intake of CAT-containing plants have been described for both man and animals. CAT inhibits mitochondrial oxidative phosphorylation through inhibition of the ANT (adenine nucleotide translocase)-mediated adenonucleotide transport through the inner mitochondrial membrane. Closely related compounds (kaurene glycosides) were later isolated from hepatotoxic plants such as *Wedelia asperrima* and *Wedelia biflora* (*Compositae*) and *Cestrum parqui* (*Solanaceae*). For structures see Fig. 16.2.

Cardeno- and bufodienolides (cardiac glycosides)

The cardiac-active steroids grouped as the 'cardiac glycosides' include two subgroups called cardenolides and bufadienolides (Fig. 16.3). While

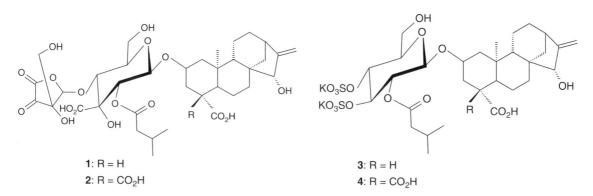

1: R = H
2: R = CO₂H

3: R = H
4: R = CO₂H

Fig. 16.2. CAT and related compounds: **1**, parquin; **2**, carboxyparquin; **3**, atractyloside; **4**, carboxyatractyloside.

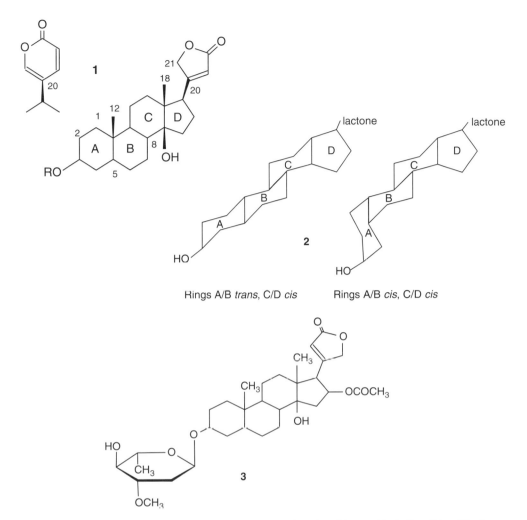

Fig. 16.3. Cardeno- and bufadienolides. **1**, The basic skeletons of cardenolides and bufadienolides differ in the structure attached to the four-fused-ring system at C-17, with the five-membered lactone characteristic of cardenolides and the six-membered lactone of all bufadienolides. **2**, The *cis* orientation of rings C and D is characteristic of cardenolides; furthermore a *cis* A/B configuration is a feature of medically important cardenolides in the plant families *Apocynaceae* and *Scrophulariaceae*, whereas *trans* A/B cardenolides are most widely distributed among *Asclepiadaceae*. **3**, Oleandrin.

bufadienolides have been recorded from not more than six plant families, and from the skin secretions of poisonous toads, cardenolides have a much wider although still restricted distribution within the plant kingdom. Thus, cardenolides have been found in at least 200 plant species representing 55 genera and 12 angiosperm families. Important families with respect to number of cardenolide-bearing species include *asclepiadaceae*, *Apocynaceae*, *Celastraceae* and *Scrophulariaceae*. Although William Withering

described the medicinal use of the cardenolide-containing foxglove (*Digitalis purpurea*, *Scrophulariaceae*) in 1785, it was not until 1890 that the toxic effects were described by Sir Thomas Fraser in his search for the sources of African arrow poisons. Some structures are shown in Fig. 16.3.

Almost every spring, some people living in the Alps in Europe who collect leaves of wild garlic (*Allium ursinum*) for culinary use mistakenly pick the young leaves of lily-of-the-valley (*Convalaria majalis*) instead. This leads to intoxications, with blurred vision, diarrhoea and irregular heart beat due to the content of close to 40 different cardenolides such as convallarin and convallatoxin in lily-of-the-valley leaves. Luckily this intoxication is seldom fatal.

The veterinary literature from Africa and North America includes many reports on the lethal effect of cardenolide-containing plants to domestic livestock, and photographic illustrations documenting that grazing cattle avoid the highly toxic milkweeds (*Asclepias* spp.). Likewise, intoxications of cattle and donkeys often occur when green leaves and branches from pruning of oleander (*Nerium oleander*) are either mixed with forage or left under a tree.

Cucurbitacins

Cucurbitacins were first characterized as the bitter compounds of cucumbers, marrows and squashes, all members of the family *Cucurbitaceae*. The cucurbitacins as a group are thought to be among the bitterest substances known to man. Thus, cucurbitacin B has been detected by taste panels in dilutions as low as 1 ppb and the glycosides of cucurbitacin E at 10 ppb. The cucurbitacins are a group of oxygenated tetracyclic triterpenes (Fig. 16.4), some of which occur as glycosides (e.g. cucurbitacin L in *Citrullus colocynthis* and carnosifloside III in *Hemsleya carnosiflora*). While most cucurbitacins, aglycones as well as glycosides, are bitter in taste, a few are tasteless or even sweet. An example of the latter is the glycoside carnosifloside

found in *H. carnosiflora* (*Cucurbitaceae*). Certain of the cucurbitacins are not only intensely bitter but also quite toxic. Thus, the LD_{10} for oral intake in mice of cucurbitacin B, which is a feeding attractant to cucumber beetles (but a feeding deterrent to other insects), was found to be around 5 mg kg^{-1} BW.

Several of the species within the family *Cucurbitaceae* that are used as human food naturally contain cucurbitacins in amounts unacceptable to the market. However, intense domestication and breeding has resulted in cultivars low in bitter compounds. Thus, breeding programmes for curcurbits are constantly aware of the bitterness.

Cyanogenic glycosides

Cyanogenic compounds are compounds that upon degradation release HCN, a highly toxic clear to pale blue liquid or gas. Naturally occurring cyanogenic compounds include the following groups: (i) cyanogenic glycosides, compound **a**; (ii) cyanogenic lipids, compound **b**; (iii) cyanohydrins (= hydroxynitriles), compound **c**; and (iv) 2,3-epoxynitriles, compound **d** (Fig. 16.5). Of these compounds **a**, **b** and **d** are chemically relatively stable, however giving rise to the formation of cyanohydrins (compound **c**) as a result of their degradation. One may classify the food-related use of cyanogenic plants as follows: the plant commodity is (i) a staple food component; (ii) a minor food component (of sporadic use); (iii) a component in the production of beverages, pastry or sweets; or (iv) used in medical

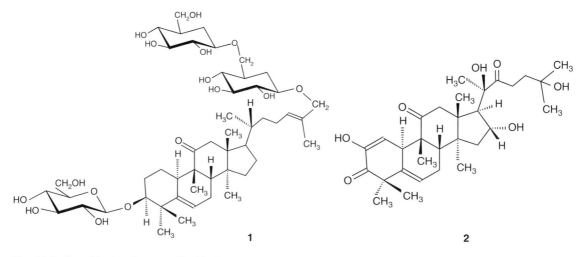

Fig. 16.4. Cucurbitacins: **1**, carnosifloside III; **2**, cucurbitacin L (occurs as the 2-*O*-β-D-glucoside).

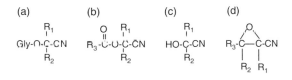

Fig. 16.5. Classes of cyanogenic compounds: **a**, cyanogenic glycoside; **b**, cyanogenic lipid; **c**, cyanohydrin (α-hydroxynitrile); **d**, 2,3-epoxynitrile (e.g. sarmentosin epoxide).

treatments, usually within the sector of green/alternative medicine. Cyanogenic plants and plant parts are also grazed by animals and relatively often deliberately included in the feedstuffs used for animal husbandry.

The HCN released from the degradation of cyanogenic glycosides may give rise to acute as well as chronic toxicity. In general, safety regulations have been implemented in the EU and in most other industrialized countries, for foods as well as feedstuffs. Food based on highly cyanogenic plant parts such as bitter cassava roots can be made safe (based on the levels accepted in existing standards) by processing. However, food safety authorities and the general population must be aware that changing food habits, e.g. as a result of new health trends, may cause risks of hitherto unseen exposure to cyanogenic glysosides, as in the case of an increased intake of linseed.

Cyanogenesis has been detected in prokaryotes, fungi, plants and animals. Cyanogenic constituents have been isolated from a great number of organisms, but the glycosides only from plants and insects. The first cyanogenic constituents to be isolated and elucidated structurally were plant glycosides like amygdalin (1830), sambunigrin (1928) and acacipetalin (1935). The cyanogenic glycosides, which are the most common cyanogens and comprise around 60 structures, were recognized early as substances poisonous to wild as well as domesticated animals. An example of a cyanogenic glycoside where the sugar moiety is glucose is the cyanogenic glucoside linamarin present in cassava roots (Fig. 16.6).

Examples of total contents of cyanogenic glycosides in plants and plant products used for or in food are (as HCN equivalents in mg kg^{-1}): lima bean, 200–3000; bitter almond, 300–3000; apricot and peach kernels, 100–500; flaxseed, up to 500.

The acute toxicity of HCN in man is well described. The information has been gained from fatal as well as non-fatal poisonings from both oral and respiratory exposure to HCN. Clinical symptoms include: anxiety and excitement, rapid breathing, faintness, weakness, headache (pulsating), constricting sensations in the chest, facial flushing, dyspnoea, nausea, vomiting, diarrhoea, dizziness, drowsiness, confusion, convulsions, incontinence of urine and faeces, irregular respiration and coma. In the case of large lethal doses, convulsions are seen immediately, followed by coma and death.

Cyanide is absorbed in the gastrointestinal tract. It is rapidly and ubiquitously distributed throughout the body, although the highest levels are typically found in the liver, lungs, blood and brain. There is no accumulation of cyanide in the blood or tissues following chronic or repeated exposure. Most cyanide is metabolized to thiocyanate in the liver by the mitochondrial sulfur transferase enzyme rhodanese and other sulfur transferases.

The toxic effects of the cyanide ion in man and animals are generally similar and are believed to result from inactivation of cytochrome oxidase, inhibition of cellular respiration and consequently histotoxic anoxia. The primary targets of cyanide toxicity are the cardiovascular, respiratory and central nervous systems.

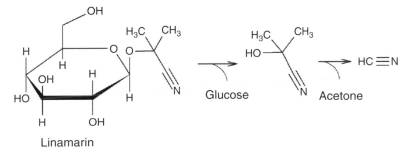

Fig. 16.6. Linamarin and its degradation to release HCN.

Chronic exposure to lower (non-fatal) concentrations of HCN is known to affect the CNS of both animals and man. In production animals, cyanide is associated with syndromes affecting the CNS and gives rise to ataxia in sheep, cattle and horses grazing on another cyanogenic crop, i.e. sorghum (*Sorghum bicolor* (L.) Moench), which contains the cyanogenic glucoside dhurrin. Histopathological examinations of affected horses and cattle have shown spheroids in the white matter of the spinal cord, mostly in the ventral funiculi, and in the cerebellar peduncles.

A restricted number of controlled long-term studies in traditional laboratory animals such as rats as well as studies in pigs and dogs have also demonstrated damage to the CNS as evidenced by findings of slower reaction time, reduced explorative behaviour, etc. Among a variety of neuropathies reported from regions of Africa with populations that consume a high level of the tuberous starchy root of cassava (*M. esculenta* Crantz), at least konzo is generally believed to be caused by cyanide from the monotonous consumption of insufficiently processed bitter cassava. The edible parts of cassava contain the two cyanogenic glucosides, linamarin and lotaustralin, the bitterness being – at least to a certain extent – a function of the content of these compounds. Konzo is a distinct upper motor neuron disease characterized by the sudden onset of varying degrees of symmetric, isolated, non-progressive spastic paraparesis.

In 2003 CAC intervened in the internationalization of cassava as a food commodity by launching a 'Codex Standard for Sweet Cassava'. According to this, sweet cassava varieties are those that contain less than 50 mg HCN kg^{-1} (fresh weight, FW, basis). In addition to the CAC standard for sweet cassava and its standard for edible cassava flour setting a maximum level of 10 mg kg^{-1} FW for the total hydrocyanic acid content, Food Standards Australia New Zealand (FSANZ) is about the only authority that has published a number of risk assessments, made a proposal for a future legislation and made publicly available some documented risk communications concerning the possible adverse health effects of intake of cassava roots and cassava root products. As a result of a process of risk assessment running from 2004 to 2009 and including cassava chips, bamboo shoots and other food items with a possible content of cyanogenic constituents, FSANZ thus concludes that: (i) 'by adequate processing (peeling, slicing and cooking) both the cyanogenic glycosides and hydrocyanic acid can be removed prior to consumption'; (ii) 'while the current users have adequate knowledge regarding the risks associated with consumption of cassava (and bamboo shoots), more widespread use in the community would increase the public health risks'; and (iii) 'a maximum level of 10 mg HCN/kg is considered to be necessary to confidently protect public health and safety' when looking at ready-to-eat-cassava chips.

Glucosinolates

In 1990 already more than 100 glucosinolates were known, the structural variations being due to various side chains and the attachment of carboxylic acids as esters to the thioglucose part, glucosinolates being thioglucosides (Fig. 16.7).

Glucosinolates are known to occur in *Capparales*, *Salvadorales*, *Violales*, *Euphorbiales* and *Tropaeolales*. Reasons for interest in glucosinolates or glucosinolate-containing plants are the various flavour, off-flavour, anti-nutritional and toxic effects, as well as positive physiological effects associated with these constituents and plants, caused by the glucosinolates themselves and byproducts thereof. The food plants of greatest interest here are different forms of cabbage, capers used as a kind of 'spice', and rapeseed from which we produce rapeseed oil for the production of margarine and for direct use as a food oil.

Among the most important crops containing glucosinolates we thus find rape, i.e. *Brassica napus*, *Brassica campestris* and *Brassica juncea*. The seeds of these three species contain about 400 g of oil and approximately 250 g of protein per kilogram. However, use of rapeseed meal (the press cake remaining after the extraction of the oil) as a protein source in livestock rations and in human diets is limited, due to the toxic and anti-nutritional compounds associated with the protein fractions. These include the glucosinolates as well as phytic acid and phenolic compounds. In addition it should be mentioned that the oil fraction also contains toxins, namely lipids of the toxic fatty acid erucic acid.

Rapeseed bred to contain less than 2% erucic acid in its oil and less than 30 µmol of aliphatic glucosinolates per gram is called 'double low'.

All pure glucosinolates tested in animal diets have proved to cause anti-nutritional and/or toxic effects even when included in concentrations relevant to levels based on the use of double-low rapeseed press

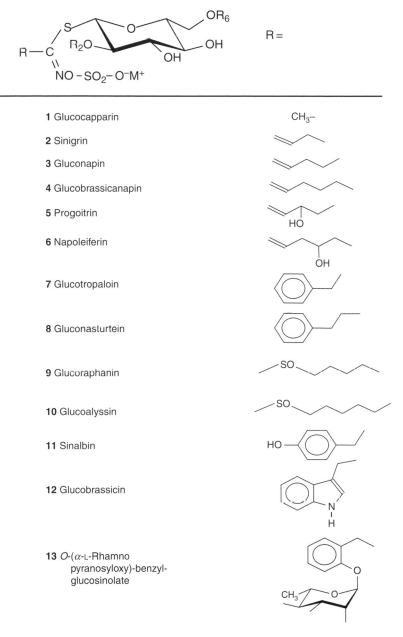

R =

1 Glucocapparin   CH₃–

2 Sinigrin

3 Gluconapin

4 Glucobrassicanapin

5 Progoitrin

6 Napoleiferin

7 Glucotropaloin

8 Gluconasturtein

9 Glucoraphanin

10 Glucoalyssin

11 Sinalbin

12 Glucobrassicin

13 O-(α-L-Rhamno pyranosyloxy)-benzyl- glucosinolate

Fig. 16.7. Glucosinolates. As shown in the general structure of glucosinolates (top), these differ at three sites: R, R₂ and R₆. R, a side chain with structural resemblance to the parent amino acids; R₂ and R₆, H or acyl derivatives; M⁺, cation. The variation in R as shown in examples **1** to **13** gives rise to the different non-acylated glucosinolates named.

cakes as the protein source. The effects are related to differences in both types of functional group in the side chains. The mechanism(s) behind the toxic and anti-nutritional effects thus are several. From the degradation of glucobrassicin (an indol glucosinolate), indolyl-3-methanol is formed in considerable amounts, but it disappears very fast, leaving appreciable amounts of thiocyanate ion. No isothiocyanates and thiocyanates are formed. In contrast, degradation of various aliphatic glucosinolates results in the formation of nitriles as well as isothiocyanates and thiocyanates. Thiocyanate inhibits the uptake of iodine in the thyroid gland and therefore may cause goitre especially if the intake of iodine already is low.

Up to the beginning of World War II, when cabbage was a major food component and iodine intake was restricted, goitre was seen especially in European countries such as England and Poland.

Glycoalkaloids

Steroidal alkaloids and alkaloid glycosides are well known to occur throughout the *Solanum* genus (*Solanaceae*). The common (Irish) potato (*Solanum tuberosum*) contains, as the main constituents in its edible tuber, the two compounds α-chaconine and α-solanine, both 3-O-glycosides of the genin solanidine (Fig. 16.8), which also may occur unglycosylated.

The potato was first cultivated by people in the Andes about 8000 years ago and was brought to Europe at the end of the 16th century with the Spanish invasion of South America. The total production of potatoes in the world today is increasing as shown in Table 16.2.

A number of investigations and literature reviews are available showing that the glycosides are concentrated just under the skin (in the peel)

and that the total content indeed varies very much from cultivar to cultivar. Thus, literature data compiled by Gelder was published in 1991. The range of solanidine glycoside content was 10–390 mg kg^{-1} FW, with a mean of 73 mg kg^{-1} FW. Another publication gives the contents shown in Table 16.3.

In other species of *Solanum* different glycosides and free genins may dominate. Thus, up to 55% of the total alkaloid content in *Solanum dulcamara* is 15-α-hydroxylated spirosolanes and solanidanes, such as 15-α-hydroxytomatidine. Gastrointestinal absorption of steroidal alkaloid glycosides seems to vary between animal species and moreover may depend on factors such as food/feed intake, as indicated by several studies made on the main potato alkaloids, α-chaconine and α-solanine. These studies further indicate that some hydrolysis of the glycosidic bond and further metabolism seem to occur in different species, as judged from analysis comparing the serum level of α-chaconine and/or α-solanine with that of total alkaloids.

The toxicity of the potato glycosides to man includes gastrointestinal upset with diarrhoea, vomiting and abdominal pain. In severe cases neurological symptoms, some of which clearly are a result of the acetylcholinesterase inhibitor activity of these glycosides, may occur. Such adverse effects are seldom seen, however. In fact, the risk almost solely arises if potatoes that have been exposed to

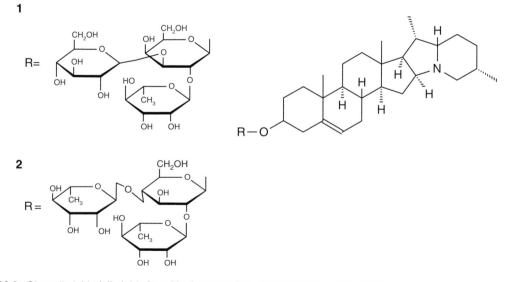

Fig. 16.8. Glycoalkaloids (alkaloids found in the potato): **1**, α-solanine; **2**, α-chaconine.

Table 16.2. The development in world potato production (million tonnes; from FAOSTAT).

Countries	Year						
	1991	1995	1999	2001	2003	2005	2007
Developed	183.13	177.47	165.93	166.93	160.97	159.97	159.89
Developing	84.86	108.50	135.15	145.92	152.11	160.01	165.41
World	267.99	285.97	301.08	312.85	313.08	319.98	325.30

Table 16.3. Content of glycoalkaloids in peel, flesh and whole potatoes of different cultivars. Adapted from Friedman (2006).[1]

Cultivar – sample	mg kg^{-1} dry weight			
	α-Chaconine	α-Solanine	Total	Chaconine:solanine ratio
Atlantic – peel	59.4	24.4	83.8	2.43
Atlantic – flesh	22.6	13.9	36.5	1.63
Russet Narkota – peel	288	138	425	2.09
Russet Narkota – flesh	3.7	2.7	6.4	1.37
Dark Red Norland – peel	859	405	1261	2.12
Dark Red Norland – flesh	16.0	6.1	22.1	2.62
Snowden – peel	2414	1112	3526	2.17
Snowden – flesh	366	226	591	1.62
Russet – whole potato	65.1	35.0	100	1.86
White – whole potato	28.2	15.3	43.5	1.84
Benji – whole potato	70.7	27.6	98.3	2.56
Lenape – whole potato	413	216	629	1.91

light (often green peel) or have sprouted are eaten in greater amounts. Light stimulates the synthesis of the glycosides and sprouts show much higher contents than the tuber.

Both α-chaconine and α-solanine, together with their aglycones, are teratogenic in one or more animal species. However, an association between the consumption of blighted potatoes by women during pregnancy and the incidences of suspected malformations such as spina bifida could not be substantiated. Turning to *S. dulcamara*, the intake of tissues from this plant has been associated with losses of cattle, horses and sheep from acute intoxication. Moreover, it was shown that tissues from this plant had an approximately sevenfold ability to induce terata compared with that seen in similar experiments with tissues of *S. tuberosum*. This was tentatively correlated to its high content of 15-α-hydroxylated alkaloids.

In Europe a guideline for new potato cultivars recommends that these have a total content of glycoalkaloids (α-chaconine + α-solanine) lower than 200 mg kg^{-1} FW, although according to Regulation (EC) No. 1881/2006 there is no legislatively set maximum for potatoes.

Glycosides of organic nitriles

A number of non-cyanogenic nitrile (= cyano) glucosides are known to occur in terrestrial plants. Seeds of *Simmondsia chinensis* Link. (syn. *Simmondsia californica*) contain approximately 50–60% (w/w) of an oil which is highly marketable due to its unique mixture of unsaturated liquid wax esters and its derived technical properties. The oil (jojoba oil) is commercially pressed (first quality) and extracted by hexane. Although they contain around 25–30% crude protein by weight, the press cakes or hexane extraction cakes have had limited use as animal feed owing to their content of a number of anti-nutritional constituents, i.e. tannins and at least four nitriles – 5-demethylsimmondsin (DMS), 4,5-didemethylsimmondsin (DDMS), simmondsin (S) and simmondsin 2'-ferulate – that have adverse effects on animals (Fig. 16.9). The unfavourable effects on a number of animal species have been known for quite a long time. The effects are apparently related to the nitrile group, since chemical treatments such as reactions with ammoniacal hydrogen peroxide to hydrate the nitrile group to an amide have been shown to effectively

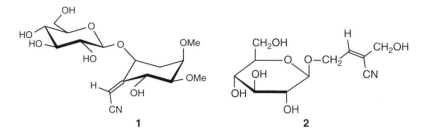

Fig. 16.9. Glycosides of organic nitriles: 1, simmondsin; 2, sarmentosin. Simmondsin is shown in the preferred configuration for the cyclohexyl ring.

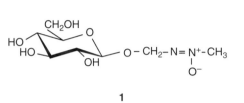 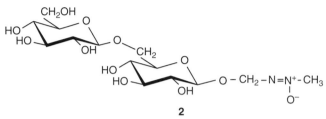

Fig. 16.10. MAM glycosides: 1, cycasin; 2, macrozamin.

reduce the toxicity of meals. In spite of this, it was not until 1983 that an apparent mechanism for the toxicity in monogastric animals, i.e. cyanide poisoning, was reported. The theory was based on the finding of cyanide and thiocyanate in mice fed with simmondsin. This implies that simmondsin, and perhaps some of the other compounds, may be degraded in the animal to form cyanide; however, the reaction sequence is unknown.

Methylazoxymethanol glycosides

Cycadales, represented today by ten genera found in all continents except Europe, together with *Ginkgoales* are included in the *Prephanerogams*, a relict group of ancient gymnosperms. Far back in time, so-called Japanese sago could be prepared from the pith of certain *Cycas* spp. (e.g. *Cycas revoluta*). Today sago everywhere is prepared from the palm *Metroxylon sagu* (*Arecaceae*).

Extensive losses of sheep have occurred in Australia as a result of consumption of *Macrozamia* and *Cycas* spp. The presence of high concentrations of glycosides of methylazoxymethanol (MAM) has been reported only in the seeds of cycads and in smaller quantity in their stems and leaves.

The first isolation of a MAM glycoside, macrozamin (the β-primeveroside of MAM), was obtained from seeds of *Macrozamia spiralis* Miq., an Australian cycad. Since then a number of other

MAM glycosides (Fig. 16.10) have been characterized, among these cycasin (the β-D-glucopyranoside of MAM), which was shown to be characteristic of, and exclusive to, all the genera of cycads. The quite limited investigations available seem to indicate that the relative concentrations of cycasin to macrozamin in ripe seeds differ within the cycad genera.

The MAM glycosides release MAM upon hydrolysis, which is catalysed by β-glycosidases. MAM is an alkylating agent which has been shown to be mutagenic and carcinogenic. A mechanism including the same alkylating end product as for dimethylnitrosamine has been proposed. Cycasin has been shown to be toxic to a number of animals, causing among other effects hepatic lesions and demyelination with axonal swelling in the spinal cord.

Cow's milk may be a vector of transmission of plant toxins. The aglycone of cycasin can pass into the milk of lactating rats, causing tumours in the offspring of such animals. The seeds of several *Cycas* spp. were traditionally eaten in Australia and on certain islands, e.g. Guam. A special neurological syndrome occurring on the island of Guam, and termed Guam ALS-PDC, has been hypothesized to be due to the intake of seeds of *Cycas circinalis*. In 1987 scientists proposed that the causative factor was the neuro-excitotoxic amino acid β-N-methylamino-L-alanine (BMAA). However, a number of subsequent investigations doubted this, as reviewed in an article concerning the gradual disappearance of this disease on the island of Guam. Thus, it may never be disclosed whether the MAM glycosides could have a role in this disease, which might not be unthinkable when looking at the spinal cord lesions reported in goats as a result of chronic intake of cycasin.

Naringin

In citrus species, bitterness arises from two distinctly different classes of chemical compound: the limonoids and the flavanone neohesperidosides. The limonoids are triterpene derivatives, of which 36 have been described to occur in or be formed during extraction of fruits from the genus *Citrus*. Of these four are known as bitter, namely limonin, nomilin, ichangin and nomilinate. Only two of these – limonin and nomilin – may present a problem to the citrus juice industry, limonin being formed in the acidic juice from the precursor limonoic acid found mainly in the albedo, the centre bundle and the segment membranes. Of several flavanone glycosides present in citrus fruits the bitter naringin (i.e. naringenin-7-β neohesperidoside; β-neohesperidose = 2-O-α-L-rhamnosyl-β-D-glucopyranose; Fig. 16.11) is the major flavonoid of grapefruit (*Citrus paradis*), pommelo (*Citrus grandis*) and sour oranges; while the non-bitter hesperidin is dominating in sweet orange (*Citrus sinensis*). Neither naringenin nor neohesperidose is bitter, and comparison with a number of closely related glycosides shows that both the aglycone and the sugar moiety are extremely important in determining whether the glycoside is bitter or not.

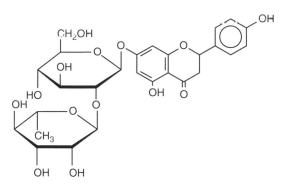

Fig. 16.11. Naringin.

Oligosaccharides (flatulence-producing)

Flatulence is a common phenomenon associated with the ingestion of legumes. Studies indicate that flatus is caused by the microbial fermentation of low-molecular-weight sugars – raffinose (Gal-Glu-Fru) and stachyose (Gal-Gal-Glu-Fru) – which are not digested because humans do not have α-galactosidase in their digestive tract. The oligosaccharides raffinose, stachyose and verbascose (Fig. 16.12) have been heavily implicated in flatus production from legumes. Soybeans contain (by weight) about 1% raffinose and 2.5% stachyose, and the winged bean 1–2% raffinose, 2–4% stachyose and 0.2–1% verbascose. However, the theories that point to these compounds as the only flatugenic agents seem to be oversimplified, in that any food polysaccharide that finds its way into the colon is a potential source of flatus.

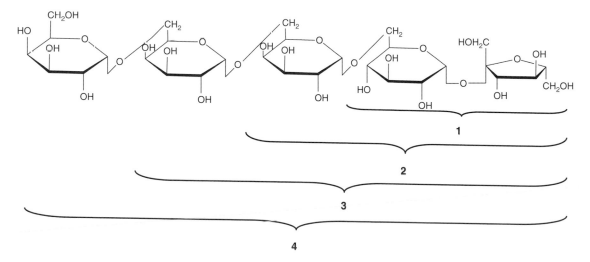

Fig. 16.12. Oligosaccharides (flatulence-producing) and their structural relationship to sucrose: **1**, sucrose; **2**, raffinose; **3**, stachyose; **4**, verbascose.

Polyphenols (cathartic)

The seeds of safflower *Carthamus tinctorius* (*Asteraceae*) contain approximately 40% oil and the meal after extraction about 25–20% protein by weight. Safflower oil, although of minor importance in the world fats and oils trade, is distinctive because of its highly polyunsaturated nature. Most safflower oil is consumed in its country of origin, but growing portions have been entering the world trade for some years now. Safflower meal is a source of high-quality protein for animal feeds, but is not used for human consumption, among other reasons owing to its bitterness and mild cathartic effect. Both the bitterness and the cathartic effect have been reported to be due to two lignan β-glucosides (Fig. 16.13): (i) 2-hydroxyarctiin (cathartic); and (ii) matairesinol monoglucoside (bitter). The aglycone of (ii), i.e. matairesinol, occurs both as free polyphenol and as glycoside in a number of plant species. Matairesinol has in screenings been shown to possess a number of biological activities such as antiviral and cytostatic. Furthermore, this compound has been shown to possess oestrogenic activity, i.e. it is a phyto-oestrogen.

Ptaquiloside

Bracken fern(s) (*Pteridium* spp.), commonly occurring throughout the world, cause cancer of the urinary bladder of ruminants, and is the only higher plant that has been shown to cause cancer naturally in animals. Enzootic haematuria, the clinical name given to the urinary bladder neoplasia of ruminants, tends to occur persistently in localized bracken-infested regions. The major carcinogen of bracken is the mutagenic and clastogenic norsesquiterpene glucoside ptaquiloside (Fig. 16.14), the carcinogenicity of which has been shown in feeding experiments on laboratory animals.

The carcinogenicity demonstrated in feeding experiments with rats, mice, hamsters, guinea pigs and cattle among other species is indeed alarming, since the young shoots are highly regarded as a tasty dish in Japan. Thus, this intake of bracken has been linked to high incidences of stomach cancer in Japan, and in Costa Rica among people exposed to milk produced in bracken-infested grasslands. The latter link was further supported by the finding of a high tumour incidence in rats and mice fed milk obtained from cows fed with dietary complements of bracken and by the subsequent demonstration of ptaquiloside in bovine milk.

Great variations may be found in the content of ptaquiloside (0–13,000 μg g^{-1}) as a result of both ecological and genetic variation, a tendency for higher contents being reported for *Pteridium esculentum* when originating in relatively colder climates.

Saponins

A great number of plants, including several food and feed resources, are known to contain saponins.

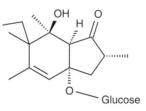

Fig. 16.14. Ptaquiloside.

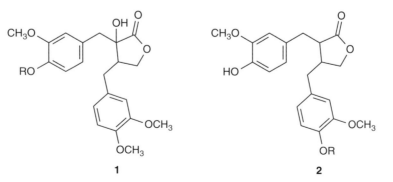

Fig. 16.13. Polyphenols (cathartic): **1**, 2-hydroxyarctiin; **2**, matairesinol monoglucoside (R = glucosyl).

Saponins may belong to the group of either pentacyclic triterpenoid saponins or steroidal saponins (including in a broad sense also the steroidal alkaloid glycosides found for example in potatoes, see above). Examples of saponin aglycones and saponins are shown in Fig. 16.15. Several steroidal saponins and alkaloids are, or have been, used as starting materials for the production of steroidal hormones. Although certain saponins, such as the earlier medicinally used quillaia saponin, have been known for centuries to be damaging to mucous membranes, and to possess piscicidal and molluscicidal effects, most saponins are in general considered quite unproblematic upon oral administration.

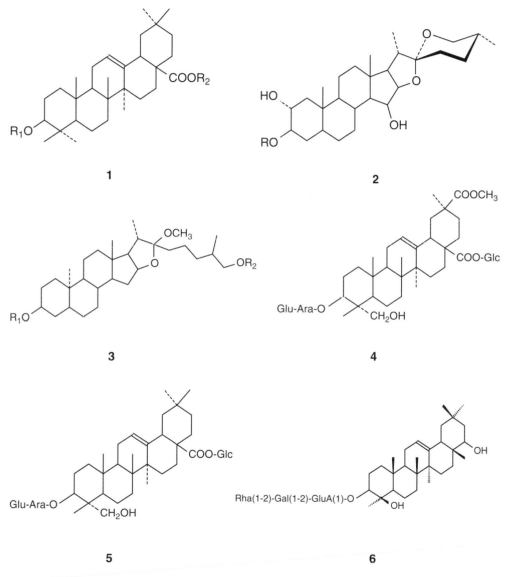

Fig. 16.15. Saponins. **1**, **2** and **3** show examples of different saponin skeletons: **1**, a pentacyclic triterpene skeleton, namely oleanolic acid (R$_1$ = R$_2$ = H); **2**, a steroid skeleton with a spiroketal side chain attached at C-17, namely digitogenin (R = H); **3**, a steroid skeleton lacking the spiro cyclization found in structure **2**; the skeleton can represent, for example, 22-methoxy-(25,*S*)-5-furostan-3,26-diol (R$_1$ = R$_2$ = H). Structures **4** and **5** represent proposed structures of quinoa saponins, while structure **6** is soysaponin I.

However, concerns have been raised about the danger that saponins in food or feed may promote oral sensitization to allergens through their membranolytic action in the gastrointestinal tract, resulting in enhanced uptake of the allergens. Besides the general ability of these compounds to damage biological membranes, this concern is also based on the fact that saponins have been shown to act as oral adjuvants. Foods and feeds containing saponins include among others soybean, guar, quinoa and balanites fruits. As well as their membranolytic action, certain of these saponins exert special effects due to the structure of their aglycone. Such effects include: (i) lowering of blood cholesterol; and (ii) reversible sodium retention and potassium loss leading to hypertension, water retention and electrolyte imbalance, as seen for example with glycyrrhizinic acid found in liquorice root (the roots and stolons from *Glycyrrhiza glabra*) and for products to which liquorice root extract, or glycyrrhizinic acid, has been added.

Actually, different saponin-containing extracts of quillaia bark are commercially available and added especially to beverage products such as beer. JECFA assessed the risk posed by such products in 2005 and derived an ADI of 0–0.1 mg quillaia saponins kg^{-1} BW. Likewise, glycyrrhizinic acid and its ammonium salt were evaluated by the EU Scientific Committee for Food (SCF) in 2003. The Committee considered that an upper limit for regular ingestion of 100 mg day^{-1} provides a sufficient level of protection for the majority of the population if it includes the intake of glycyrrhizinic acid via all products, liquorice confectionery as well as products flavoured with glycyrrhizinic acid or ammonium glycyrrhizinate. At the same time, SCF underlined that there are population subgroups for which this upper limit might not offer sufficient protection.

These subgroups comprise people with decreased 11-β-hydroxysteroid dehydrogenase-2 activity (the target enzyme of glycyrrhizinic acid, for which genetic polymorphisms resulting in reduced basal activity have been described), people with prolonged gastrointestinal transit time, and people with hypertension or electrolyte-related or water homeostasis-related medical conditions.

A number of saponins are bitter. The occurrence of bitter saponins in 'palmyrah' (*Borassus flabellifer* L.) fruit pulp thus reduces the use of juices based on this fruit. Likewise, seeds of *Chenopodium* spp. that are used for human consumption, namely *C. quinoa* (quinoa), *Chenopodium pallidicaule* (canihua) and *Chenopodium berlandieri* ssp. *nuttaliae* (Safford) Wilson and Heiser (huauzontle), contain bitter saponins of the aglycones oleanoic acid, hederagenin, phytolaccagenic acid and possibly other sapogenols, most of which is concentrated in the outer layers of the grain. Besides the seeds, leaves of quinoa are consumed as a vegetable with a protein content of approximately 2.8–4.2% (w/w, FW basis). As for other plant tissues containing secondary constituents, quinoa cultivars vary concerning the quantitative content, and the tradition has, as for other crops containing toxic or anti-nutritional agents, been working with so-called sweet and bitter varieties.

Vicine and convicine

Faba bean (*V. faba* L.) contains the two glycosides vicine and convicine (Fig. 16.16), substances that after hydrolysis in the intestine and uptake of the genins (divicine and isouramil) cause haemolytic anaemia (favism) in G6PD-deficient individuals. Together with condensed tannins these two glycosides also limit the use of the proteinaceous raw faba beans

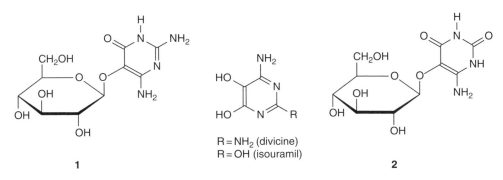

R = NH$_2$ (divicine)
R = OH (isouramil)

Fig. 16.16. Vicine (**1**) and convicine (**2**). In the middle, the structures and names for the aglycones.

as feed for monogastric animals. Vicine and convicine contents of cultivars used in the 1990s were reported to be around 7 and 2.5 mg g[-1], respectively.

G6PD deficiency is one of the genetically determined enzymatic abnormalities most often seen, with over 80 variants. More than 400 million people, of whom about 90% are male, are affected. A fatality rate of up to about 8% was the norm for G6PD-deficient persons consuming favic agents. The availability of blood transfusions has reduced this significantly today. The symptoms of favism are fatigue, nausea, abdominal pain, fever, haemoglobinuria, jaundice and acute renal failure.

Phyto-oestrogens

Phyto-oestrogens are a group of plant secondary constituents of different basic structure that can act like the hormone oestrogen. Phyto-oestrogens have been characterized from plant foods such as beans, seeds and grains. Foods made from soybeans have some of the highest levels of phyto-oestrogens and therefore have been studied the most. It is not clear – in spite of initial optimism – whether eating foods rich in phyto-oestrogens decreases breast cancer risk, and potential adverse effects have not been thoroughly characterized either.

Around 300 foods have been shown to contain phyto-oestrogens. The compounds regarded as important for investigation in future research are from one of three chemical classes: the isoflavonoids, the lignans and the coumestans. Isoflavonoid phyto-oestrogens are found in beans from the legume family; soybeans and soy products are the major dietary source of this type of phyto-oestrogen. Lignan phytoestrogens are found in high-fibre foods such as cereal brans and beans; flaxseeds contain large amounts of lignans. The coumestan phyto-oestrogens are found in various beans such as split peas, pinto beans and lima beans; alfalfa and clover sprouts are the foods with the highest amounts of coumestans.

Here we take a short look at the soy phyto-oestrogens which are of isoflavonoid structure. One important compound currently being investigated is the isoflavonoid glycoside daidzin (Fig. 16.17), which in the gastrointestinal tract is hydrolysed to release the aglycone daidzein. In the intestine this may further be metabolized to equol (4′,7-isoflavandiol). However, only about 30–50% of the general population seems to have the intestinal bacterial flora that make equol. Structural

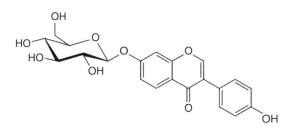

Fig. 16.17. Daidzin.

similarity of equol to the human oestrogen oestradiol means that equol competes against oestradiol for binding to endocrine receptors.

16.3   Conclusion

The glycosides naturally present in plants are numerous. As described in this chapter some may be toxic as parent compounds, while others may be so only after hydrolysis to their aglycones or even to derivatives of these.

Notes

[1] Friedman, M. (2006) Potato glycoalkaloids and metabolites: roles in the plant and in the diet. *Journal of Agricultural and Food Chemistry* 54, 8655–8581.

Further Reading

Backshall, S. (2007) *Venomous Animals of the World*. Johns Hopkins University Press, Baltimore, Maryland.

Bevan-Jones, R. (2009) *Poisonous Plants: A Cultural and Social History*. Windgather Press/Oxbow Books, Oxford, UK.

Cheeke, P.R. (1997) *Natural Toxicants in Feeds, Forages, and Poisonous Plants*, 2nd edn. Prentice Hall, Upper Saddle River, New Jersey.

Dauncey, E.A. (2010) *Poisonous Plants. A Guide for Parents and Childcare Providers*. Kew Publishing, London.

EFSA (2009) Marine biotoxins in shellfish – Summary on regulated marine biotoxins. Scientific Opinion of the Panel on Contaminants in the Food Chain. *EFSA Journal* 1306, 1–23.

EFSA (2009) Scientific Opinion. Influence of processing on the levels of lipophilic marine biotoxins in bivalve molluscs. Statement of the Panel on Contaminants in the Food Chain (Question No EFSA-Q-2009-00203). Adopted on 25 March 2009. *EFSA Journal* 1016, 1–10.

Juneja, V.K. and Sofos, J.N. (eds) (2010) *Pathogens and Toxins in Foods: Challenges and Interventions*. ASM Press, Washington, DC.

Wagstaff, D.J. (2008) *International Poisonous Plants Checklist: An Evidence-Based Reference*. CRC Press, Boca Raton, Florida.

17 Naturally Inherent Toxins: Mushrooms, Algae (Marine Biotoxins) and Animals

- Some mushrooms, algae and fish are (or may be) toxic.
- We discuss false morel mushrooms and marine biotoxins causing shellfish poisonings.
- We further discuss the very toxic puffer fish and problems caused by escolar and oilfish waxes.

17.1 Toxicants from Mushrooms

The vegetative part of a fungus is always a threaded mycelium or single cells, i.e. microscopic in nature. Nevertheless we can go to the forest and pick mushrooms. Mushrooms are the reproductive structures of higher *Ascomycetes* and *Basidiomycetes*, which produce copious amounts of microscopic spores but are themselves macroscopic.

Many mushrooms are known as edible and for several of these the scientific name already indicates this impression of the character of the mushroom, like those with the species name '*esculenta*', which in Latin means *edible*. Additionally the common names often indicate that a mushroom is edible or even delicious. However, probably no adult person doubts also that a number of mushroom species are indeed very toxic; in English these are sometimes denoted *toadstools* (from the German word *todesstuhl*).

Among the very toxic we find *Amanita phalloides* and *Amanita virosa* together with *Galerina autumnalis* that all form the easily absorbed cyclic octapeptides, the so-called *amatoxins* (Fig. 17.1), which inhibit RNA polymerase II, a vital enzyme in the synthesis of mRNA. Without mRNA, protein synthesis – and hence cell metabolism – stops and the cell dies. The estimated minimum lethal dose is $0.1 \, mg \, kg^{-1}$ BW or about 7 mg of toxin for an adult. The liver is the primary target organ followed by the kidneys. Effects are hepatitis with centrolobular necrosis and hepatic steatosis, as well as acute tubulointerstitial nephropathy, which altogether induce a severe hepato-renal syndrome. Intoxications will often be fatal.

Another often discussed group of toxic mushrooms are those that cause neurological effects, especially those where the symptoms may include hallucinations. These include mushrooms deliberately sought for use as hallucinogens such as *Psilocybe cubensis* and *Psilocybe mexicana*, both of which form the alkaloid psilocybin and have been used by Indians in southern Mexico in magico-religious ceremonies. Other neurotoxic mushrooms are the two *Amanita* species *Amanita muscaria* and *Amanita pantherina*; both of these contain the psychotropic isoxazole derivatives ibotenic acid and muscimol. The symptoms of intoxication appear within an hour or two and are characterized by an initial state of excitement followed by muscular twitching and depression. For all types of neurotoxic mushroom, death is seldom seen.

A relatively large number of mushrooms are gastrointestinal irritants giving rise to symptoms such as nausea, vomiting, abdominal pain and diarrhoea. For most species the irritants remain unidentified with respect to their chemical structure.

While the mushrooms described above are not normally added to food deliberately, it is different when we come to the species of *Gyromitra* (false morel mushrooms). Indeed, *G. esculenta* according to its name should be edible; however, together with the related species *Gyromitra ambigua* and *Gyromitra infula* it can cause fatal poisonings. *Gyromitra* spp. fruit in the spring and most poisonings occur during this part of the year. The mushrooms are found on the ground or on rotten wood, are orange-brown to brown, have no gills, and have convoluted brain-like caps that are

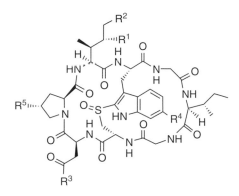

Fig. 17.1. The basic structure of the nine amatoxins.

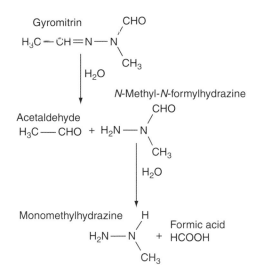

Fig. 17.2. The formation of MMH from gyromitrin.

occasionally saddle-shaped. The toxic agent is gyromitrin (*N*-methyl-*N*-formylhydrazone), which rapidly decomposes in the stomach to form acetaldehyde and *N*-methyl-*N*-formylhydrazine. This in turn is converted to monomethylhydrazine (MMH) by hydrolysis (Fig 17.2). MMH is a water-soluble toxin that causes gastroenteritis, haemolysis, methaemoglobinaemia, hepato-renal failure, seizures and coma. MMH has an LD$_{50}$ (in rat) of 33 mg kg^{-1} BW and is carcinogenic. MMH is employed in rocket fuel and causes similar toxicity in aerospace industry workers. Cooking can render these mushrooms less toxic, although not reliably so.

17.2 Algal Toxicants

As already stressed in the introductory chapters and dealt with further in Chapter 26 on analysis of food contaminants, a number of micro-algae may – depending on the environmental conditions – biosynthesize one or more toxic organic constituents called *algal toxins/toxicants* or *marine biotoxins*. Shellfish such as oysters, scallops and blue mussels live by filtering plankton including algal plankton. Thus, the shellfish can take up and concentrate these toxic compounds, especially during blooms of such algae. The shellfish show no apparent ill effects from large amounts of toxin and such marine algal toxins can occur in shellfish in all seasons. The algal toxins do not affect the taste of the shellfish and in general are not destroyed by freezing or cooking. People therefore have no possibility of checking whether the shellfish are toxic on their own.

Traditionally, the algal toxins were divided into groups based on their effects as follows.

- Paralytic shellfish toxins (PSTs) (= PSP; paralytic shellfish poisons) which cause paralysis. The most prominent compound is STX.
- Diarrhoetic shellfish toxins (DSTs) causing diarrhoea. Chemically we speak of the group consisting of okadaic acid (OA) and analogues.
- Amnesic shellfish toxins (ASTs) causing amnesia. First and foremost of these is domoic acid (DA).
- To these have come three additional groups of compounds: (i) the azaspiracid (AZA) group of toxins (causing vomiting, stomach cramps and diarrhoea); (ii) the pectenotoxin (PTX) group of toxins (causing intestinal effects); and (iii) the yessotoxin (YTX) group of toxins (which seem to affect different organs, with the heart as a prominent target organ).

As an example let us look at the present regulation in the EU concerning algal toxicants; there, we find the accepted maximum limits to vary from 160 µg to 20 mg per kilogram of shellfish meat. The differences of course reflect the different toxicities of the different single compounds and compound groups. Furthermore, if we calculate the possible 95th percentile of high exposure and compare it with the acute reference dose (ARfD), we find that there are differences from country to country concerning exposure (Table 17.1). All calculated exposures are below the respective ARfDs. We also see, however, that for the AZA group, exposure can be relatively close to the ARfD.

Table 17.1. Current EU limits and exposure levels from consumption of shellfish.

Toxin group[a]	Acceptance limit[a] (per kg shellfish meat)	Exposure from eating a 400g portion at the EU limit (per kg BW)	Exposure from eating a 400g portion at the 95th percentile of the concentrations in samples marketed in the EU (per kg BW)	ARfD (per kg BW)
OA	160 µg	1 µg	1.6 µg	0.3 µg
AZA	160 µg	1 µg	0.3 µg	0.2 µg
PTX	160 µg	1 µg	0.5 µg	0.8 µg
YTX	1 mg	6.7 µg	5.3/2.1 µg (Italy/Norway)	25 µg
STX	800 µg	5.3 µg	4.3 µg	0.5 µg
DA	20 mg	130 µg	17 µg	30 µg

[a] The mixture of accumulated compounds was calculated as if it all were in the form of the compound giving name to the group, using relative toxicity factors.

Paralytic shellfish toxins

STX and its derivatives were found as a result of a poisoning affecting over 100 people along the California coast near San Francisco in 1929. The poisoning was found to stem from shellfish that had accumulated the dinoflagellate *Gonyaulax catenella* (later moved to the genus *Alexandrium*). Six people died but the group of tricyclic diguanidinium compounds named STXs was found and characterized, a group that today is known to be made up of more than 20 individual compounds. The compounds bind to site 1 of the voltage-activated sodium channel, stopping the normal passive influx of sodium ions through the channel and thereby the propagation of action potentials along nerve and muscle membranes. The symptoms start with peripheral tingling that develops into muscular paralysis, in severe cases resulting in death from suffocation.

Diarrhoetic shellfish toxins

In the late 1970s a large outbreak of diarrhoea and other gastrointestinal symptoms was seen among shellfish consumers in Japan. The outbreak was soon traced to the uptake of dinoflagellates by the shellfish. The dinoflagellates synthesized the compound OA and some derivatives, which had caused the diarrhoetic shellfish poisoning. Today we know that the most important flagellates in this respect are those belonging to the genera *Dinophysis* and *Prorocentrum*. OA is a potent inhibitor of protein phosphatase.

Amnesic shellfish toxins

DA (or DOM) binds strongly to glutamate receptors in the hippocampus, leading to sustained activation of the associated neurons. The toxicity of DA is in part because of this strong binding and in part because the mechanisms that scavenge glutamate, keeping its concentration low and its stimulation brief, do not act on DA. The primary source of DA in seafood comprises diatoms belonging to the genus *Pseudonitzschia*.

17.3 Venomous Animals in Food

Worldwide a number of venomous animals are used in the preparation of food. In this chapter we only consider the use (mostly in Japan and Hong Kong) of puffer fish (in Japanese 'fugu', normally species of *Takifugu*, *Lagocephalus* or *Sphoeroides*), which may contain a potent and deadly toxin called tetrodotoxin (Fig. 17.3). In puffer fish, the toxin is found mainly in the eggs, liver and skin. The puffer fish must be cleaned and prepared properly so that the organs containing the toxins are carefully removed and do not cross-contaminate the flesh of the fish. The toxin cannot be destroyed by cooking, drying or freezing. The toxin can affect a person's CNS and, in extreme cases, can cause death. There is no antidote.

Tetrodotoxin is a potent marine neurotoxin, named after the order Tetraodontiformes with which it is commonly associated. Puffer fish and porcupine fish are common examples of fish containing tetrodotoxin under this order. Tetrodotoxin has also been isolated from other animal species including goby,

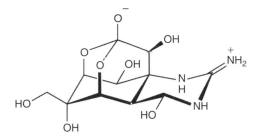

Fig. 17.3. Tetrodotoxin.

shellfish, California newt, parrotfish, frogs of the genus *Atelopus*, the blue-ringed octopus, starfish, angelfish and xanthid crabs. Tetrodotoxin is considered likely to be produced by marine bacteria that are often associated with marine animals.

One should avoid purchasing and dressing puffer fish, porcupine fish or unknown fish for consumption on one's own. Since 1958, only specially licensed chefs in Japan can prepare and sell 'fugu' to the public.

17.4 Escolar and Oilfish Waxes

Some fish can provoke diarrhoea. Escolar and oilfish thus call for special preparation to avoid the strong purgative effect of these fish species. Escolar (*Lepidocybium flavobrunneum*) and oilfish (*Ruvettus pretiosus*), which is sometimes wrongly sold as escolar, can give diarrhoea if not correctly prepared. The reason is the natural content of wax (instead of lipid/fat), which is indigestible. The two species do not metabolize wax esters that occur naturally in their diet and, as a consequence, these wax esters are stored in the body of these fish. The oil content of the muscle meat of escolar and oilfish amounts to 18–21% and the oil contains >90 % wax esters. The effect can be compared with that of castor oil. The fish must be boiled or fried very thoroughly to ensure that the oil content – and with that the wax – is melted from the fish. The boiling water and/or the frying fat/oil must not be used for preparation of sauces. Escolar and oilfish must under no circumstances be smoked by cold methods because the temperature will not reach

that needed to ensure the wax melts off the fish. The Danish food authorities in 1999 produced a special information pamphlet to fish-importing companies, so as to ensure that consumers get information about how to prepare these fish. In 2004 EFSA published an opinion recommending better information on this problem.

17.5 Conclusion

In our daily life we do not normally think of the mushrooms we buy in the supermarket or the shellfish or fish we buy at the same place or at a specialized fish market as possible sources of natural compounds that can lead to poisoning/discomfort, whether as paralysis or diarrhoea. However, as we have seen in this chapter, this can be the case if food control and communication (refer to escolar) from production to consumption is not in place.

Further Reading

Backshall, S. (2007) *Venomous Animals of the World.* Johns Hopkins University Press, Baltimore, Maryland.

Bevan-Jones, R. (2009) *Poisonous Plants: A Cultural and Social History.* Windgather Press/Oxbow Books, Oxford, UK.

Cheeke, P.R. (1997) *Natural Toxicants in Feeds, Forages, and Poisonous Plants,* 2nd edn. Prentice Hall, Upper Saddle River, New Jersey.

Dauncey, E.A. (2010) *Poisonous Plants. A Guide for Parents and Childcare Providers.* Kew Publishing, London.

EFSA (2009) Marine biotoxins in shellfish – Summary on regulated marine biotoxins. Scientific Opinion of the Panel on Contaminants in the Food Chain. *EFSA Journal* 1306, 1–23.

EFSA (2009) Scientific Opinion. Influence of processing on the levels of lipophilic marine biotoxins in bivalve molluscs. Statement of the Panel on Contaminants in the Food Chain (Question No EFSA-Q-2009-00203). Adopted on 25 March 2009. *EFSA Journal* 1016, 1–10.

Juneja, V.K. and Sofos, J.N. (eds) (2010) *Pathogens and Toxins in Foods: Challenges and Interventions.* ASM Press, Washington, DC.

Wagstaff, D.J. (2008) *International Poisonous Plants Checklist: An Evidence-Based Reference.* CRC Press, Boca Raton, Florida.

18 An Introduction to Food Contaminants and About Metals, Metalloids and Other Elements

- We look at the question – what is a food contaminant?
- We discuss the most important elements the presence of which may have an adverse effect.
- We look at the different forms in which such elements can occur and the influence of the form on target organs and adverse effects.

18.1 Introduction to Food Contaminants

According to the definition laid down by the EU, contaminants in relation to food are substances that have not been intentionally added to food. These substances may be present in food as a result of the various stages of its production, packaging, transport or holding. They also might result from environmental contamination.

Most countries worldwide have pieces of legislation that set maximum accepted levels for contaminants in food. The compounds regulated and the levels accepted vary and, especially for smaller countries that are not members of one of the greater regional political communities such as the EU, levels often can be those recommended by CAC. However, let us for a moment turn to the EU as an example of how a complex system of regulations together can build consumer protection against toxic food contaminants no matter what their origin.

The basic principles of EU legislation on contaminants in food are found in the Council Regulation 315/93/EEC of 8 February 1993. This legislation states that:

- food containing a contaminant to an amount unacceptable from the public health viewpoint, and in particular at a toxicological level, shall not be placed on the market;
- contaminant levels shall be kept as low as can reasonably be achieved following recommended good working practices; and

- maximum levels must be set for certain contaminants in order to protect public health.

By 2009 community measures had been taken for the following contaminants: mycotoxins (aflatoxins, OTA, *Fusarium* toxins (e.g. DON, zearalenone, fumonisins), patulin), metals (cadmium, lead, mercury, inorganic tin), dioxins and PCBs, PAHs, 3-monochloropropane-1,2-diol (3-MCPD) and nitrates, while investigations to lay down the basis for future measures are ongoing for acrylamide, organotins, furan and ethyl carbamate.

The measures taken are with regard to the maximum levels described in the Commission Regulation (EC) No. 1881/2006, which entered into force on 1 March 2007 and has been amended by: (i) Commission Regulation (EC) No. 1126/2007 of 28 September 2007 setting maximum levels for certain contaminants in foodstuffs as regards *Fusarium* toxins in maize and maize products; (ii) Commission Regulation (EC) No. 565/2008 of 18 June 2008, which regards the establishment of a maximum level for dioxins and PCBs in fish liver; and (iii) Commission Regulation (EC) No. 629/2008 of 2 July 2008.

The latter states that:

- 'On the basis of new information, good agricultural and fisheries practices do not allow keeping levels of lead, cadmium and mercury in certain aquatic species and fungi as low as required in the Annex of Commission Regulation (EC) No 1881/2006. It is therefore necessary to revise the maximum levels fixed for those contaminants while maintaining a high level of consumer health protection.'

- 'It has been shown that certain food supplements can contribute significantly to human exposure to lead, cadmium and mercury. In order to protect public health, it is therefore appropriate to set maximum levels for lead, cadmium and mercury in food supplements. These maximum levels must be safe and as low as reasonably achievable based upon good manufacturing practices.'

- 'Seaweed accumulates cadmium naturally. Food supplements consisting exclusively or mainly of dried seaweed or of products derived from seaweed can therefore contain higher levels of cadmium than other food supplements. To take this into account, a higher maximum level for cadmium is needed for food supplements consisting exclusively or mainly of seaweed.'

The amendments clearly demonstrate the dilemma that food safety managers have to deal with: to ensure a low overall exposure of the population to harmful substances while at the same time taking into consideration the possibilities for a viable economic sector with a varied production.

In 2007 the European Commission through its Health and Consumer Protection Directorate-General published a 4-page factsheet on food contaminants entitled 'Managing food contaminants: how the EU ensures that our food is safe'. This pamphlet (which is available at http://ec.europa.eu/food/food/chemicalsafety/contaminants/fs_contaminants_final_web_en.pdf) describes in a relatively easy-to-approach form and simple language the overall system of consumer protection against food contaminants as this is established and carried out in the EU. The headings include 'Overview of EU rules', 'Control and response', 'Promoting best practice' and 'Research'.

Following this small overview let us now turn to the different groups of contaminants. We start by treating the metals and metalloids in the present chapter, while in the following chapters (Chapters 19–23, respectively) we look at mycotoxins, pesticides and POPs, contaminants from processing machinery and packaging materials, toxic compounds formed during processing or improper storage and, finally, veterinary drugs.

18.2 Metals, Metalloids and Other Elements

A number of metals and metalloids can occur at non-safe levels as contaminants in feed and food products. Taking the EU as an example the maximum concentration in food of lead, cadmium, mercury and tin is regulated by the Commission Regulation (EC) No. 1881/2006 of 19 December 2006 setting maximum levels for certain contaminants in foodstuffs.

One route into food products is by migration during contact with materials containing metals and metalloids. Metals and alloys are found as food contact materials mainly in processing equipment, containers and household utensils but also in foils for wrapping foodstuffs. Such containers and foils play a role as a safety barrier between the food and the exterior. In particular, containers and foils for the final distribution to consumers may be covered by a surface coating which reduces the migration of metals into foodstuffs. When they are not covered these food contact materials can give rise to migration of metal ions into foodstuffs, therefore endangering human health if the total content of the metals exceeds the sanitary recommended exposure limits.

At the time of writing this text the EU had established a number of strict rules for the migration of individual chemical components from plastic and into food through Commission Directive 2002/72/EC of 6 August 2002 relating to plastic materials and articles intended to come into contact with foodstuffs and its amendments. For metals and alloys no such common European legislation is in place. However, acknowledging the problem, a policy statement was launched entitled 'Council of Europe's policy statements concerning materials and articles intended to come into contact with foodstuffs – policy statement concerning metals and alloys – technical document – guidelines on metals and alloys used as food contact materials of 13.02.2002'. These guidelines cover the following elements and alloys: aluminium, cadmium, chromium, cobalt, copper, iron, lead, manganese, mercury, nickel, silver, tin, titanium, zinc, alloys other than stainless steel, and stainless steel.

For a number of elements analysis of the content in either hair or nails (or for birds, feathers) can give a good impression of the mid- and long-term (historical) exposure. This is true for lead for example, where a recent study of the level in hair and rib bone of 59 persons post-mortem showed a mean concentration of 3.0 µg Pb g^{-1} in bone and 5.2 µg Pb g^{-1} in hair. A positive correlation between the lead content in bone and hair was found in this study ($P<0.05$). Also for arsenic, mercury and selenium chemical analysis of hair may be of value for the purpose of disclosing the medium- to long-term exposure.

For many of the essential elements a *life window* exists, defined by the minimum requirements on the one hand and the lower limit for adverse (toxic) effects on the other. Obviously this window is slightly different depending on the age and status of the individual. We can get an impression of the requirements as well as the maximum tolerable intakes for a number of essential as well as non-essential elements (including non-metals, metals and metalloids) by looking at recent figures from the USA.

The National Research Council of the US National Academy of Sciences has for decades taken responsibility for establishing guidelines on what quantities of the various nutrients should be eaten by human males and females at various ages. These were called Recommended Dietary Allowances (RDAs). In August 1997 the Institute of Medicine of the National Academy published a report that: (i) set new standards for calcium intake (as well as for vitamin D, fluoride, magnesium and phosphorus); and (ii) dropped the name RDA in favour of Dietary Reference Intakes (DRIs). Furthermore three new categories were added, namely:

- Adequate Intake (AI), where no (more precise) RDA/DRI has been established;
- Estimated Safe and Adequate Daily Dietary Intake (ESADDI), expected to satisfy the needs of 50% of the people in that age group; and
- Tolerable Upper Intake Level (UL), to caution against excess intake of nutrients – like vitamin D – that can be harmful in large amounts.

Let us now take a short look at a number of elements, their generally accepted function(s) if any and the requirements (as the DRI or AI value) and maximum tolerable intake (UL value) as reflected by the US figures.

- Arsenic: no biological function in humans although animal data indicate a requirement.
- Boron: no clear biological function in humans although animal data indicate a functional role.

- Calcium: essential role in blood clotting, muscle contraction, nerve transmission, and bone and tooth formation.
- Chromium: helps maintain normal blood glucose levels. DRI/AI (µg day^{-1}): infants aged 0–6 months, 0.2; infants aged 7–12 months, 5.5; children aged 1–3 years, 11; children aged 4–8 years, 15; males aged 9–13 years, 25; males aged 14–50 years, 35; males aged >50 years, 30; females aged 9–13 years, 21; females aged 14–18 years, 24; females aged 19–50 years, 25; females aged >50 years, 20; pregnant women, 30; lactating women, 45.
- Copper: component of enzymes in iron metabolism. DRI/AI (µg day^{-1}): males and females aged 19–70 years, 900. UL (tolerable daily intake, µg day^{-1}): males and females aged 19–70 years, 10,000.
- Iron: component of haemoglobin and numerous enzymes; prevents microcytic hypochromic anaemia. DRI/AI (mg day^{-1}): males aged 19–70 years, 8; females aged 9–13 years, 8; females aged 14–18 years, 15; females aged 19–50 years, 18; females aged >50 years, 8; pregnant women, 27; lactating women, 9. UL (tolerable daily intake, mg day^{-1}): males and females aged 19–70 years, 45.
- Selenium: defence against oxidative stress, regulation of thyroid hormone action, reduction and oxidation status of vitamin C and other molecules. DRI/AI (µg day^{-1}): infants aged 0–6 months, 15; infants aged 7–12 months, 20; children aged 1–3 years, 20; children aged 4–8 years, 30; males aged 9–13 years, 40; males aged 14–50 years, 55; males aged >50 years, 55; females aged 9–13 years, 40; females aged 14–50 years, 55; females aged >50 years, 55; pregnant women, 60; lactating women, 70. UL (tolerable daily intake, µg day^{-1}): males and females aged 19–70 years, 400.
- Fluoride: inhibits the initiation and progression of dental caries and stimulates new bone formation. DRI/AI (mg day^{-1}): males aged 19–70 years, 4; females aged 19–70 years, 3. UL (tolerable daily intake, mg day^{-1}): males and females aged 19–70 years, 10.

The requirements for adults are seen to range from about 30 µg day^{-1} for chromium to nearly 30 mg day^{-1} for iron (in pregnant women). The life window (defined here as the interval between the

RDA and the UL) for copper is 900–10,000 μg day^{-1}, corresponding to approximately a 1:10 relationship; fluoride has a window between about 3 and 10 mg day^{-1}, corresponding to a 1:3 relationship only; while for selenium the interval of 55 to 400 μg day^{-1} defines a window with a relationship between the requirement and the toxic level of around 1:7. So, certain elements are necessary but soon become toxic at higher levels.

18.3 Arsenic

Arsenic exists in several forms in nature, lead arsenate ($PbAsO_4$) being the most abundant. Arsenic has historically always been associated with poisoning, particularly murder cases, up until the late 19th century. Trivalent arsenic trioxide (As_4O_6) is odourless and tasteless and seems to be the compound most often employed in arsenic homicides. The oxidation states for arsenic include −3 (arsenides; often alloy-like intermetallic compounds), +3 (arsenites and most organoarsenic compounds) and +5 (arsenates; the most stable inorganic arsenic oxycompounds). When it comes to oral intake the oxidation state +3 is particularly toxic, largely due to a more full absorption.

Our knowledge about arsenic poisoning and its symptoms stems not only from industrial exposures and homicides but certainly also from the fact that several different arsenic compounds have been used in human as well as veterinary medicine. Examples of inorganic arsenic compounds used are sodium arsenate ($AsHNa_2O_4$), arsenic trioxide (As_2O_3) and arsenic triiodide (AsI_3), all of which have been used against a number of skin diseases and malaria. Also synthetic organic compounds containing arsenic have been used pharmacologically. Among aliphatic compounds we find 'sodium cacodylate' (sodium salts of dimethylarsenic acid, $(CH_3)_2As(O)OH$, used in both human and veterinary medicine against anaemia) and among aromatic compounds 'arsphenamin' (used against feline syphilis and heartworms in dogs).

Arsenic binds to the sulfhydryl groups of many proteins, resulting in 'non-specific' toxic effects such as weakening the integrity of structural proteins or partly inactivating some enzymes. The acute lethal effect of arsenic is due to two different specific molecular interactions between arsenic and enzymes of importance for biochemical energy production and storage in cells.

- Arsenic inhibits the formation of acetyl coenzyme A from the pyruvic acid arising from glucose metabolism. Acetyl coenzyme A should enter the Kreb's cycle which – working together with oxidative phosphorylation – is responsible for over 90% of the biochemical energy production. More specifically, arsenic inhibits the action of the pyruvate dehydrogenase complex by binding to an enzyme–lipoic acid complex.
- Another mechanism is arsenate replacement of phosphate in the phosphorylation of ADP to ATP. This leads to the formation of arsenophosphoglycerate, which spontaneously dissociates, and no ATP is formed.

Depending on the form of arsenic ingested, the dose and the duration of exposure, symptoms of poisoning with arsenic may vary. However, acute poisoning after ingestion results in gastrointestinal damage with vomiting, bloody diarrhoea, nausea, intense abdominal pain, 'ricewater stolls' (tissue sloughed off from the walls of the gastrointestinal tract), muscular cramps, cardiac depression and coma. In cases surviving long enough, liver and renal failure resulting in jaundice and followed by liver cirrhosis and ascites are seen. Chronic arsenic poisoning leads to hair loss (alopecia), blush of the skin from vasodilation of the facial capillaries, dermal hyperkeratosis and hyperpigmentation. Furthermore, an increased incidence of cancer of the liver, skin and lungs (reported from workers exposed to arsenic in plants manufacturing arsenic-containing pesticides) has been seen.

The mechanism behind the suspected carcinogenicity of arsenic in man is not well understood. Arsenic is not mutagenic and has not been shown to be carcinogenic to laboratory animals.

For most people worldwide the major exposure to arsenic is through food, which in general contains less than 1 mg kg^{-1}, a level that is regarded as non-problematic. However, the level in seafood has been reported to reach up to about 5 mg kg^{-1}. Fortunately, most arsenic in bivalves and crabs has been shown to be in organic forms, i.e. to occur as arsenocholine or arsenobetaine, which is almost non-toxic (Fig. 18.1). Some complex arseno sugars are present in edible seaweeds. In fish the majority of arsenic present is in the form of arsenobetaine, according to the relatively few studies with speciation of the content of total arsenic.

In certain parts of Taiwan, South America, West Bengal and Bangladesh, the water may naturally

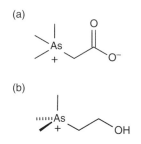

(a)

(b)

Fig. 18.1. Arsenocholine (a) and arsenobetaine (b).

contain hundreds of milligrams of arsenic per litre. Populations depending on such water supplies for drinking water as well as for preparing their food have been shown to suffer from the aforementioned hyperkeratosis and to have an elevated occurrence of cancer of the skin. Apart from being a severe local health problem, obviously such water cannot be used for the industrial processing of foods or for the production of beverages.

18.4 Cadmium

Human use of the metallic element cadmium is relatively new, it being discovered in 1817 by the German chemist F. Strohmeier. Most cadmium in nature occurs as an atomic substitution for zinc in zinc minerals, making up less than 1% of the mineral. Only a few relatively pure cadmium minerals are known. The best known is the mineral greenockite (cadmium sulfide, CdS). The most common oxidation state of cadmium is +2, although rare examples of +1 exist.

Until the beginning of the 1960s when a phasing out of the use of cadmium for many purposes started, a considerable amount was used for colours: red (cadmium selenide, CdSe) and yellow (cadmium sulfide, CdS). In the beginning these cadmium pigments were mostly used by artists for enamels on metal and ceramics, but later they were employed to a much greater extent in colours for different kinds of plastic ware. Also some popular stabilizers for certain types of plastic product contained cadmium. From a technical point of view, cadmium organic salts such as cadmium stearate or cadmium laurate are the most effective stabilizers for many polymers especially for PVC and its related products. These stabilizers retard the degradation caused by UV and heat.

Due to the serious health-impairing effects of cadmium described below its use was gradually

restricted in most countries. Thus, Council Directive 91/338/EEC of 18 June 1991 limited the use of cadmium compounds in PVC products. Except in a very few applications, placing on the market products manufactured from plastic materials coloured or stabilized with cadmium was prohibited if the cadmium content exceeded 0.01% by mass of the plastic material. In Europe the use was subsequently even more restricted as part of the Voluntary Commitment 'Vinyl 2010'. This agreement meant that no member of ESPA (the European Stabiliser Producers Association) could any longer sell such products in the EU, Norway and Switzerland, and that EuPC (the European Plastics Converters) should communicate to its members not to use cadmium-based stabilizers. For the EU, Annex XVII to the REACH chemical legislation further specifies the present restrictions in the import and use of materials containing cadmium. According to this Annex cadmium still can be present in colour pigments for ceramics; however, the cadmium weight percentage in pigments for ceramics intended for contact with food must not exceed 0.002.

Today a major part of the world's production of cadmium is used in batteries, especially as an ingredient in rechargeable batteries of the nickel–cadmium type. Other uses include cadmium as a component in certain alloys characterized by a low melting point, as a surface cover on certain metallic products such as musical instruments and for precision instruments within optics.

The first report on cadmium toxicity appeared in 1858. Persons using cadmium carbonate as a polishing agent showed acute gastrointestinal and delayed respiratory symptoms. In line with these observations, a branch of the US Public Health Service in 1942 reported on acute gastrointestinal effects with vomiting and diarrhoea in persons consuming cadmium-contaminated food and drinks. As the industrial production and use of cadmium grew, lung emphysema (an unnatural distension of the lung tissue with air, followed by breathing difficulties) and proteinuria were repeatedly reported persons working with cadmium. In 1952 it was shown that rabbits given daily injections of cadmium sulfate excreted only minimal amounts during the first 2 months, after which the excretion suddenly increased at least 50-fold. At the same time proteinuria appeared.

After World War II a disease was seen in Fuchu, Japan, that was characterized by pseudo-fractures in the long bones, changes characteristic of osteomalacia.

The disease was found mostly in postmenopausal women. Upon further investigation elevated levels of cadmium in the urine were demonstrated as was a decrease in serum levels of calcium and phosphate. The bone disease caused severe pain in the patients and was therefore named 'itai-itai' (Japanese for 'ouch-ouch'). In 1968 the Japanese Government officially declared the disease to be related to pollution of the Jinzu River with cadmium from mining activities. The water from the river was used for the irrigation of rice fields and the rice plants took up the cadmium through their roots.

Today we know that both plants and certain mushrooms used in food can take up cadmium from the soil. Thus, an investigation from a metal-liferous region in Bulgaria where the content of lead, cadmium and zinc in soil was respectively 3500 mg kg^{-1}, 280 mg kg^{-1} and 30 mg kg^{-1} found the seeds of plants grown there to accumulate the three metals as follows: groundnut (peanut) and maize (corn) seeds mainly Pb (5.2–9.6 mg kg^{-1}), pea seeds Cd (1.0–1.2 mg kg^{-1}) and wheat seeds Zn (59.4–73.2 mg kg^{-1}). Sunflower seeds also are known to accumulate cadmium. Within food of animal origin, crabs especially are known to show a high content of cadmium, up to as high as 30–50 mg kg^{-1}. Also organs from cattle and especially the kidney may contribute to food-related cadmium exposure: the kidneys of clinically healthy fattened cattle from different localities in East Slovakia slaughtered in 1980 showed a mean content of 7.93×10^{-1} mg Cd kg^{-1} (n=39), but with a strong region-specific variation.

An estimate from the year 2000 showed that an average person in the USA consumed approximately 30 µg Cd day^{-1} through food materials. However, cigarette smoking was shown to be another major source for human exposure as the tobacco plant selectively accumulates cadmium from the soil. One cigarette contains about 1–2 µg Cd, of which roughly 10% is inhaled with an approximate 50% absorption in the lung. In full agreement with this it is fairly well established that the blood cadmium level of smokers is significantly higher than that of non-smokers.

The absorption of cadmium after ingestion is relatively low. In rats it has been shown to be of the order of about 1%; however, in man it seems to be higher, i.e. from approximately 3% up to about 10%. Cadmium absorption increases when calcium or iron status is poor. Comparisons of cadmium concentrations in human kidneys, livers and other tissues obtained at autopsy with measured levels of cadmium in urine and estimations of total excretion indicate that cadmium has a biological half-life in man of 10–30 years, which is very long compared with most other elements and compounds. After absorption into the blood, cadmium is initially bound to albumin and soon an even higher concentration occurs in the erythrocytes where the cadmium is bound partly to a high-molecular-weight protein and partly to a protein with a lower molecular weight.

The albumin-bound cadmium is taken up in the liver where it is degraded. The released cadmium induces the synthesis of new metallothioneins (MTs; see Box 18.1). The MTs effectively bind cadmium in the liver cells. However, slowly a small proportion of the liver Cd-MT is released into the blood plasma and filtered through the glomerular membrane, thus carrying cadmium into the kidney tubules. In the proximal tubules reabsorption of the low-molecular-weight Cd-MT takes place, as does the reabsorption of other small proteins. Upon entering the tubule cells the Cd-MT is degraded. At low concentrations, however, the cadmium ions formed

---

Box 18.1. Metallothioneins

The first MT was isolated from horse kidneys and characterized as a cadmium- and zinc-containing protein, rich in sulfhydryl (–SH) groups, by scientists from Harvard University, Boston, in the late 1950s MTs are low-molecular-mass proteins with M_W of about 6–7 kDa. Four major forms have been described and named MT1 to MT4. As a group of proteins the MTs have been conserved during the evolution of the mammals with an amino sequence that varies among MT1 to MT4 only between amino acids 61 and 68. MTs are characterized by a content of not less than 20 cysteine residues (30%), an N-terminal acetylmethionine and alanine as the C-terminal residue. As the name indicates, the MTs can bind metals, the single metal ion being bound by several sulfhydryl groups. The metals in question are zinc, cadmium, mercury and copper. MT1 and MT2 are the major forms that are inducible by cadmium. They occur in many tissues.

---

are quickly bound to new MT synthesized by the kidney tubular cells and stored as such in these cells. In conclusion, following absorption, cadmium is stored in the liver from where it is translocated to its final storage in the cells of the proximal tubules of the kidneys.

The S1 segment of the kidney proximal tubule is a major target of chronic cadmium intoxication, the damage to this segment leading to the previously described proteinuria as well as loss of calcium and phosphorus leading to osteoporosis. We have already seen that Cd^{2+} complexed to the high-affinity metal-binding protein MT is the major form by which cadmium is delivered to the kidneys from the liver. The mechanisms of Cd-MT uptake and the molecular processes underlying Cd-MT toxicity in proximal tubule cells are still not fully understood, however, although lysosomal release of toxic free Cd^{2+} inside the tubular cells is often mentioned.

Early investigations in rats showed that when the cadmium concentration in the renal cortex reached a level of approximately 100 mg kg^{-1} low-molecular proteinuria started to occur. This is due to the fact that the small proteins filtered through the glomerular membrane are not reabsorbed by the damaged tubules. Proteins found in the urine include β_2-microglobulin, α_1-microglobulin (protein HC) and retinol-binding protein (RBP). Also there is increased activity of some tubular enzymes such as N-acetyl-β-D-galactsidase (NAG).

However, it seems very important to stress that a recent Swedish study – which included approximately 1000 persons of whom many were occupationally exposed to cadmium – concluded that renal tubular damage develops at lower levels of body cadmium burden than earlier expected. This study also quantified for the first time the risk in humans as a function of the cadmium concentration in the urine, i.e. the results showed an increased prevalence of 10% tubular proteinuria (taking into account a background prevalence of 5%) at a urinary cadmium concentration of 1.0 nmol mmol^{-1} creatinine. These findings are especially important when one takes into consideration that the kidney cadmium concentration seems to have increased in modern communities, as demonstrated by another Swedish investigation comparing the content of 30 adult kidneys from the 19th century with that from 42 autopsy samples from 1972/73 (age span 20–79 years). The geometric means were found to be 15.1 and 57.1 mg of cadmium per kilogram of renal cortex (dry weight) for the old and the new samples, respectively.

Cadmium is also classified by IARC as a human carcinogen, causing tumours of the lung, prostate and testes.

Commission Regulation (EC) No. 1881/2006 sets the maximum limits for the content of cadmium in food commodities including products of animal as well as plant origin; the level (in mg kg^{-1} wet weight) ranges from 0.050 in meat (except for horse meat, where the limit is 0.2) to 1.0 in bivalve molluscs to 3.0 in food supplements consisting exclusively or mainly of dried seaweed or products derived from seaweed.

18.5 Chromium

Chromium is a metal that occurs as Cr^{3+} and Cr^{6+}. Chromium is found in the environment mainly in the trivalent form. It occurs in ores, and its production as well as industrial uses tend to increase its environmental levels if extreme care is not taken. The general levels in air, water and food are, however, normally very low. Thus, most foodstuffs contain less than 0.1 mg kg^{-1} and mainly as Cr^{3+}. The main food sources of chromium are cereals, meat, vegetables and unrefined sugar. Fish, vegetable oil and fruits contain smaller amounts. Under non-polluted environmental conditions chromium normally causes no food safety problems.

The data available on the metabolism of chromium are in general sparse. The speciation of chromium is of great importance for the toxicity, however. By the oral route Cr^{3+} has a low toxicity due to low absorption (about 0.5%). Indeed, Cr^{3+}, the most stable oxidation state in biological material, appears to have a beneficial role in the regulation of insulin action, metabolic syndrome and cardiovascular disease. There is growing evidence that chromium may facilitate insulin signalling, and chromium supplementation therefore may improve systemic insulin sensitivity. Tissue chromium levels of subjects with diabetes are lower than those of normal control subjects, and a correlation exists between low circulating levels of chromium and the incidence of type 2 diabetes. Controversy still exists, however, as to the need for chromium supplementation. In contrast, Cr^{6+} is highly toxic due to its high absorption, easy penetration of the cell membranes, genotoxicity and oxidizing properties. Thus, Cr^{6+} ions which have entered the cell are reduced by intracellular enzymes, a process during which free radicals are formed.

Cr^{6+} is characterized by IARC as carcinogenic to humans, inducing lung cancer among workers exposed during industrial processes such as welding, and plasma- and industrial laser processing of chromium-containing stainless steel. Cr^{6+} is also corrosive and causes ulceration of the nasal passages and the skin while at the same time it can induce hypersensitivity reactions of the skin. The hypersensitivity reaction is the reason why the EU in Directive 2003/53/EC of 18 June 2003 states that cement and cement-containing preparations may not be used or placed on the market if they contain, when hydrated, more than 0.0002% of soluble chromium(VI) per total dry weight of the cement.

Acute intoxication with Cr^{6+} can lead to renal tubular necrosis with inhibited glucose reabsorption by damaging the proximal convoluted tubule.

Chromium-containing stainless steels (alloys) are important food contact materials used for transportation (e.g. in milk trucks), for processing equipment (e.g. in the dairy and chocolate industry), in the processing of fruit, for containers such as wine tanks, for the processing of dry food such as cereals, in slaughterhouses, in the processing of fish, for brew kettles, and for nearly all of the equipment in big kitchens. Chromium is also used to coat other metals. Chromium does not migrate from stainless steel or surface-treated metals to any significant degree, however, and any released chromium is Cr^{3+} with a low toxicity.

A considerable industry using chromium salts is the leather tanning industry. Due to problems of pollution and subsequent political demands from governments in the richer parts of the world for control measures regarded as being expensive by the industry (among other reasons), this industry is to a great extent concentrated in developing countries. Chromium-polluted wastewater, coming from such industries, may result in elevated and generally unacceptable levels of chromium in some sources of seafood. For example, an investigation in 2001 of the concentration of heavy metals in the edible bivalves and gastropods available in major markets of the Pearl River Delta in China showed that, among the 14 edible molluscs investigated, only three species (*Ruditapes philippinarum*, *Perna viridis* and *Hemifusus tuba*) had cadmium, lead, nickel, chromium, antimony and tin concentrations within the local regulatory limits. Over 60% of

bivalve species exceeded maximum permitted levels of cadmium ($2 \mu g\ g^{-1}$) and chromium ($1 \mu g\ g^{-1}$); while over 40% of gastropod species exceeded the maximum levels of antimony ($1 \mu g\ g^{-1}$) and chromium ($1 \mu g\ g^{-1}$). In general, the molluscs purchased in Guangdong markets had higher metal contents than those purchased from Hong Kong markets. No information was given concerning the speciation of the chromium, however.

Cases of contamination of drinking water resources with Cr^{6+} resulting in impairment of health are known and described. Beyond any doubt the best described is the case from the southern California town of Hinkley. Between 1952 and 1966, a facility called the Hinkley Compressor Station, part of a natural gas pipeline connecting to the San Francisco Bay Area, was corrosion protected by the use of Cr^{6+} compounds. The wastewater was discharged to unlined ponds at the site. Some of the wastewater percolated into the groundwater, affecting an area near the plant approximately 2 miles long and nearly a mile wide. In 1993 Erin Brockovich-Ellis (born 22 June 1960) was instrumental in constructing a case against the company responsible for the pollution, the Pacific Gas and Electric Company (PG&E) of California. The case was settled in 1996 for US$333 million, the largest settlement paid in a direct action lawsuit in US history. The story was later told in the film *Erin Brockovich* starring the American actress Julia Roberts in the leading role, for which she received an Oscar.

18.6 Copper

Copper is a metal which is found at a concentration of $70\ mg\ kg^{-1}$ in the Earth's crust. It generally occurs in the oxidation states Cu^{1+} (cuprous) and Cu^{2+} (cupric), although under special conditions it also can occur in a trivalent state. Copper is essential to man. While iron is a component of haemoglobin, copper facilitates the utilization of iron in the synthesis of haemoglobin. Deficiency of either metal results in hypochromatic, microcystic anaemia. Copper is naturally present in most foodstuffs in the form of salts. Generally, the concentration in foodstuffs is about $2\ mg\ Cu\ kg^{-1}$. The main sources are meat, offal, fish, pecans and green vegetables. High levels up to about $40\ mg\ Cu\ kg^{-1}$ have been reported for liver and cocoa.

In general copper is not very toxic, the oral LD_{50} of cupric sulfate to the male rat being about

1500 mg kg^{-1} BW. In man semi-acute intoxications characterized by gastrointestinal distress may be seen with copper intakes of about 5 mg day^{-1}, however. Chronic copper intoxications occur once the capacity of the liver to bind copper (as Cu-MT) is exceeded, with weakness, listlessness and anorexia as early signs. In severe cases these symptoms will be followed by hepatic necrosis, vascular collapse, coma and death. It should be noted that a genetic disease (Wilson's disease) results in excess copper storage in the body, i.e. in the brain, liver, kidney and cornea. This results in a number of clinical manifestations in each of the target organs for the accumulation. There is a relatively high concentration of zinc and copper bound to the protein MT in the neonate (kidney, liver). This is consistent with the need for an effective buffer against the toxicity of these metals while there is a need for these elements during active cell proliferation.

Copper vessels are traditionally used in many specialized industrial food processing activities, such as in breweries and distilleries, for cheese-making, and for the production of chocolate, jam and sweets. Food utensils such as cooking vessels and saucepans can be made of copper but will normally be lined inside with tin (traditional) or stainless steel. The lining protects the food product from migration of copper from the kitchen utensil. Acidic foodstuffs in particular can attack copper surfaces. Therefore, copper may be present in food due to migration from food contact materials (e.g. copper utensils) or from using drinking water from copper pipes for food preparation. In some cases, high copper migration can even induce some product discoloration. Migration of copper into sugar confectionery cooked at 125–140°C and at pH 5.1–6.0 on average increases the copper concentration in the confectionery from about 0.1 to 0.25 mg kg^{-1}.

JECFA has established a Provisional Maximum Tolerable Daily Intake (PMTDI) of 0.5 mg kg^{-1} BW while the daily requirement is about 0.05 mg kg^{-1} BW. WHO has set a provisional health-based guideline value for copper in drinking water of 2 mg l^{-1} as a result of uncertainties in the dose–response relationship between copper in drinking water and acute gastrointestinal effects in man.

In general copper is of no great concern in a food context today. However, it should be mentioned that acute oral poisonings with gastrointestinal symptoms have been reported after consuming improperly canned vegetable juices containing excessive amounts of copper. So too have vomiting and diarrhoea in small children given water or breast-milk substitutes prepared from water that had been stagnant for a long time in copper pipes. Such a situation might occur when a family arrives at a summerhouse and uses water from the tap immediately, without flushing the pipes, for drinking or for preparing baby food.

18.7 Lead

Lead has been known to mankind for thousands of years. Lead water pipes were found in the preserved Roman towns of Pompeii and Herculaneum (southern Italy) and an estimated 12,000 t of lead were used in the building of one section of the great lead-lined aqueduct at Lyon (now France). However, even more interesting is the fact that lead – in the form of lead acetate (so-called *sugar of lead*) – was used as a 'food' additive by the Romans who added it to wine to prevent spoilage by further microbial growth and at the same time improve the taste. Since then lead has been used for a number of purposes and been found in a number of products including lead solders, lead-based paints, lead-glazed glasses, lead-covered roofs, storage batteries, cables and leaded gasoline, i.e. gasoline with added TEL. This use has meant that in general the lead exposure of human populations worldwide has steadily increased, as can be documented from investigations of the lead content in bones from skeletons from different historical periods.

In its inorganic form lead is found in the oxidation states +2 and +4. The Pb(II) oxidation state is the more stable, and there is a strong tendency for Pb(IV) compounds to react to give Pb(II) compounds. Inorganic lead is absorbed from the gastrointestinal tract by one or more specialized transport systems. This is evident from the findings that blood lead levels often are negatively correlated with blood iron levels, that lead–zinc interaction has been observed at the gastrointestinal absorptive site, and that the extensive experimental literature on interaction of lead with calcium rather consistently supports the observations that ingestion of diets low in calcium increases lead absorption and toxicity.

Under normal conditions about 10% of ingested soluble lead is absorbed in adults while in children this figure may be higher, sometimes even up to 30–40%. In the case of ingestion of a considerable dose of a lead salt (accidental or suicide attempt) gastrointestinal upset and inflammation will occur followed by renal damage. The person may ultimately die of cardiovascular collapse.

Lead is a non-essential so-called heavy metal which affects a number of organs and biochemical pathways in the body. After absorption into the blood it is distributed to a number of soft tissues. However, as a result of redistribution, ultimately the major part (up to about 90%) of the lead burden of our body is accumulated in the bones, where divalent lead ions replace the chemically similar calcium ions. Here the lead causes little harm, and the storage in the bones means that lead under normal conditions has a long half-life (greater than 25 years) in the body. However, if bone tissue is degraded during pregnancy or illness lead ions enter the bloodstream and may cause poisoning, or, in the case of pregnancy, reach the unborn child.

Like many other metals discussed in this book for their toxicity, lead binds to sulfhydryl (–SH) groups of proteins. Since sulfhydryl groups often play important roles in the active centre of enzymes, such metals thereby can impair their function. Lead more specifically also inhibits the activity of the zinc-dependent enzyme δ-aminolaevulinic acid dehydratase (= aminolaevulinate dehydratase; δ-ALAD) by displacing zinc. δ-ALAD catalyses the second step in the porphyrin and haem biosynthetic pathway. The production of haem is a multi-step process that requires eight different enzymes. δ-ALAD is responsible for the second step in this process, which combines two molecules of δ-aminolaevulinic acid (δ-ALA; the product of the first step) to form a compound called porphobilinogen. Furthermore,

the ability to generally impair the function of proteins combined with the ability to readily pass the placental barrier means that lead can reach and damage the endothelial cells of capillaries in the developing brain, resulting in brain oedema and impairment of the blood–brain barrier with lead entering the nervous tissue of the CNS. This can happen even in young children or (at very high levels) in adults.

Thus, apart from the already discussed acute damage to the gastrointestinal tract and kidneys happening as a result of a large single dose of a lead salt, the haematopoietic system and the nervous system, together with the kidneys, are targets for the subchronic and chronic toxicity of lead in the fetus, child and adult.

The *haematopoietic (blood forming) system* and the erythrocytes are the first to show signs of lead poisoning. The inhibition of δ-ALAD and (later in the biochemical pathway leading to the formation of haem) also of the incorporation of a ferrous ion into protoporphyrin IX as catalysed by ferrochelatase thus means accumulation of different intermediate products of this pathway (Fig. 18.2). Laboratory investigations of possible lead poisoning therefore can focus on the determination of increased urinary excretion of δ-ALA and coproporphyrin or accumulation of protoporphyrin IX in the erythrocytes. The physiological effect of lead inhibition of this pathway is anaemia of the type known as microcystic (small cells) hypochromic (with a low content of haemoglobin) anaemia with fatigue and weakness.

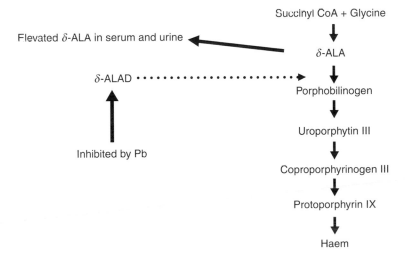

Fig. 18.2. Inhibition of the biosynthesis of haem by lead.

Both peripheral and central nervous system effects have been attributed to chronic exposure to lead.

Toxic injuries to the nervous system may be classified into neuropathies, axonopathies, myelinopathies and toxic degeneration of the synapse. Lead seems to possess the ability to cause both neuropathic and myelinopathic injuries. Lead ions thus can damage the dendritic processes (dendrites bring information into the neuron body (soma) and are hence critical elements in the communication processes of the nervous system) and cause destruction of myelin sheaths around the axons. In agreement with these basic effects of lead, occupational exposure previously often led to lead palsy, which is due to demyelination of the median nerve. Since this nerve supplies the extensor muscles of the hand, any damage to the nerve results in a 'wrist-drop' phenomenon.

Concerning CNS effects it has for decades also been known that really severe work-related lead poisoning may be associated with encephalopathy in which brain tissue becomes necrotic. The mechanism is the aforementioned damage to the blood–brain barrier formed by the endothelial cells of the brain capillaries, resulting in brain oedema and diffusion of lead ions into the CNS. Minor symptoms like lethargy are initially present and they proceed to delirium, convulsions and coma.

While encephalopathy is seldom seen in adults it is more easily induced in small children as a result of a longer-lasting lead exposure. As a follow-up on this knowledge research has tested the hypothesis that long-term low-level lead exposure during fetal life and/or infancy may also result in subclinical neurobehavioural deficit in otherwise asymptomatic children. Various psychological tests have been used while lead concentrations in blood and teeth have served as markers of current and past exposure of the test individuals. The alarming conclusions are that: (i) lead-related intellectual deficits seem to occur worldwide; (ii) the fetus will be affected by a high lead concentration in the maternal blood since lead passes the placental barrier and the fetal blood–brain barrier; (iii) early postnatal lead exposure is, however, the most damaging; and (iv) no clear-cut effect threshold can be established so far.

Severe acute lead poisoning will result in kidney damage as already mentioned. However, medium- to low-level exposure over a long period may also give rise to adverse effects on the kidneys. Generally speaking lead as Pb^{2+} has been the most abundant nephrotoxic metal throughout industrial history, although clinical toxicity was observed only after relatively high occupational exposure giving rise to a blood concentration of $600 \mu g \, l^{-1}$. Reaching the kidneys the lead first binds to high-affinity lead-binding proteins that are present in the tubule cells. This complex is translocated into the cell nucleus, where *de novo* synthesis of a unique acidic protein results in lead precipitation to form intranuclear inclusion bodies which may be seen microscopically. In the long run the accumulation of lead in the cells of the proximal tubules results in cell damage and impairment of the normal reabsorption of small proteins and ions, the same effect as seen for cadmium intoxication. Hence, early signs of lead-induced kidney damage also are identical, i.e. the presence of NAG as well as α_1-microglobulin and RBP in the urine.

From a food perspective lead is special. The intense pollution with lead along heavily trafficked roads of former times, due to the addition to gasoline of the synthetically produced organometallic compound TEL $((CH_3CH_2)_4Pb)$, has stopped in Europe and the USA as well as in many other countries worldwide. The effect of this abandonment of leaded petrol was seen as a decrease in blood lead levels in both these geographical regions. TEL was used as an antiknock additive in gasoline and is degraded in the motor to give micro-particulate lead oxides, which leave with the combustion gas. Since plants do not take up lead through the roots – in contrast to the situation with cadmium – the problem mainly is (was) one of surface contamination of fruits and vegetables.

Furthermore, it should be mentioned that if dairy cattle have been poisoned with lead – not an infrequent incident – the concentration of lead in the milk normally will be high. Hence, milk from such cows must be discarded until the level is acceptable again.

Lead was still used as a petrol additive, for example in China, for years after the termination of its use in the USA and Europe. With the strong growth in car ownership this fact gave rise to an increasing problem with lead exposure of the population, a development that could be followed and documented through an increase in blood lead levels in the bigger cities. This situation may still exist elsewhere, especially since non-leaded gasoline is more expensive. Available information indicates that TEL remains in use as an additive in aviation fuel for piston engine-powered aircrafts.

This, together with the fact that local lead contamination may be a result of industrial activities, means that lead still lingers.

The EU limit set by Commission Regulation (EC) No. 1881/2006 for lead in food commodities (mg kg^{-1} wet weight) ranges from 0.02 (milk) to 1.5 (bivalve molluscs).

18.8 Mercury

According to many sources archaeologists found mercury in an Egyptian tomb dating back to 1500 BC. In this context it cannot be a surprise that it has been known for a long time that high concentrations of mercury can be toxic to humans; the first account of mercury poisoning was recorded as early as 50 BC.

Mercury (chemical symbol Hg; from the Latinized Greek *hydrargyrum*, *hydr* = watery or runny, and *argyros* = silver) has atomic number 80. Mercury is the only metal that is liquid at normal temperatures and atmospheric pressure. With a melting point of −38.83°C and a boiling point of 356.73°C, mercury has one of the narrowest ranges of its liquid state of any metal. Mercury occurs in deposits mostly as cinnabar (mercuric sulfide). About half of the world production is from Spain and Italy.

Mercury occurs as elemental Hg^0 and as inorganic ions Hg^{1+} and Hg^{2+} forming mercurous and mercuric salts, respectively. Furthermore, organic mercury compounds are known such as methylmercury $CH_3Hg^+X^-$ (actually monomethylmercuric cation) and dimethylmercury $(CH_3)_2Hg$. Elemental mercury easily forms alloys with other metals such as gold, silver, zinc and cadmium. Such alloys are called *amalgams*. Amalgams are used to help extract gold from its ores and to create dental fillings (in the case of silver).

When the world production was at its maximum (around 1970) it amounted to approximately 20,000 t per annum. In addition to this source of mercury to be spread in the environment, the annual release from the burning of fossil sources of energy amounts to about 5000–10,000 t while natural degradation of the Earth's crust/volcanoes releases approximately 1000 t per annum. Traditional uses were by dentists for amalgam, as a component in thermometers and barometers, as a chemical component in fluorescent tubes and, until abandoned, in so-called *mercury fungicides* used for the protection of seeds for sowing as well as by the paper industry to protect the pulp from fungal degradation. Furthermore, mercury served as a catalyst in many processes in the chemical industry.

Elemental mercury is easily absorbed through the pulmonary alveoli. Once absorbed to the blood circulation it is oxidized in the erythrocytes to mercuric (Hg^{2+}) ions. Most mercurous salts in general are not water-soluble and therefore mercurous ions are relatively non-toxic; in contrast many salts of the mercuric ion are soluble and thus Hg^{2+} is readily absorbed from the duodenum.

Organic mercury in general is well absorbed. Aside from occupational exposure to special organic mercury compounds, the compound of relevance to discuss further in a food and environmental context is the monomethylmercuric cation, in the following called methylmercury.

Methylmercury is formed in nature. Although the first reports on this formation date back to the 1960s and much research has been conducted since then, the processes are still not fully understood. Until recently it was often just stated that mercury is methylated in the aquatic sediment as a result of biological processes, primarily involving sulfate-reducing bacteria. First of all it has to be pointed out that the processes described in general start with Hg^{2+} ions and not (elemental) mercury. This being said, however, it is important also to note that very recently a scientific group based in Canada and the USA stressed that, according to their calculations, these processes cannot account for all of the methylmercury that is formed naturally. The group presented several new models for additional non-biological formation of methylmercury in the aquatic environment. Of special interest is the process for formation of methylmercury from elemental mercury:

Hg(0) + MeI → HgMeI

This process may account for quite some production and for the first time also involves elemental mercury in the total environmental 'mercury circle' (Fig. 18.3). In order for this process to be realistic a substantial concentration of methyl iodide must be present in the water milieu. This is often the case since methyl iodide plays an important role in the biogeochemical cycle of iodide in seawater. Thus, marine organisms such as seaweed, marine algae and fungi produce methyl iodide as a defence compound or as a by-product of the production or breakdown of larger-molecular-weight defence compounds. Concentrations of methyl iodide in open ocean waters range from

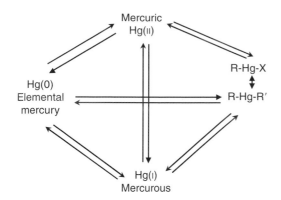

Fig. 18.3. The environmental 'mercury circle'. All processes can take place in the environment, some as biological processes, others as non-biological (some as both).

1.2 to 235 ng l⁻¹, but levels can be thousands of times higher in coastal areas with intensive biomass production. For example, in the waters off southwest Ireland, concentrations between $3.4\,\mu g\,l^{-1}$ and $0.12\,mg\,l^{-1}$ have been detected.

Mercury and mercury compounds are believed to be toxic primarily due to the affinity of particularly Hg^{2+} for –SH groups in proteins, as already described for cadmium and lead. The toxicity of different mercury species differs to a great extent, however, which is due very much to differences in their distribution in the body after systemic absorption. Table 18.1 lists some mercury species and the main targets for their toxicity.

What we can learn from Table 18.1 is that the non- or medium lipophilic compounds are toxic to the gut surface and to the extent they are absorbed to the proximal tubules. This is in agreement with the fact that mercuric ions are excreted primarily into the urine, although with a long half-life of

about 60 days. The mercury induces the formation of Hg-MT1 and Hg-MT2 in the kidney; it is bound specifically to these proteins in the cytosol of the kidney cells as recently demonstrated in an investigation where the distribution of mercury (after exposure to elemental Hg) was compared between wild-type and MT-null mice.

Toxicity to the CNS is seen for methylmercury and elemental mercury, both of which pass the blood–brain barrier.

The Mad Hatter, made famous in Lewis Carroll's *Alice in Wonderland*, was 'mad' as a result of mercury poisoning. A process called 'carroting' was used in the making of felt hats that were fashionable from the mid-18th to the mid-19th century, in which mercury nitrate was used to preserve the beaver felt. Workers in beaver felt factories of the time did, in fact, go mad as a result of breathing toxic mercury fumes formed, some effects of which are irreversible. Irritability is one of the early symptoms of mercury poisoning and this may also account for the description of 'mad' hatters. Today, we know that elemental mercury and especially organic mercury compounds such as methylmercury are neurotoxins and that high levels of exposure can lead to serious illness and, in extreme cases, death. The US Public Health Service banned the use of mercury in the felt industry in December 1941.

The mad hatter history demonstrates the CNS toxicity of elemental mercury. Unfortunately we also have examples with several victims that demonstrate the CNS toxicity of methylmercury.

The town of Minamata is located on the western coast of Kyushu, Japan's southernmost island. In 1932 the Chisso Corporation began to manufacture acetaldehyde, used to produce plastics. The chemical reaction used mercury sulfate as a catalyst. A side reaction of the catalytic cycle led to the production

Table 18.1. The effects and main target organs for the toxicity of different types of mercury compound.

Type of mercury compound	Main target organs	Effects
Inorganic salts	Gastrointestinal tract and kidneys[a]	Corrosive ulcerations in the gastrointestinal tract (gastroenteritis, colic, diarrhoea, shock, collapse)
Alkyloxyalkyl-Hg	Gastrointestinal tract and kidneys[a]	Corrosive ulcerations in the gastrointestinal tract (gastroenteritis, colic, diarrhoea, shock, collapse)
Aryl-Hg	Gastrointestinal tract and kidneys[a]	Corrosive ulcerations in the gastrointestinal tract (gastroenteritis, colic, diarrhoea, shock, collapse)
Elemental (metallic) Hg	CNS and kidneys[a]	CNS symptoms
Alkyl-Hg (e.g. methyl)	CNS and kidneys[a]	CNS symptoms

[a] Proximal tubule damage.

of a small amount of methylmercury. Together with other spill products this highly toxic compound was released into Minamata Bay. At that time, Minamata residents relied almost exclusively on fish and shellfish from the bay as a source of protein.

In 1956 when the production was still ongoing, a 5-year-old girl was examined at the Chisso Corporation's factory hospital. Her symptoms were difficulty walking, difficulty speaking and convulsions. Soon after her sister exhibited the same symptoms and was hospitalized. A survey in the town disclosed eight more patients. About 2 weeks later the hospital director reported to the local public health office the discovery of an 'epidemic of an unknown disease of the central nervous system', marking the official discovery of *Minamata disease*. To investigate the epidemic, the city government and various medical practitioners formed the Strange Disease Countermeasures Committee. The investigation, which included interviews with the townsfolk, soon disclosed some very uncommon phenomena. People reported that for some time they had observed cats to have convulsions, go mad and die. Locals called it the 'cat dancing disease', owing to their erratic movement.

This incident is the so-called *Minamata poisoning*, which researchers from Kumamoto University finally concluded was caused by organic mercury in July 1959. Years later, 2123 previously unrecognized victims were granted one-off payments of 2.1 million yen (US$23,000) each from the company and a monthly state medical allowance of up to 17,700 yen as a compensation for their suffering.

Another methylmercury poisoning happened in Canada in 1970, when excessive levels of mercury – as well as such symptoms as vision loss, chronic pain and tremors – were recorded in many residents of the two settlements Grassy Narrows and Wabaseemoong, about 90 km north-east of Kenora, Ontario, Canada. Residents found to have the illness were compensated in the 1980s by the Mercury Disability Board as well as by the pulp mill deemed responsible for dumping mercury compounds into the Wabigoon River between 1962 and 1970. The paper pulp mill had discharged inorganic mercury compounds which, however, had been biologically methylated in the river and given rise to methylmercury intoxications in local people consuming fish and shellfish from the river.

From the Minamata tragedy we had already learned something about the adverse effects caused by poisoning with methylmercury. However, the very peculiar situation that mankind soon synthesized the compound and used it intensively as a surface fungicide meant that unfortunately we got more mass intoxications to learn from. Thus, an outbreak of poisoning happened in Iraq in the winter of 1971/72 in a rural region where farmers ingested home-made bread made from seed wheat treated with a methylmercury fungicide. Analysis of the flour used gave an estimated amount of 1–4 mg of mercury per loaf of bread. The bread was eaten over a period from 2 weeks to 2 months depending on the family in question. Out of 49 children clinically investigated 2 years after the incident, 40 still had symptoms relating to the nervous system. The symptoms noted are shown in Fig. 10.3 as a function of the mercury concentration in the hair of the poisoned victim.

Unfortunately it is now confirmed that mercury (in the form of methylmercury ingested with food) resembles lead in that it also impairs brain development. A prospective study of mercury-exposed children was started by Professor Grandjean and colleagues almost 20 years ago. The scientists identified 1022 Faroese children who were particularly vulnerable to mercury due to the fact that their mothers' diets included pilot whale meat, a traditional – and often highly contaminated – Faroese food. The mercury level in the pregnant women's hair was measured before the children were born; some had up to 50 times more mercury than an average US mother. When the children were 7 years old, the scientists measured the mercury levels in their hair and blood, measured their heart rates, and tested developmental variables like the speed at which their brain responded to auditory signals. All of these examinations were repeated at age 14 years. The research group reported that mercury seems to slow the brain's response to sound. Somewhere along the transmission line from ear to auditory nerve to brain the signal is delayed. Some children's autonomic systems also seemed less able to regulate heart-rate variations. The changes seem irreparable. At age 7 years, it was found that the more mercury the children were exposed to in the womb, the worse off they were in terms of language skills, attention span and motor speed. Seven years later there was no evidence that the children's bodies had recovered or compensated for the damage. What is more, the data suggested that, as the children matured and began eating mercury-tainted whale meat and other seafood themselves, the brain damage continued – even at relatively low exposure levels.

Today there is in general no risk of exposure to inorganic mercury from any food commodity, and probably no risk to meeting, for example, methylmercury as an accidental pollution of food. However, there certainly are risks of being exposed to relatively high concentrations of methylmercury when eating predator fish on a high trophic level, since these may have accumulated high levels through a combined bioaccumulation and biomagnification. As is obvious from the above study from the Faroe Islands, mammal predators such as seals and predator whales also pose a risk.

In view of this, in the USA, FDA and EPA advise women of childbearing age, nursing mothers and young children to completely avoid swordfish, shark, king mackerel and tilefish (golden bass), to limit consumption of albacore ('white') tuna to no more than 6 oz (170 g) per week and to limit consumption of all other fish and shellfish to no more than 12 oz (340 g) per week.

Examples of the EU maximum limits for mercury in food commodities (Commission Regulation (EC) No. 1881/2006) are (mg kg^{-1} wet weight):

- fishery products and muscle meat of fish and crustaceans, excluding the brown meat of crab and excluding head and thorax meat of lobster and similar large crustaceans (*Nephropidae* and *Palinuridae*), 0.50;
- halibut (*Hippoglossus hippoglossus*), kingklip (*Genypterus capensis*), marlin (*Makaira* spp.) and megrim (*Lepidorhombus* spp.), 1.0.

18.9 Selenium

Selenium was deemed an essential nutrient only in 1957, but was discovered in 1817 by Berzelius in the sludge of sulfuric acid vats. Selenium toxicity was, however, first reported by the explorer Marco Polo (1254–1324) who was born on the island of Curzola in Croatia, at that time governed by the Italian Republic of Venice. Marco Polo made a number of journies for the Mongolian ruler Kublai Khan inside Mongolia and to China. During these he referred in his journals to 'a poisonous plant ... which if eaten by (horses) has the effect of causing the hoofs of the animal to drop off'. The plant Marco Polo described in the 13th century is today known to be one of several *specifically selenium-accumulating plant species*, which store toxic amounts of selenium.

In modern veterinary medicine, the toxicity of selenium has been known since the early 20th century when *blind stagger* of livestock was recognized as acute toxicity and *alkali disease* as chronic toxicity following ingestion of seleniferous grains, grasses or weeds. Blind stagger is characterized by signs of CNS impairment. Alkali disease, on the other hand, is characterized by retarded growth, emancipation, deformed hoofs, hair loss, arthritis and eventual death. In experimental animals symptoms of hepatic damage such as yellow liver atrophy and anaemia follow repeated oral administration of selenate or selenite.

In 1964, the existence was noted of a coincidence between the endemic distribution of the fatal so-called *keshan disease* (discovered in 1935 and named after Keshan County, Heilongjiang Province, China) in humans and that of the *white muscle disease* of domestic animals already known to be due to selenium deficiency. Soil in Keshan region is very low in selenium and a special type of cardiomyopathy is part of the keshan disease pattern. Treatments with Na_2SeO_3 were shown not only to reduce the morbidity and mortality of keshan disease but also to alleviate its clinical course.

Today we know that the range between adequate selenium and toxicity is narrow, i.e. from about 0.1 to 2 mg kg^{-1} diet, respectively. This life window is for humans who can also suffer from selenosis due to too high an exposure from food as described below.

The intestinal absorption of selenium depends on the chemical form; to some extent, so too does the retention and hence the body distribution. Thus, the retention from organic selenium compounds such as SeMet has been demonstrated to be high at about 80–90%. Organic selenium may not only be incorporated into selenium-specific proteins such as glutathione peroxidase (GSH-Px) and iodothyronine deiodinase, but also non-specifically into blood proteins such as albumin and haemoglobin due to homology between SeMet and methionine. For the inorganic forms it has been shown that they are equally well utilized for incorporation into GSH-Px but organic selenium still gives higher plasma and erythrocyte selenium levels.

An investigation of 75 corpses showed a general distribution of selenium levels in tissues which decreased in the following order: kidney > liver > spleen > pancreas > heart > brain > lung > bone > skeletal muscle. Nevertheless, the highest proportion of the total body selenium was found in skeletal muscles (around 27%); much less selenium was found in bones (16%) and blood (10%).

The metabolic pathway of various selenium compounds as disclosed so far is shown in Fig. 18.4.

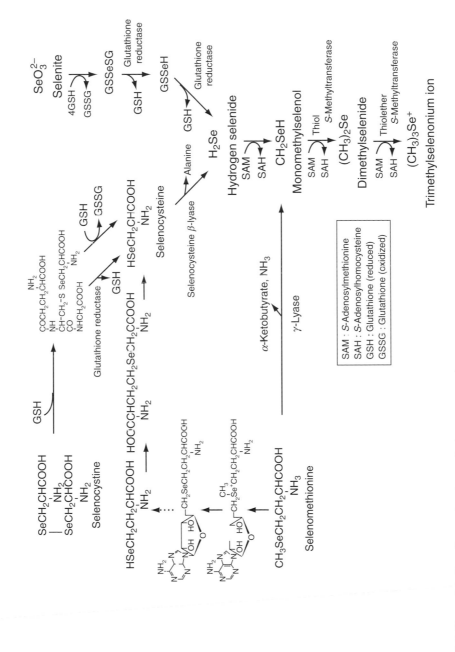

Fig. 18.4. The metabolic pathway of various selenium compounds.

Selenite is metabolized to hydrogen selenide (H_2Se) via selenodiglutathione and glutathionylselenol intermediates. H_2Se is subject to sequential enzymatic methylation resulting in the formation of mono-, di- and trimethylated derivatives. The trimethylselenonium ion (TMSe) is excreted in urine, whereas dimethylselenide (DMSe) is a volatile product and is exhaled via the lungs giving rise to *garlic breath odour*.

Selenium occurs in a number of proteins in the human body. Thus, it is an integral part of several enzymes, among others GSH-Px, an enzyme involved in cellular protection against oxidative damage (destruction of hydrogen peroxide and lipid peroxides), and iodothyronine deiodinase, which catalyses the conversion of thyroxine into triiodothyronine. Several other selenoproteins, such as selenoprotein P, have been isolated, but their physiological role is still not fully elucidated. In addition, selenium has been reported to play a role in maintenance of an optimal immune response. In its function as a part of the cellular antioxidative system it is closely related to the action of vitamin E. This relationship is reflected in the fact that the minimal daily intake of selenium in rats is $0.01\,mg\,kg^{-1}$ BW; however, if there is a vitamin E deficiency, a higher intake will be needed to avoid cellular damage.

Plant foods are the major dietary sources of selenium in most countries throughout the world. The content of selenium in food depends on the selenium content of the soil where plants are grown or animals are raised. Thus, the concentration of selenium in plant tissues depends both on the concentration and availability of selenium in the soil where the plants are grown. Selenium-accumulator plants grow only in soil containing high levels of selenium – 1–50 ppm – and can accumulate concentrations as high as from 1000 to $10,000\,mg\,Se\,kg^{-1}$. In many countries and regions with a low soil selenium concentration, selenium deficiency has caused health problems to livestock (white muscle disease); however, the problems are today often eliminated by selenium supplementation.

In China a national survey from 2002 showed that the distribution of the two human diseases keshan disease and the so-called *Kashin–Beck disease* (an osteoarthropathy) is linked to a topsoil selenium concentration below $0.125\,mg\,kg^{-1}$, while excessive levels of more than $3\,mg\,kg^{-1}$ (corresponding to blood levels of selenium greater than $1\,mg\,l^{-1}$) are associated with human selenosis, in the form of chronic nutritional selenium intoxication. Symptoms of the latter include nausea, weakness/irritability and diarrhoea, followed by hair loss, white blotchy nails, mottling of the teeth, skin lesions and garlic breath odour. The different selenium compounds show different LD_{50} values as found for rats (Fig. 18.5). Note that two different values are given for selenomethionine, which reflects that there are only two studies reported, which found two slightly different values for this compound.

The molecular mechanism(s) behind the different toxic effects of the various selenium compounds, acutely as well as chronically, is (are) not well understood however. For hepatic toxicity induced by SeCys it has been suggested that H_2Se accumulated in the tissues due to an observed inhibition of the methylation process may be the toxic molecular species. However, the mechanism for the toxicity of this compound remains to be established.

Overexposure to selenium has also been described in certain regions in the USA. Soils in the high plains of northern Nebraska and the Dakotas have very high levels of selenium. People living in these regions generally have the highest selenium intakes in the US population. A major part comes from maize, which, although not a specific selenium-accumulator plant, still can accumulate selenium to a considerable extent. This ability was also demonstrated by a growth experiment showing that the selenium content of maize grain produced in central New York could be increased by up to 670% following the application of fly ash containing 6.5 ppm Se to the soil. Fat-extracted maize produced from untreated soil contained 0.038 ppm Se while maize produced from fly ash-amended soil contained 0.296 ppm Se.

While selenosis was formerly seen relatively frequently in the northern regions of Nebraska and

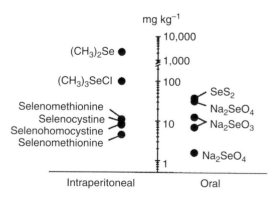

Fig. 18.5. The different selenium compounds show different LD_{50} values.

Dakota, this is not the case today due to the more varied and industrially processed diet of most people in these regions as elsewhere.

Because of the growing public interest in selenium as a dietary supplement and the occurrence of environmental selenium contamination, medical practitioners in the USA during the 1990s were asked to be familiar with the nutritional, toxicological and clinical aspects of this trace element by the Western State Public Health Departments. Finally it should be noted that deaths are seen as a result of the use of selenium compounds with homicidal intent, as was the case for two persons from Kentucky, USA, reported to be fatally poisoned with selenium in 2007.

18.10 Tin

The metal tin has the chemical symbol Sn from the Latin name *stannum* and atomic number 50. After gold, copper and silver, tin seems to be the earliest known metal. In Egypt tin items dating back nearly 6000 years have been excavated. Tin occurs in the Earth's crust with an average abundance of $2\,mg\,kg^{-1}$ mainly as cassiterite or tinstone (SnO_2); the main source of tin production. Tin occurs in most foodstuffs in small quantities of complex-bound Sn(II) ions; in unprocessed foodstuffs generally at levels less than $1\,mg\,kg^{-1}$.

Tin has long been used for items in contact with food and beverages. Thus, plates and mugs of tin were common and later foil made from a thin leaf of tin became commercially available. In the late 19th century and early 20th century, tin foil was in common use, e.g. for wrapping food products. Today it has been replaced by its more durable aluminium counterpart. This happened after World War II and aluminium foil is therefore sometimes confused as 'tin foil' because of its similarity to the former material. Tin is still used to coat kitchen utensils especially pots and pans made of copper, which is a very good heat conductor but relatively toxic.

The present major source of tin in the diet is food contact materials, especially the release from tin cans to acidic foodstuffs. A tin can is actually a steel can with a thin coating of metallic tin. Today there is often an internal resin-based coating on the tinplate, which of course reduces the diffusion of tin into the foodstuff.

The use of cans has in recent decades been decreasing in Europe, North America and other more highly industrialized nations, where among others distribution chains based on cold stored or frozen foods have taken over.

Inorganic tin compounds, especially tetravalent tins, are poorly absorbed from the gastrointestinal tract. Tin compounds act as an irritant for the gastrointestinal tract mucosa, causing nausea, vomiting, diarrhoea and fatigue. Cases of tin poisoning have been reported as a result of consumption of canned fruit juices, tomato juice, cherries, asparagus, herrings and apricots. The concentrations of tin in the products thought to have been associated with the incidents of acute poisoning were probably in the range of $300–500\,mg\,kg^{-1}$. Chronic exposure to high levels of tin has been described to result in growth depression and altered immune function, possibly due to interactions between tin and zinc or selenium.

The resulting tin content in foodstuffs stored in tin cans depends on: (i) whether the tin cans are lacquered; (ii) the presence of any oxidizing agents or corrosion accelerators (nitrate, for example); (iii) the acidity of the product in the can; and (iv) how long, and at what temperature, the tin cans have been stored before being opened.

In the EU, Commission Regulation (EC) No. 1881/2006 of 19 December 2006 setting maximum levels for certain contaminants in foodstuffs gives maximum levels for tin as follows ($mg\,kg^{-1}$ wet weight):

- canned foods other than beverages, 200;
- canned beverages, including fruit juices and vegetable juices, 100;
- canned baby foods and processed cereal-based foods for infants and young children, excluding dried and powdered products, 50;
- canned infant formula and follow-on formula (including infant milk and follow-on milk), excluding dried and powdered products, 50; and
- canned dietary foods for special medical purposes intended specifically for infants, excluding dried and powdered products, 50.

Tin may also occur as part of organometallic compounds, in general termed organotin compounds (OTCs). In 2004 the EFSA Scientific Panel on Contaminants in the Food Chain (CONTAM) was asked to assess the possible risks to human health from the consumption of food contaminated with such compounds based on intake estimates for Europe.

OTCs in general are synthetic compounds used in a number of different products and for a number of different purposes. The main source of OTC in food is likely to be tri-substituted compounds – e.g. tributyltin (TBT) and triphenyltin (TPT) – which have been used extensively as biocides in wood preservatives and in antifouling paints for boats and as pesticides. Mono- and di-substituted compounds – e.g. monomethyltin (MMT), dimethyltin (DMT), dibutyltin (DBT), mono-*n*-octyltin (MOT) and di-*n*-octyltin (DOT) – are used in mixtures in various relative amounts as PVC stabilizers; actually dialkyltins have been approved as PVC stabilizers for food contact materials. OTCs may accumulate in fish and other aquatic organisms. The CONTAM Panel focused on the most toxic compounds, i.e. TBT, DBT and TPT, primarily found in fish and fishery products and for which the exposure databases were available.

OTCs are for different reasons considered to be endocrine disruptors, and reproductive and developmental toxicity in rodents at daily doses of about 1 mg Sn kg^{-1} BW supports such endocrine activity. The critical toxicological endpoint for risk assessment was considered to be immunotoxicity, however. Making intake calculations based on fish and seafood consumption in Norway, the Panel noted that the consumption of fish, mussels and other marine animals gathered from highly contaminated areas, such as in the vicinity of harbours and heavily used shipping routes, may lead to an OTC intake that exceeds the group Tolerable Daily Intake (TDI) for these compounds.

18.11 Fluorine

Approximately 99% of the fluoride in the body is associated with calcified tissues. Fluoride is incorporated into bones and teeth where, as a result of similarities in size and charge, it replaces the hydroxyl ion in the crystal lattice of apatite.

The natural fluorine level in most feed and food recourses is in general of no concern with regard to any negative influence on human health. Indeed, in regions where the fluorine intake is very low, *water fluoridation*, i.e. the controlled addition of fluoride to a public water supply to reduce tooth decay, has been or is used. Fluoridated water has fluoride at a level that is effective for preventing teeth cavities.

Fluoridated water operates on tooth surfaces: drinking it creates low levels of fluoride in saliva, which reduces the rate at which tooth enamel demineralizes and increases the rate at which it remineralizes in the early stages of cavities. A level of around 1 ppm is the desired. However, in certain geographical regions the natural fluorine content of soil and thereby water may be so high that adverse effects of fluoride are seen as dental fluorosis. In this case the enamel of the teeth is weakened, resulting in surface pitting. An example described in the scientific literature is from San Luis Potosi, Mexico, where a study was carried out in 1992. The prevalence and severity of dental fluorosis in children (11–13 years) increased dramatically as the concentration of water fluoride increased above the level of 2.0 ppm.

Although the fluorine levels in food, beverages, etc. in most cases do not give rise to adverse effects such as the mentioned dental fluorosis, it has been shown that certain Tibetan people living in nomadic or semi-nomadic areas and regularly consuming so-called *brick tea* (both as a beverage and in food) may have a fluoride intake up to about 7 and 15 mg day^{-1} for children and adults, respectively. This can be compared, for example, with the *maximum level of daily nutrient intake that is likely to pose no risk of adverse effects* for fluorine as established by the US authorities. This ranges from 0.7 to 2 mg day^{-1} for children of different ages and up to 10 mg day^{-1} for adults. Black brick tea has a high fluorine content due to the fact that the tea plant concentrates fluorine and that the highest levels are found in older leaves, which are used to make the beverage.

Further Reading

Klaassen, C.D. (2008) *Casarett & Doull's Toxicology: The Basic Science of Poison*, 7th edn. McGraw-Hill Companies, New York, New York.

Lu, F.C. and Kacew, S. (2009) *Lu's Basic Toxicology: Fundamentals, Target Organs, and Risk Assessment*, 5th edn. Informa Healthcare, New York, New York.

Ross, S.M. (ed.) (1994) *Toxic Metals in Soil–Plant Systems*. John Wiley & Sons, Chichester, UK.

Siegel, F.R. (2002) *Environmental Geochemistry of Potentially Toxic Metals*. Springer-Verlag, Berlin.

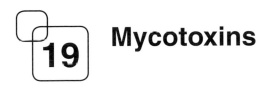

Chapter 18

19 Mycotoxins

- We define mycotoxins as a concept.
- We describe a number of classes of mycotoxins, their formation and adverse effects.
- We look at the legislation meant to reduce the human exposure to mycotoxins.

19.1 Introduction

The term *mycotoxin* is derived from the Greek word *mykes* = fungus and the Latin word *toxicum* = poison. The study of *mycotoxicology* began in 1891 in Japan, when Sakaki demonstrated that ethanol extracts from mouldy, unpolished yellow rice were fatal to dogs, guinea pigs and rabbits. Yellow rice is undried rice fermented by the native microbial flora present at harvest. During the fermentation the grains acquire a yellowish-brownish colour that remains. The poisonings that affected the nervous system causing paralysis were later demonstrated to be due to the formation of toxins by species of *Penicillium* such as *Penicillium citreonigrum* among the flora. The toxins include citrinin with an oral LD_{50} of about 100 mg kg^{-1} BW in the mouse, which affects the kidneys by causing tubular damage, and citreoviridin with an LD_{50} of approximately 30 mg kg^{-1} BW, shown to cause paralysis of hind limbs. Sakaki's findings meant that the sale of yellow rice was banned in Japan in 1910.

Other food-related intoxications caused by mycotoxins were described relatively early in history. These include *ergotism*, the first Western reference to which dates back to the 9th century. An epidemic of so-called gangrenous ergotism, wherein 'a great plague of swollen blisters consumed the people by a loathsome rot so that their limbs were loosened and fell off before death' was seen. A mixed epidemic, i.e. with gangrenous as well as convulsive manifestations, was described in the 11th century. In 1676, it was recognized that epidemic ergotism resulted from eating foods, usually breads or cereals, made from rye which was contaminated with the fungus nowadays called *Claviceps purpurea*.

19.2 Aflatoxins

Aflatoxins are mycotoxins shown to be produced by the following species of *Aspergillus*: *Aspergillus flavus*, *Aspergillus parasiticus*, *Aspergillus nomius*, *Aspergillus pseudotamarii*, and *Aspergillus bombycis*. Chemically they are difuranocoumarins. *A. flavus* is ubiquitous and attacks mostly the aerial parts of plants, while *A. parasiticus* is more adapted to the soil environment. While *A. flavus* and *A. pseudotamarii* produce the B type aflatoxins only, *A. parasiticus*, *A. nomius* and *A. bombycis* also produce the so-called G type (Fig. 19.1). *A. flavus* populations are genetically diverse and phenotypic variations have been well documented. Isolates also vary considerably in their ability to produce aflatoxins and colonize plants. They generally can be grouped into two *schlerotial morphotypes* (strains): the L strains and the S strains. L strain isolates produce abundant conidiospores and schlerotia that are usually larger than 400 μm in diameter, whereas S strain isolates produce fewer conidiospores and numerous schlerotia that are usually smaller. The S strain isolates typically produce higher amounts of aflatoxins than do the L strain isolates on the same media.

The aflatoxins are beyond any doubt the group of mycotoxins feared the most for their health-impairing effects of various kinds. Therefore harmonized maximum levels for aflatoxins have been

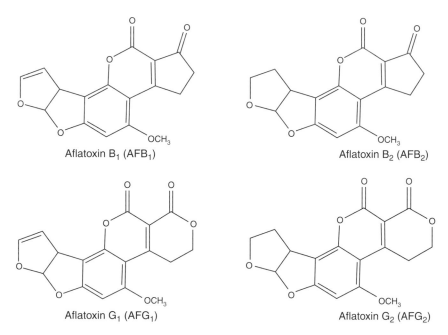

Fig. 19.1. Structures of the aflatoxins biosynthesized by *Aspergillus* spp.

in place in the EU since 1999 and are at present to be found in the Annex of Commission Regulation (EC) No. 1881/2006 setting the maximum levels for certain contaminants in foodstuffs. The Commission safeguard decision 2006/504/EC sets stricter controls on a number of products for which it is considered especially important to perform a constant monitoring. For Brazil nuts in the shell from Brazil, groundnuts (peanuts) from China and Egypt, pistachios from Iran, and figs, hazelnuts and pistachios from Turkey, extra safety assurances based on a stricter sampling procedure thus are required.

IARC classifies the aflatoxins as carcinogenic. For the compounds belonging to Group 1, i.e. the fungal metabolites AFB_1 and aflatoxin G_1 (AFG_1) together with the metabolite AFM_1 which is excreted in milk, IARC found sufficient evidence for carcinogenicity in experimental animals. Based on this and the fact that AFB_1 consistently is genotoxic *in vitro* and *in vivo*, an overall conclusion was that aflatoxins must be considered as carcinogenic to man. In accordance with this classification JECFA in 1998 concluded that aflatoxins are among the most potent mutagenic and carcinogenic substances known.

Based on epidemiological data it has been estimated that AFB_1 exposure gives rise annually to 0.3/100,000 cancers per ng AFB_1 kg^{-1} BW in hepatitis

B virus (HBV) antigen-positive individuals and 0.01/100,000 cancers in HBV antigen-negative persons. Hereby we have already indirectly pointed to the main target organ for the carcinogenicity of aflatoxins, which is the liver.

Aflatoxins have been shown to produce acute necrosis, cirrhosis and carcinoma of the liver in many animal species. All species tested were susceptible to acute poisoning, with LD_{50} values varying but being in the range from 0.5 to about 10 mg kg^{-1} BW. Concerning the tumorigenicity of AFB_1, mice are much more resistant to the compound than are rats.

The aflatoxins were isolated and their structures elucidated for the first time in the early 1960s as a result of a deeper investigation on a major intoxication of turkeys. Early chemical analysis was based on TLC separation of the compounds in an extract. Subsequent identification and quantitative estimation of the compounds on the plate was based on fluorescence of the aflatoxin spots under long-wave UV light. This analysis gave rise to the naming of the compounds. Thus, B and G refer to blue and green fluorescence, respectively, while the numeric designation refers to the distance the compound travelled on the chromatographic plate as compared with the other within the same fluorescence group.

A wide range of food commodities and products can be contaminated with aflatoxins. However, with regard to human exposure various tree nuts, groundnuts, figs (and other dried fruits), spices (such as chilli), crude vegetable oils, cocoa beans, maize (corn) and rice must be considered the most important sources.

The aflatoxin-producing species grow best under warm conditions. As already mentioned, A. *flavus* exists in two morphotypes (S and L strains) of which the S strain isolates typically produce higher amounts of aflatoxins than do the L strains on the same media. However, a significant portion of A. *flavus* L strain isolates do not produce aflatoxins at all due to lack of the enzymatic setup needed. In contrast, the aflatoxigenic trait of the S strain isolates seems very stable. Very recent investigations have shown that, while maize most often supports the formation of aflatoxins (if infested), a root crop such as cassava seldom (or never) does.

Exposure and mechanism of toxicity

From the above list of commodities and the summary of the characteristics of A. *flavus* it is clear that one can expect a variation in aflatoxin exposure depending on geographical region.

Indeed, exposure estimates around the world show such variations. Thus, data from Austria show an average daily intake of $0.15\,ng\,kg^{-1}$ BW, the 95th percentile reaching twice that level. In contrast to this, some Chinese reports have come up with daily intake estimates ranging from zero to $91\,\mu g\,kg^{-1}$ BW for AFB_1. Also some estimates of intakes in certain parts of Africa show high exposure, groundnut and maize being the major sources.

Taking a special look now at the carcinogenic metabolite AFM_1, an overview of its occurrence in European commercial milk and milk product samples in the 1990s and up to 2006 also demonstrates variation. Just 34 milk samples out of about 11,000 analysed by the EU member states in the period 1989–1995 had AFM_1 levels above the maximum of $0.05\,\mu g\,kg^{-1}$. On the other hand, a subsequent Italian submission of 789 results from the testing of milk and cheese from 2002 to 2006 showed that about 6% contained more than this level, most positive results coming from a testing of cheeses in 2004. However, it must be emphasized that the estimated overall daily intake of 0.03–$1.3\,ng\,kg^{-1}$ BW for AFB_1 in Europe from all sources is indeed very low compared with what

is seen in several other regions of the world, as already demonstrated by the figures given above for China.

As shown in the rat, absorption of aflatoxins in the small intestine is a rapid process. Absorbed toxins reach the liver through the portal system. The biological activity is mainly dependent on the presence of a double bond at the 8,9-position of the molecule(s), which among the genuine compounds makes AFB_1 and AFG_1 the most toxic. These are metabolized by cytochrome P450-dependent monooxygenases to form a very reactive 8,9-epoxide (Fig. 19.2).

In the liver the formation of the epoxide is carried out predominantly by cytochrome P4503A4, which catalyses the formation of AFB_1-8,9-*exo*-epoxide, which is able to bind to DNA and thereby give rise to mutations as cell divisions occur. Some AFB_1-8,9-*endo*-epoxide, which cannot bind to DNA, is also formed, however, through the reaction catalysed by cytochrome P4501A2. Since the *exo*-epoxide is very reactive (unstable) it will react predominantly with molecular targets within the cell or tissue where it is formed, which is why the liver is the most important target organ.

The AFM_1 formed (Fig. 19.3) is to a limited extent excreted into the milk of lactating animals and humans. Since this compound has retained the double bond at the 8,9-position it still is a substrate for the cytochrome P4503A4-catalysed formation of AFB_1-8,9-*exo*-epoxide, and hence it represents a risk upon intake.

As already noted above there are data to suggest that liver infection with HBV alters the susceptibility to aflatoxin exposure and hence the toxicity, with focus especially on the carcinogenic effect. Many theories have been presented on the nature of this interaction. However, all that can be said so far is that it possibly has to do with the effects of HBV infection on aflatoxin metabolism inducing an altered balance between activation and detoxification.

DNA and protein adducts (mechanism of mutagenicity and marker compounds)

Which macromolecular adducts are formed and in which relative amounts in a given organism exposed to aflatoxins depends on the balance between the rate of production of the 8,9-*exo*-epoxide compared with other oxidized metabolites and on the rate of epoxide detoxification. The detoxification in turn

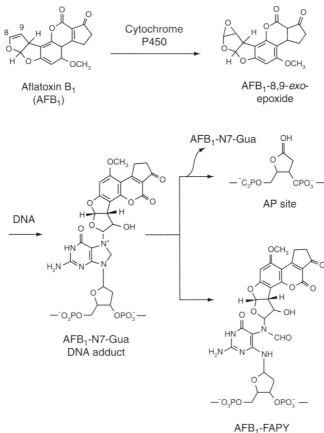

Fig. 19.2. Metabolism of AFB$_1$ resulting in formation of epoxide and subsequently DNA adduct.

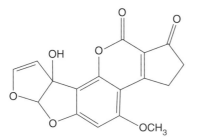

Fig. 19.3. Structure of AFM$_1$.

involves several biochemical pathways including conjugation to glutathione and hydrolysis to the 8,9-dihydrol.

The primary DNA adduct formed from the 8,9-epoxide produced is the AFB$_1$-8,9-dihydro-8-(N7-guanyl)-9-hydroxy adduct (if we take AFB$_1$ as the example). However, this adduct is further converted into others such as the imidazole-ring-opened AFB$_1$-formamidopyrimidine (AFB$_1$-FABY) adduct. Recent studies seem to support a theory that points to this adduct being the most likely candidate for the actual mutagenicity of AFB$_1$ after activation.

Aflatoxins can also form adducts with proteins; among which albumin is of importance when we look for markers for aflatoxin exposure. To date the only adduct structurally identified for albumin is based on an AFB$_1$–lysine bond. This adduct together with urinary aflatoxin metabolites are valuable markers in exposure studies. Thus, a high correlation has been demonstrated between aflatoxin–DNA adducts in the liver, the urinary excretion of metabolites/adducts and the serum aflatoxin–albumin adduct level. Urinary and serum levels reflect recent (1–2 days) and chronic (2–3 months) exposure, respectively.

Legislatively set maximum concentrations of aflatoxins

Regulations for aflatoxins have been over time and still are different between, for example, the USA and the EU as two major players in the world import and export market. The current EU regulations with respect to maximum levels of aflatoxins (AFB_1, AFB_2, AFG_1, AFG_2 and AFM_1) are laid down in Commission Regulation (EC) No. 1881/2006 as amended by Commission Regulation (EU) No. 165/2010 (Table 19.1). Interestingly, the amendment includes an increase in the levels accepted for certain commodities, such as the opinion (EFSA) adopted on 25 January 2007 on almonds, hazelnuts and pistachios and derived products. This increase was adopted after a discussion with CAC.

19.3 Ochratoxins

Ochratoxin A is one of three mycotoxins, named OTA to OTC. OTA is the most common, toxic and abundantly formed in foods. OTA contains a dihydrocoumarin moiety linked to a molecule of L-β-phenylalanine via an amide bond (Fig. 19.4). As the structural formula shows, OTA contains a chlorine atom – a relatively uncommon feature for natural organic compounds that is, however, shared with OTC and the well-known broad-spectrum antibiotic chloramphenicol.

In contrast to the aflatoxins which are produced by fungi within only one genus, OTA is produced by several fungal species from the *Penicillium* and the *Aspergillus* genera, primarily *Penicillium verrucosum* and *Aspergillus ochraceus*, together with some species of aspergilli from the section *Nigri* such as *Aspergillus carbonarius*.

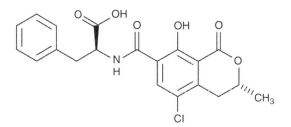

Fig. 19.4. Structure of OTA.

Table 19.1. Levels of aflatoxins in foodstuffs allowed in the EU (examples as accompanied with a simplified description of the single foodstuff).

Foodstuff	Maximum aflatoxin level (μg kg^{-1})		
	B_1	Sum of B_1, B_2, G_1, G_2	M_1
Groundnuts (peanuts) and other oilseeds to be subjected to sorting or other physical treatment before consumption	8	15	–
Almonds, pistachios and apricot kernels to be subjected to sorting or other physical treatment before consumption	12	15	–
Hazelnuts and Brazil nuts to be subjected to sorting or other physical treatment before consumption	8	15	–
Groundnuts (peanuts) and other oilseeds and processed products thereof intended for consumption	2	4	–
Dried fruit to be subjected to sorting or other physical treatment before human consumption	5	10	–
All cereals and all products derived from cereals	2	4	–
Maize and rice to be subjected to sorting or other physical treatment before human consumption	5	10	–
Raw milk, heat-treated milk and milk for the manufacture of milk-based products	–	–	0.05
Spices: *Capsicum* spp. (dried fruits, chilli powder, etc.) *Myristica fragrans* (nutmeg) and others	5	10	–
Processed cereal-based foods and baby foods for infants and young children	0.1	–	–

P. verrucosum is important in the contamination of grains in cooler regions of Northern Europe while *A. carbonarius* is the key species responsible for OTA contamination of grapes, wine and vine fruits. It is known that *A. ochraceus* infects cereals, coffee, cocoa and edible nuts. However, confirmation of actual ochratoxin production by *Aspergillus* strains on cereals has not been reported.

OTA has been found in many different commodities worldwide in warm as well as more temperate climates. Examples include raw materials such as cereals, pulses, coffee, grapes/raisins and cocoa, together with nuts and many spices. This occurrence means that OTA, which is a very stable compound requiring temperatures above 250°C for several minutes to reduce the concentration, also must be found in processed commodities including beer, grape juice, wine and cocoa products.

ADME and toxic effects

OTA is absorbed rapidly following oral intake although the absorption fraction varies from species to species: from 40% in chickens up to about 70% in pigs. In the blood OTA is extensively bound to plasma proteins including albumin. Bacterial transformation in the gastrointestinal tract yields a cleavage product called ochratoxin *α*, which can be absorbed from the lower gastrointestinal tract. The absorbed genuine OTA is to a lesser extent hydroxylated in the liver giving rise to *R*- and *S*-epimers of 4-OH-OTA. The major route of excretion differs between species with renal elimination being the most important in monkeys and man, whereas biliary excretion is important in rodents.

OTA has proved to be a potent renal toxin in all species and has for decades been known as a problem in the production of pigs. The pig is the most sensitive species for the toxicity of OTA. The compound gives rise to a typical karyomegaly and a progressive nephropathy in a dose-dependent manner, which is also associated with the duration of exposure, since OTA accumulates in renal tissue.

The possible carcinogenicity of OTA with the kidney as the target organ has been discussed for many years and a number of experiments as well as analyses of epidemiological data of different natures have been performed. In 1993 IARC evaluated OTA and classified it as possibly carcinogenic to humans (Group 2B), based on sufficient evidence for carcinogenicity in animal studies and inadequate evidence in humans.

However, tumour formation has been seen only at very high doses exceeding the doses inducing severe kidney damage. The mechanism for the carcinogenesis is not yet clear but seems to be attributed to DNA damage and a genotoxic effect caused by cellular oxidative damage. On the basis of this conclusion and the fact that even advanced chemical analytical methods recently failed to demonstrate the existence of any specific OTA–DNA adducts, EFSA in a risk assessment from 2006 concluded that hazard characterization must be based on the nephrotoxicity of the compound.

Strong sex- and species-specific differences have been observed in sensitivity to the nephrotoxic action of OTA. Thus, in the rat the male has been demonstrated to be the most sensitive sex.

Occurrence, exposure and limits

The strong renal toxicity to pigs, and the fact that – especially in humid summers in temperate climates – it has been difficult to avoid too high an OTA contamination of, for example, barley fed to pigs, has meant for decades that traditional slaughterhouse meat inspection has been looking for pale swollen kidneys as a sign of OTA poisoning. If observed, analysis is then done for OTA in the kidneys; only if this proves negative or results in a concentration under a given level can the meat from the pig in question be released for consumption.

In general, contamination of animal feeds with OTA results in the presence of residues in edible tissues and meat products. The higher concentrations are found in certain local specialties such as blood puddings and sausages prepared with pig blood serum.

As we can understand from the discussion so far, exposure can result from a variety of both plant and animal products. The three most recent exposure assessments for OTA have been done in Europe in 1998, 2001 and 2006. The last was a part of the aforementioned risk assessment from EFSA and concluded that in Europe exposure of high consumers varies between 40 and 60 ng OTA kg^{-1} BW week^{-1}. Exposure is predominantly due to the intake of contaminated plant-derived products and only to a minor extent to foods of animal origin, although regular consumption of a product such as Swedish blood pudding based on pig blood will increase exposure significantly.

EFSA in their risk assessment from 2006 used the Lowest Observed Adverse Effect Level (LOAEL) of $8\,\mu g\;kg^{-1}$ BW day^{-1} for early markers of renal toxicity in pigs and a composite uncertainty factor of 450 to account for uncertainties in the extrapolation of experimental data derived from animals to humans as well as for intra-species variability, to derive a Tolerable Weekly Intake (TWI) for OTA of $120\,ng\;kg^{-1}$ BW.

The present maximum limits for OTA in different products as set by the EU in Commission Regulation (EC) No. 1881/2006 of 19 December 2006 setting maximum levels for certain contaminants in foodstuffs are ($\mu g\;kg^{-1}$):

- unprocessed cereals, 5.0;
- products derived from unprocessed cereals, 3.0;
- dried vine fruit (currants, raisins and sultanas), 10.0;
- roasted coffee beans and ground roasted coffee, excluding soluble coffee, 5.0;
- soluble coffee (instant coffee), 10.0;
- wine, 2.0; and
- processed cereal-based foods and baby foods for infants and young children, 0.50.

19.4 Trichothecenes

The trichothecenes make up a very large family of chemically related toxins produced by various fungal species of the genera *Fusarium*, *Myrothecium*, *Trichoderma*, *Cephalosporium*, *Verticimonosporium* and *Stachybotrys*. The compounds are markedly stable under different environmental conditions. The distinguishing chemical feature of trichothecenes is the presence of a trichothecene ring, which contains an olefinic bond between C-9 and C-10 and an epoxide group between C-12 and C-13 (Fig. 19.5).

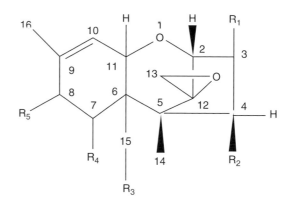

Fig. 19.5. General structure, numbering system and variable side groups of the tetracyclic trichothecene nucleus.

There are four groups of trichothecenes (A–D), of which the compounds belonging to groups A and B are the most important in a food context. The type A compounds include some of the most acutely toxic agents such as T-2 toxin, HT-2 toxin, diacetoxyscirpenol, monoacetoxyscirpenol and neosolaniol. The type B compounds, which have a carbonyl group at the C-8 position, include nivalenol (NIV), DON (deoxynivalenol or vomitoxin), fusarenon X and diacetylnivalenol. For important individual structures see Table 19.2.

This group of mycotoxins as such has been shown to cause multi-organ effects including emesis and diarrhoea, weight loss, nervous disorders, cardiovascular alterations, immune depression, haemostatic derangements, skin toxicity, decreased reproductive capacity and bone marrow damage.

Human intoxications due to trichothecenes were seen in Russia during World War II, the so-called *alimentary toxic aleukia*, with mortality rates as high as 80%. These incidents of intoxication arose

Table 19.2. Specific side groups of the most abundant trichothecene mycotoxins.

Trichothecene	R_1	R_2	R_3	R_4	R_5
T-2 toxin	–OH	–OCOCH$_3$	OCOCH$_3$	–H	–OCOCH$_2$CH(CH$_3$)$_2$
HT 2 toxin	–OH	–OH	–OCOCH$_3$	–H	–OCOCH$_2$CH(CH$_3$)$_2$
DAS^a	–OH	–OCOCH$_3$	–OCOCH$_3$	–H	–H
Nivalenol	–OH	–OH	–OH	–OH	=O
Deoxynivalenol	–OH	–H	–OH	–OH	=O
Macrocyclics^b	–H	–O-R′–O–		–H	–H

^{a} DAS is also called anguidine and 4,15-diacetoxyscirpenol.

^{b} R′, macrocyclic ester or ester–ether bridge between C-4 and C-15. The most abundant macrocyclic trichothecenes are verrucarins, roridins and satratoxin H.

because cereals not were harvested due to warfare and instead were left on the ground for longer periods, often at oscillating temperatures, which led to the growth of fusarium and the formation of trichothecenes.

The acutely highly toxic T-2 mycotoxin has, together with some closely related compounds, been the causative agent of a number of illnesses not only in humans but also in domestic animals.

During the 1970s and 1980s, the trichothecene mycotoxins gained some notoriety as putative biological warfare agents when, according to published studies from US intelligence, they were implicated in 'yellow rain' attacks in South-East Asia (Laos and Kampuchea). In these attacks the mycotoxins seem to have been spread by using among others 60-mm mortar shells, 120-mm shells, 107-mm rockets and M-79 grenade launchers containing chemicals.

The trichothecenes are cytotoxic to most eukaryotic cells. Protein synthesis is inhibited as demonstrated in a number of different cell lines such as Vero and HeLa cells. The inhibition is seen within minutes of administration of, for example, T-2 toxin, while it takes from 24 to 48 h before cell viability is affected. The inhibition of protein synthesis is thought to be due to interference with either the initiation or the elongation process.

Trichothecenes are commonly found on cereals grown in the temperate regions of Europe, America and Asia:

- T-2 and HT-2 are generally found in various cereal crops such as wheat, maize, barley, oats and rye, and in processed grains (malt, beer and bread). T-2 and HT-2 have been reported to be produced by *Fusarium sporotrichioides*, *Fusarium poae*, *Fusarium equiseti* and *Fusarium acuminatum*. *F. sporotrichioides* grows at −2 to 35°C and only at high water activities. The optimum temperature for occurrence of T-2 is relatively low (8–14°C), with yields being much lower or negligible at temperatures of 25°C and above. Products contaminated with T-2 can cause severe, even fatal effects in humans/animals. General signs of T-2 intoxication include nausea, emesis, dizziness, chills, abdominal pain, diarrhoea, dermal necrosis and irreversible damage to the bone marrow, resulting in a reduction in the number of leucocytes (white blood cells) (aleukia). Thus, the immune system is the main target of T-2, and secondary infections may be the result.

- DON is generally found in various cereal crops such as wheat, barley, oats, rye, rice and maize. It is produced mainly by two important cereal pathogens: *Fusarium graminearum* Schwabe and *Fusarium culmorum* Sacc., which cause ear rot in maize and head blight in wheat. DON is also called vomitoxin because of its strong emetic effects and its action as a feed refusal factor; it was first characterized and named following its isolation from *Fusarium*-infected barley in Japan. *F. graminearum* and *F. culmorum* have different optimum temperatures for growth (25 and 21°C, respectively) and this probably affects geographical distribution. In developed countries where grains are dried to ≤13% moisture content to prevent mould growth, DON is mostly an important preharvest problem.

- NIV may generally occur together with fusarenon X. *Fusarium cerealis* and *F. poae* are the main producers of NIV, but isolates of *F. culmorum* and *F. graminearum* are also able to produce NIV. *F. poae* is reported as the main NIV producer in Sweden. NIV occurs in various cereal crops such as wheat, maize, barley, oats and rye.

In the EU (Commission Regulation (EC) No. 1881/2006), DON, T-2 and HT-2 are regulated. Maximum levels of DON range from 200 to 1750 µg kg⁻¹ depending on the commodity.

19.5 Ergot Alkaloids

The mycotoxins discussed in this section are, as the heading indicates, alkaloids. Alkaloids are most often found in plants and are discussed as a group under naturally inherent plant toxicants in Chapter 15. However, the group of compounds termed *ergot alkaloids* are produced by a number of mould genera such as *Acremonium*, *Balansia* and *Aspergillus*, and by species of the fungal genus *Claviceps*. While the specific mould species doing this synthesis is not relevant when discussing food, the species of *Claviceps* certainly is, and in particular the species *C. purpurea*, also called *ergot*.

The word ergot is derived from the old French word *argot* = cock's spur. The use of this term is related to a disease caused by fungi belonging to the genus *Claviceps* on plants belonging to the grass family (*Graminaceae*). The fungi parasitize the seed heads of living plants at the time of flowering.

The fungus replaces the developing seed (grain) with its alkaloid-containing wintering body (a sclerotium), known as an ergot or ergot body. The ergot, which consists of fungal mycelium cells, is longer than the normal seed and is dark grey to violet in colour. Hence, the ergot can be seen with the naked eye on the grass/grain seed head (Fig. 19.6).

C. purpurea grows on rye (*Secale cereale*) and triticale (×Triticosecale Wittmack), which have open florets, as its most important hosts, but may also be found on wheat (*Triticum* spp.), sorghum (*Sorghum vulgare*), pearl millet (*Pennisetum* spp.) and barley (*Hordeum vulgare*). Strains adapted to a plant species or group of species have been described. While *C. purpurea* is the most important in a chemical food safety context, perhaps *Claviceps africana* – which was recently described to attack sorghum species, principally *Sorghum bicolor* – should be mentioned too. *C. africana* produces primarily dihydroergosine with lesser amounts of dihydroelymoclavine and festuclavine.

C. purpurea seldom causes serious yield losses although yield reductions of up to about 5% in rye and 10% in wheat have been reported from North America. However, the alkaloids that its sclerotia ('ergots') contain are toxic both to humans and animals, and ergot contamination of grain lots greatly reduces their economic value.

The compounds and the poisoning

According to general alkaloid classifications, the ergot alkaloids belong to the class of indole derivatives.

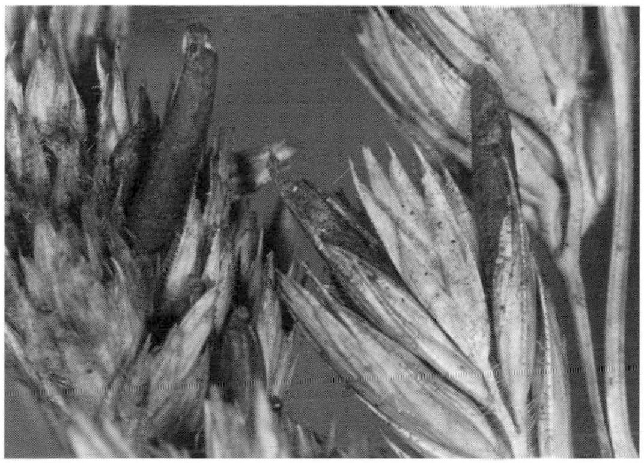

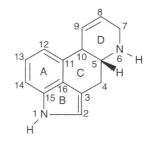

Fig. 19.6. The genus *Claviceps* is spread worldwide and includes around 40 species that together are known to parasitize about 600 plant species, most of which belong to the *Graminaceae*. With permission from http://www.naturefg.com

The structure is built around a tetracyclic ring system, which can be exemplified by ergoline (Fig. 19.7). Depending on the finer structural details of ring D and the types of substituents at C-8, all ergot alkaloids can be divided into three biogenetically related classes: (i) clavine ergot alkaloids; (ii) simple lysergic acid derivatives; and (iii) peptide ergot alkaloids (ergot peptides).

Within the group of ergot alkaloids all of the interesting, strongly physiologically active compounds are actually derivatives of the specific tetracyclic structure lysergic acid (LA; Fig. 19.8). Thus, they are either simple LA derivatives such as ergometrine (= ergonovine) where the substituent is 2-aminopropanol or peptide ergot alkaloids where the substituent is a tripeptide. The LA molecule shows two chiral centres (C-5 and C-8): these centres have the stereoconfiguration 5R,8R in the bioactive molecule.

Peptide ergot alkaloids contain the LA nucleus and a tripeptide group (Fig. 19.9) linked through an amidic bond. The classification of the ergot peptides into ergotamine, ergostine and ergocristine groups is based on the tripeptide structure. The LA fragment is responsible for the basic biological activity of the compounds, while the substituent imparts certain specificity to this general activity.

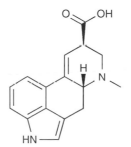

Fig. 19.7. Ergoline.

Fig. 19.8. Lysergic acid in the 5R,8R configuration.

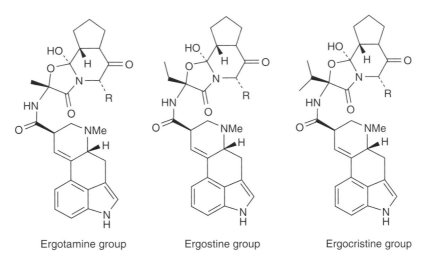

Fig. 19.9. Structure of three groups of ergot alkaloids: the ergotamine group, the ergostine group and the ergocristine group.

According to literature the first recorded outbreak of ergotism dates back to AD 857 and occurred in what now is Germany. Numerous epidemics in Europe occurred between the 9th and the 18th centuries. Overall the intoxication can cause pronounced peripheral vasoconstriction of the extremities, disruption in functions of the CNS, contraction of the uterus, gangrene (induced by vasoconstriction) and even death. In the Middle Ages epidemics of ergotism, caused by the ingestion of rye bread contaminated by *C. purpurea*, occurred frequently and were popularly known as 'St Anthony's Fire'.

Two distinctive forms of ergotism are often described: gangrenous and convulsive (neurological). In *gangrenous ergotism* tingling effects are felt in the fingers and toes, followed in many cases by dry gangrene of the limbs and finally loss of the limbs. In *convulsive ergotism* the tingling is followed by hallucinations, delirium and epileptic-type seizures. Historically the gangrenous type was mostly seen in France and the convulsive one in Germany. The two distinct types of ergotism may be considered as acute and chronic varieties according to modern theories, although differences in the relative concentration of the different alkaloids probably also may be of importance, as we may understand by looking at the medicinal use of ergot alkaloids.

A number of ergot alkaloids and semi-synthetic derivatives have been and are used in medicine. Among the natural alkaloids we find ergotamine and ergometrine, while methysergide and bromo-criptine are examples of derivatives. Ergotamine is a non-selective agonist of the serotonin type 1 sub-family (5-HT$_1$) of receptors. Its oral absorption is 60–70%. It is metabolized in the liver by P450 cytochromes and is excreted in the faeces and urine. Ergotamine can constrict coronary blood vessels and inhibit the trigeminal sensory nerves through pre-junctional 5-HT$_{1D}$ receptors. It is widely used for the treatment of severe migraine attacks. Ergometrine is an amide derivative of D-LA and is used in the treatment of postpartum haemorrhage. It is rapidly absorbed after oral administration.

Ergotamine can cause adverse effects, like ergotism, stroke, gangrene, diarrhoea, swollen fingers, generalized weakness, peripheral and coronary vasoconstriction, and also death. The main adverse effects of ergometrine are nausea, vomiting, abdominal pain, diarrhoea, headache, chest pain, palpitations, bradycardia, hypertension, dyspnoea, leg cramps and haematuria. The acute toxicity of ergometrine has been reported as 93 mg kg^{-1} BW (LD$_{50}$, oral, in the rat).

Taking a look at the pharmacological and adverse effects of these two major ergot alkaloids, it is not difficult to identify elements of the previously described food-related ergotism.

Modern times and ergot as a chemical food safety issue

Today, modern production methods reduce the content of sclerotia in grain products as discussed later and thus one could think that alertness towards ergot is no longer important. However, human poisoning from ergot has occurred in more recent times in France, India and Ethiopia. The Ethiopian case followed two years of drought. During this time, the locally grown barley had become dominated by wild oats heavily contaminated with *C. purpurea* sclerotia. A total of 93 cases of ergotism were reported during the spring of 1978. More than 80% of affected persons were between 5 and 34 years of age. Examination of 44 patients out of 93 registered revealed ongoing dry gangrene of the whole or part of one or more limbs.

Decontamination

In industrialized agricultural production with a technically well equipped and knowledgeable flour-producing sector, most problems with ergot are under control nowadays. This is due to a number of procedures.

Ergot bodies remain intact during grain storage. They are largely removed with the dockage during conventional grain cleaning (about 80% from dirty wheat). The sclerotia most often are larger than cereal grains and are removed by mechanical means with the conventional grain cleaning equipment such as sieves and separators used already during the harvesting process. However, the mechanical separation methods become less reliable when dry seasons result in the production of smaller sclerotia than usual. Thus, ergot alkaloids have been detected in Canadian, Danish, German and Swiss surveys of cereals and cereal products, with total ergot alkaloid toxin levels of up to 7.255 μg kg^{-1} in German rye flours.

Other methods to further clean a grain batch include: (i) gravity separation and electronic separators since ergot bodies are less dense than wheat grains; and (ii) flotation in 20% (w/v) sodium chloride or 32% (w/v) potassium chloride solutions. Today effective clearing techniques at mills generally enable the removal of up to about 80% of ergots from grain. During milling ergots pass into flour fractions used for human consumption with relatively little in the break flours and 18–36% in the bran fractions.

Legislation

No country has yet set limits for individual ergot alkaloids in food. In the EU also no regulatory limits apply to ergots in grain for human consumption. However, according to Commission Regulation (EC) No. 1572/2006, amending Commission Regulation (EC) No. 824/2000, a maximum value of 500 mg ergot bodies kg^{-1} grain (0.05% w/w) has been set for intervention grain, but not for consumption grain. The EU has established an intervention system in order to stabilize the markets and ensure a fair standard of living for the agricultural community in the cereals sector (EU Council Regulation 1784/2003). Through this system, the EU dictates certain standards in grain for intervention affairs within the common market, which individual countries can also accept for consumption grain.

19.6 Patulin

The mycotoxin patulin is produced by certain species within the three fungal genera of *Penicillium*, *Aspergillus* and *Byssochlamys*. In a chemical food safety context the spp. *Penicillium expansum* is the most important. This fungus, as well as other *Penicillium* spp. which produce patulin, are plant pathogens that invade damaged tissue of many different fruits including apricots, grapes, peaches, pears, apples and olives to produce mould-damaged fruits. In certain instances internal growth of moulds may result from insect or other invasions of otherwise healthy tissue, resulting in occurrence of patulin in fruit which appears undamaged externally. Although the focus is on fruits and especially apples for regulations and recommendations to food product producers, patulin has also been found in vegetables, cereals and other foods.

The structurally quite simple patulin molecule (Fig. 19.10) has been investigated for several decades. Yet it is still not easy to describe its total profile of toxic effects in a few words. From a number of tests for acute toxicity in different animal species it is obvious that patulin is toxic. Among studies available in the literature, two short-term (14 days) studies in mice and rats both showed patulin to produce histopathological lesions in the gastrointestinal tract, including epithelial degeneration,

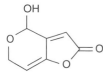

Fig. 19.10. Patulin.

haemorrhage, ulceration of gastric mucosa, and neutrophil and mononuclear cell infiltration.

These effects are in good correlation with the established fact that patulin has strong affinity for –SH groups and therefore inhibits a broad pallet of enzymes. At the moment IARC classifies the compound in Group 3, i.e. IARC considers the evidence for carcinogenicity in experimental animals inadequate.

Patulin is relatively thermostable, particularly at acid pH. Thus, short-term high-temperature (150°C) treatments have been reported to reduce patulin concentrations by only approximately 20%. Since alcoholic fermentation of fruit juices destroys patulin, fermented products such as cider and perry will not contain the mycotoxin. Even so, patulin has been found in fermented products to which apple juice has been added after fermentation.

In the EU, at its meeting of 8 March 2000, SCF endorsed a PMTDI of $0.4\,\mu g\,kg^{-1}$ BW for patulin. Subsequently an assessment of the dietary intake of patulin by the population of EU member states was performed in 2001. On the basis of these facts, Commission Regulation (EC) No. 1881/2006 set the following maximum limits for the content of patulin in different products ($\mu g\,kg^{-1}$):

- fruit juices, concentrated fruit juices as reconstituted and fruit nectars, 50;
- spirit drinks, cider and other fermented drinks derived from apples or containing apple juice, 50;
- solid apple products, including apple compote and apple purée intended for direct consumption, 25;
- apple juice and solid apple products, including apple compote and apple purée, intended for consumption by infants and young children (aged <16 years) and labelled and sold as such, 10; and
- baby foods other than processed cereal-based foods for infants and young children, 10.

In order to help industries reduce the patulin content of especially apple products, the EU published a recommendation in 2003 on the prevention and reduction of patulin contamination in apple juice and apple juice ingredients in other beverages (2003/598/EC).

19.7 Fumonisins

Fumonisins are mycotoxins produced by the moulds *Fusarium moniliforme* (= *Fusarium verticillioides*), *Fusarium proliferatum* and other *Fusarium* spp.

that are common natural contaminants of maize. More than ten fumonisins have been characterized. Of these, fumonisin B_1 (FB_1), fumonisin B_2 (FB_2) and fumonisin B_3 (FB_3) are the major fumonisins produced in nature. The most prevalent of these mycotoxins in contaminated maize is FB_1, which is believed to be the most toxic.

Fumonisins cause leucoencephalomalacia in horses and pulmonary oedema in pigs. Furthermore they have been linked to a variety of significant adverse health effects in other livestock and experimental animals. Dietary FB_1 levels of 50 ppm and above induced kidney tumours in male rats and liver tumours in female mice.

Although human epidemiological studies are inconclusive at this time, based on a wide variety of significant adverse animal health effects the association between fumonisins and human disease is possible. This is why both FDA and EFSA, in the USA and Europe, respectively, have already decided to regulate the content of these compounds in food, awaiting more detailed knowledge to be produced. FDA launched their 'Guidance for Industry Fumonisin Levels in Human Foods and Animal Feeds' in 2001.

Studies in the USA in particular have revealed that the extent of contamination of raw maize with fumonisins varies with geographic location, agronomic and storage practices, and the vulnerability of the plant to fungal invasion during all phases of growth, storage and processing. High levels of fumonisins seem to be associated with hot and dry weather, followed by periods of high humidity.

In conjunction with the guidance document, FDA set the following maximum limits for total fumonisins ($FB_1+FB_2+FB_3$) in maize and maize-derived products:

- de-germed dry milled maize products (e.g. flaking grits, maize grits, maize meal, maize flour with fat content of <2.25%, dry weight basis), 2 ppm;
- whole or partially de-germed dry milled maize products (e.g. flaking grits, maize grits, maize meal, maize flour with fat content of >2.25%, dry weight basis), 4 ppm;
- dry milled maize bran, 4 ppm;
- cleaned maize intended for mass production, 4 ppm; and
- cleaned maize intended for popcorn, 3 ppm.

In the EU, SCF established in 2000–2003 a TDI for fumonisins of $2\,\mu g\,kg^{-1}$ BW. On this basis the following shows the maximum limits ($\mu g\,kg^{-1}$, FB_1+FB_2):

- unprocessed maize, 2000;
- maize flour, maize meal, maize grits, maize germ and refined maize oil, 1000;
- maize-based foods for direct human consumption, 400; and
- processed maize-based foods and baby foods for infants and young children, 200.

19.8 Zearalenone

Commission Regulation (EC) No. 1881/2006, which we have mentioned so often, also sets maximum limits for the level in foodstufffs of the mycotoxin zearalenone biosynthesized by several *Fusarium* spp. These vary from 200 µg kg^{-1} for unprocessed maize to 20 µg kg^{-1} for processed maize-based foods for infants and young children.

Zearalenone (Fig. 19.11) is a non-steroidal oestrogenic mycotoxin that for decades has been recognised as being implicated in numerous mycotoxicoses in farm animals, especially in pigs. The compound was shown in the early 1980s to be produced on maize in Australia, Europe, North America, New Zealand, the Philippines, Thailand and Indonesia. Also findings from South America, Africa, China and the former USSR are described in the scientific literature, in these cases in different food and feed products. The ubiquitous occurrence of zearalenone is underlined by the reported fact that *Fusarium* isolates from bananas were shown to produce zearalenone and that a number of cereal crops other than maize – i.e. barley, oats, wheat, rice and sorghum – also support its formation, with the result that this heat-stable mycotoxin may be found in bread products.

The concentrations in different food commodities vary over a wide range, depending first of all on climatic conditions. Thus, zearalenone was found in 11–80% of wheat samples and 7–68% of barley samples for feed use collected randomly in south-west Germany in 1987 and 1989–1993, with mean yearly contents of 3–180 µg kg^{-1} in wheat (highest value, 8000 µg kg^{-1}) and 3–36 µg kg^{-1} in barley (highest value, 310 µg kg^{-1}). On the other hand, wheat for human consumption collected from all regions of Bulgaria (140 samples) after harvest in 1995, a year characterized by heavy rainfall in spring and summer, showed lower values. Thus, the frequency of contamination with zearalenone was 69%, but with an average concentration in positive samples of only 17 µg kg^{-1} and a maximum of 120 µg kg^{-1}.

Zearalenone is rapidly and extensively absorbed after oral administration. At high oral doses zearalenone and its metabolites can be excreted into the milk of lactating animals. The maximum concentrations in the milk of one cow given an oral dose of 6000 mg zearalenone (equivalent to 12 mg kg^{-1} BW) were found to be 6.1 µg l^{-1} for zearalenone, 4 µg l^{-1} for α-zearalenol and 6.6 µg l^{-1} for β-zearalenol. Neither zearalenone nor its metabolites were found in the milk (<0.5 µg l^{-1}) of three lactating cows fed 50 or 165 mg zearalenone (equivalent to 0.1 or 0.33 mg kg^{-1} BW) for 21 days.

Several oestrogenic effects of zearalenone have been observed in short-term and long-term studies of toxicity and in studies of reproductive toxicity in a number of mammalian species. In the year 2000 JECFA made a very comprehensive risk assessment of zearalenone based on more than 300 scientific articles and very detailed exposure models. The Committee concluded as follows (WHO Food Additives Series No. 44):

> the safety of zearalenone could be evaluated on the basis of the dose that had no hormonal effect in pigs, the most sensitive species. Using a safety factor of about 100, the Committee established a provisional maximum tolerable daily intake (PMTDI) for zearalenone of 0.5 µg/kg bw. This decision was based on the NOEL of 40 µg/kg bw per day in the 15-day study in pigs. The Committee also took into account the lowest-observed-effect level of 200 µg/kg bw per day in this study and the previously established ADI of 0–0.5 µg/kg bw for the metabolite alpha-zearalanol, evaluated as a veterinary drug. The Committee recommended that the total intake of zearalenone and its metabolites (including alpha-zearalanol) should not exceed this value.

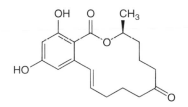

Fig. 19.11. Zearalenone.

Further Reading

Barug, D., Bhatnagar, D., van Egmond, H.P., van der Kamp, J.W., van Osenbruggen, W.A. and Visconti, A. (eds) (2006) *The Mycotoxin Factbook; Food & Feed Topics*. Wageningen Academic Publishers, Wageningen, The Netherlands.

Diaz, D. (ed.) (2004) The *Mycotoxin Blue Book*. Nottingham University Press, Nottingham, UK.

20 Pesticides and Persistent Organic Pollutants

- Pesticides and POPs (persistent organic pollutants) are defined.
- The history of the development of the different classes of pesticides is told.
- The importance of POPs in the modern world and their way into foods are discussed.

20.1 Introduction

A *biocide* by definition is any substance used with the intention of killing living organisms whether these are pests or not. *Pesticides* are compounds that man uses to control, meaning to reduce in number or to eradicate, organisms that interact negatively with his activities such as crop production and gardening, or to control disease in people, animals, etc. The total pallet of biocides/pesticides made available to man through decades of research and development may be classified into the following groups (group of target organisms): algaecides (algae), avicides (birds), fungicides (fungi), herbicides (plants), insecticides (insects and different arachnids, the latter belonging to the class Arachnida of joint-legged invertebrate animals with eight legs, including mites, ticks and spiders), molluscicides (molluscs, e.g. slugs, snails), nemat(od)icides (nematodes) and rodenticides (rodents, e.g. rats, mice). A great proportion of the fungicides used worldwide are incorporated in products for the protection of wood materials used in buildings and other constructions.

In a chemical food safety context the compounds that are used to control pests interfering with our food production activities, and therefore are deliberately administered to crops or production animals, are of greatest relevance. Although molluscs can damage certain food crops such as strawberries, here we concentrate on the groups of insecticides, herbicides and fungicides, in that order.

The ideal pesticide is one that is toxic only to the target pest(s) and is rapidly inactivated in the environment to non-toxic substances. To develop such agents is not an easy task, however. Examples of wanted target specificities could be (toxic to/non-toxic to):

- insects/all other animals;
- most insects/bees and all other animals; and
- dicotyledonous plants (broadleaved weeds)/ monocotyledonous plants (cereals).

Looking at these examples already illustrates the size of the problem and one could think that it simply is not possible to develop pesticides with a reasonable specificity, allowing more widespread use. However, as difficult as it seems, we immediately also can point to examples of striking specificities. For instance, early experiments showed that spraying species of cereal growing in a field with a dilute solution of sulfuric acid can eradicate several broadleaved weeds relatively effectively without harming the cereal crop. The mechanism behind this specificity can more or less be classified as physical and consisting of two important general differences between the two groups of plants. Most cereals (and many monocotyledonous plants in general) have a relatively thick wax layer on the leaf surface and very few leaf hairs, two characteristics that facilitate an immediate runoff of the applied acid. In the case of several broadleaved plants, the hair cover can entrap the acid on the leaf surface and the thin wax cover provides only a very weak barrier to damage by the acid of the leaf cells.

A number of preparations containing strychnine, or extracts of tobacco or of chrysanthemum were widely used in the past as pesticides together with agents such as sulfur and formulations containing arsenic or mercury compounds. While the use of some was discontinued quite early due to their limited effect or high immediate toxicity to man and animals, others like the mercury compounds were only gradually taken out of use and mostly due to their chronic toxicity and ability to accumulate in the body.

As we shall see later, the specificities of today's pesticides rely more on differences in the biochemical makeup of different organisms than on the physical ones just described for sulfuric acid used as a herbicide. However, we must also realize that there are always limits to our ability to target just the organism(s) that we want to combat. Thus, even today our most-used agents to kill rats, i.e. the modern rodenticides, actually show no or very little specificity between the rat and all other mammals including man, which is only natural since our basic biochemical makeup is indeed very similar.

The reason for our interest in pesticides is mainly grounded in the fact that both feed and food commodities are at risk of containing residues of such agents used during the production or of being contaminated with such agents because of their use in neighbouring fields. Pesticide residues in feedstuffs may represent a risk to chemical food safety in the case that they are absorbed by the production animal and concentrated in tissues used for the production of food, excreted in milk or found in eggs.

20.2 Insecticides

The early history of the insecticides used by man for crop protection and that of ectoparasiticidal drugs used in veterinary practice is more or less identical. This general history of the insecticides was reviewed by the USDA Agricultural Research Service in 1954 and can also be found at a web page from the Department of Entomology, Soils and Plant Sciences at Clemson University, South Carolina, USA (http://entweb.clemson.edu/pesticid/history.htm). Browsing this resource we find that the very first development worthy of mention is the introduction of sulfur–tobacco dip for control of sheep scab caused by the sheep scab mite, *Psoroptes ovis*; this took place in 1854. In 1867 the first use of arsenical insecticides in plant production was noted in the USA, where 'Paris green' (copper(II) acetoarsenite) was used to control the Colorado potato beetle.

Around 1870 a commercial producti California of 'pyrethrum'. 'Pyrethru 'pyrethrum flower heads' or 'insect flow of the dried flower heads of *Tanacetum lium* (Trevir.) Schultz-Bip., previously within the genus *Chrysanthemum* and with the still commonly used name *Chrysanthemum cinerariaefolium*. Also a few other species at that time denoted *Chrysanthemum coccineum* and *Chrysanthemum marschallii*, all belonging to the plant family *Asteraceae* (= *Compositae*), were used. These plants have insecticidal effect due to their content of around 0.5% by weight of so-called *total pyrethrins* – consisting mainly of the two compounds pyrethrin I and II (Fig. 20.1a). Pyrethrin-containing flowers are known to have been used as insecticides for centuries by Caucasian tribesmen and the Armenians. The powdered form was manufactured on a commercial scale in 1828 and first introduced into the USA in 1855. The importance of pyrethrum preparations before the advent of synthetic contact insecticides is demonstrated by the tremendous expansion of their importation into the USA: 270 t in 1885 rising up to 8100 t in 1945. The use in veterinary medicine included among others control of blood-sucking flies in cattle

(a)

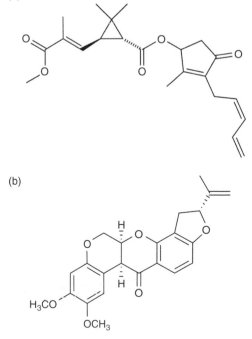

(b)

Fig. 20.1. Structural formula of pyrethrin II (a) and rotenone (b).

production (as oils to spray on the animal) and of fleas, ticks or lice on dogs (e.g. as dips).

In 1918 the insecticidal value of *derris* – yet another plant remedy – was pointed out. Derris is a collective name for a number of plant species (legumes) such as *Derris elliptica*, *Derris malaccensis* and *Derris ulignosa* found mainly in Malaysia, Indonesia and the Philippines. Extracts are insecticidal due to their content of the compound rotenone (Fig. 20.1b). In agreement with this, rotenone-bearing insecticides were reported as effective for the control of cattle grub (*Hypoderma* spp.) and cattle louse in 1922.

Organochlorines

Early insecticides included the above-mentioned extracts of chrysanthemum and other plant extracts, as will be discussed further below in connection with the pyrethroids. However, the first mass-produced synthetic compounds to be used as insecticides were the so-called *organochlorine insecticides*. These include what is possibly the most controversial compound of the 20th century: DDT (*p,p'*-DDT; dichlorodiphenyltrichloroethane) (Fig. 20.2).

DDT was synthesized originally by the German chemist Othar Zeidler in 1874. However, its insecticidal effect was not described until 1938/39, when the Swiss chemist Paul Herman Müller during a screening of existing compounds for this activity found it indeed very effective. Müller was an employee of the Swiss chemical company J.R. Geigy (later Ciba-Geigy and, after merging with Sandoz, nowadays named Novartis), which soon marketed the compound.

Quickly the compound was used worldwide in the combat of malaria and yellow fever, two diseases that are spread by mosquitoes. Soon it was also widely used to treat humans as well as husbandry for lice and to combat the spreading of typhus infections caused by *Rickettsia prowazekii* as spread by a lice vector. In 1948 Müller was given the Nobel Prize in physiology and medicine for his discoveries.

For decades DDT was regarded as being close to the *ideal* insecticide. In the 1960s the world production of DDT was almost 80 million kg, which was used to spray around 300 commodities and in the combat of a number of diseases spread by insect vectors. Over a period of about 10 years starting soon after World War II, WHO thus used more than 400,000 t of DDT to combat malaria-spreading mosquitoes. The enormous effect of DDT usage in this respect can be exemplified by comparing the situation in Ceylon (now Sri Lanka) before the start of DDT campaigns with that during the years when these were running and the situation when they were terminated. In 1948 around 2,800,000 malaria cases were reported on the island, while the numbers for 1962 and 1963 with large-scale DDT usage were 31 and 17, respectively. By 1969 – some years after the spraying had been discontinued – the number was back to around 2,500,000.

Due to the great efficiency and popularity of DDT soon a number of other organochlorine insecticides were developed and marketed. Thus, TDE (*p,p'*-TDE; 1,1-dichloro-2,2-bis(*p*-chlorophenyl) ethane) (Fig. 20.2) was introduced commercially in the USA in 1945 shortly after the introduction of DDT. Although lacking the broad-spectrum insecticidal activity of DDT, TDE did possess equal or greater potency against the larvae of some mosquitos and *Lepidoptera*. Also DDD (*p,p'*-DDD; dichlorodiphenyldichloroethane) (Fig. 20.2) was used to kill pests and to medically treat cancer of the adrenal gland.

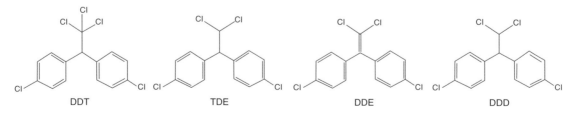

Fig. 20.2. Structural formula of DDT (*p,p'*-DDT), together with a number of other related organochlorine pesticides and/or metabolites of DDT.

Synthesized and marketed as pesticides, both TDE and DDD at the same time are also metabolites of DDT, formed in the environment and in the intestines by the action of microorganisms, and at least for TDE also in the liver (shown for rats). Furthermore, both of these compounds as well as DDE (p,p'-DDE; dichlorodiphenyldichloroethylene) also occur as impurities of the synthesis in commercial DDT preparations (see Box 20.1).

Even though TDE was added to DDT in the pallet of commercially available organochlorine insecticides, in general the introduction of the group of *cyclodienes* including aldrin, dieldrin, endrin, chlordane and heptachlor (Fig. 20.3), also dating back to the period from just after 1945, was of greatest importance. Others introduced were methoxychlor (Fig. 20.3), the structure of which resembles that of DDT (Fig. 20.2), and benzene hexachloride (hexachlorocyclohexane), a compound originally synthesized in 1825. The latter exists in 16 possible stereoisomers. The so-called γ-isomer is the most effective and was marketed and used for years under the name of lindane (Fig. 20.3).

The toxicity of the organochlorines

The success of the organochlorine insecticides originates to a great extent in their strong to relatively strong specificity towards insects and related organisms as compared with mammals and birds. Thus, the LD_{50} value of DDT to the honeybee was found to be about 2 mg kg^{-1} BW and that of lindane towards the cockroach about 4 mg kg^{-1} BW, while it is lower for the housefly, i.e. about 1 mg kg^{-1} BW. The oral LD_{50} value to the rat was shown to be about 90 mg kg^{-1} BW for DDT and the same for lindane. In general most of the cyclodienes are somewhat more toxic to warm-blooded animals than the two examples just given, with an oral LD_{50} value for the rat to aldrin and dieldrin of about 40–50 mg kg^{-1} BW. The interspecies differences seen for the acute oral toxicity in general are relatively small, although the hamster seems to be very resistant to the toxic effects of DDT when administered orally. The ratio between the LD_{50} reported for cutaneous versus oral administration may, however, vary to quite a degree among species (Table 20.1).

Despite the long time we have had these compounds in focus for research, details about their mechanism of action generally still seem to be lacking. However, it is known that DDT affects the transmission of impulses through the axon probably as a result of the compound's ability to interfere with the movement of ions over the neuron membrane by delaying the closing of the sodium channels, slowing the opening of the potassium gates, and blocking the calcium transport into the neuron. These interferences with the normal membrane function give rise to hyperexcitability of the neuron, resulting in repetitive firing of the neuron cell and leading to paralysis. The cyclodienes and lindane also are neurotoxins with slightly different mechanisms of action, however. These involve among others antagonism to the action of the inhibitory neurotransmitter GABA.

As already stated the organochlorines are *contact insecticides*, meaning that they are absorbed over the body surface of the insect. The compounds are strongly lipophilic and therefore they pass easily through the chitin surface (exoskeleton) of insects, which also is very lipophilic. This, together with the fact that insects in general are small and therefore have a high surface area in

---

Box 20.1. The identity of a pesticide (what is DDT?)

All chemical compounds contain impurities. Therefore, it is of major importance that the quality used in assays for toxicity is the same as the quality used in preparations marketed. This is as true for pesticides as it is for all other compounds in use and which can enter the food chain, another example being food additives. Most lay people today would probably think that when we say 'mankind has used DDT as an insecticide for decades', we are talking about a near to 100% pure quality. This was not the case. The WHO specification for technical DDT intended for use in public health programmes required that the product contain a minimum of 70% p,p'-DDT. A typical sample analysed when DDT was used in greater amounts actually had a composition as follows: 77.1% p,p'-DDT, 14.9% o,p'-DDT, 0.3% p,p'-TDE, 0.1% o,p'-TDE, 4.0% p,p'-DDE, 0.1% o,p'-DDE and 3.5% unidentified products.

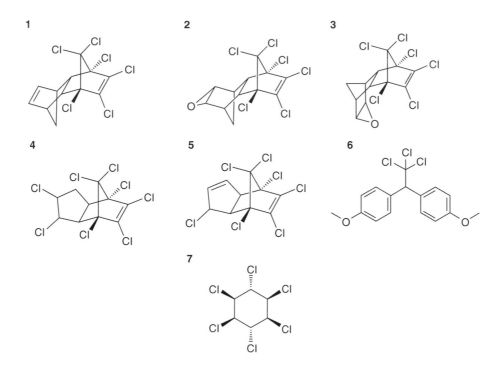

Fig. 20.3. Structural formula of some organochlorine insecticides: **1**, aldrin; **2**, dieledrin; **3**, endrin; **4**, chlordane; **5**, heptachlor; **6**, methoxychlor; **7**, lindane.

Table 20.1. Interspecies difference in LD_{50} to DDT and dieldrin by various routes (in mg kg^{-1} BW). Data extracted from ChemIDplus Dictionary.[1]

	DDT			Dieldrin		
Species	Oral LD_{50}	Cutaneous LD_{50}	Ratio cutaneous:oral	Oral LD_{50}	Cutaneous LD_{50}	Ratio cutaneous:oral
Cat	250	–		500	750	1.5
Dog	150	–		65	–	
Goat	300	–		–	–	
Guinea pig	150	1000	6.7	49	–	
Hamster	5000	–		60	–	
Monkey	200	–		3	–	
Mouse	135	–		38	–	
Rabbit	250	300	1.2	45	250	5.6
Rat	87	1931	22.2	38	56	1.5

relation to their body weight, means that a high concentration can easily and rapidly build up in the nervous system of the insect leading to paralysis. In most other animals – including man – the major fraction of the compounds will be distributed rapidly to the adipose tissue, where they are biologically inactive, thereby reducing the risk of an immediate (acute) toxic manifestation. Mobilization of body fat due to disease, fasting or extensive breast-feeding will lead to redistribution of the compounds and may give rise to serum values that result in toxic effects and/or to excretion into breast milk. The clinical signs of organochlorine poisoning are referable to the nervous system.

Chapter 20

Early signs are salivation, nausea and vomiting. Behavioural changes may be seen, as may disturbances in sensation and equilibrium. High exposure causes convulsions and coma. Fatal ventricular arrhythmias can occur.

On the basis of animal studies, in 1991 IARC classified DDT as possibly carcinogenic to man (Group 2B), i.e. there is inadequate evidence in humans for the carcinogenicity of DDT while there is sufficient evidence in experimental animals. This is a classification that is disputed, however. Several authors state that a missing link between heavy occupational long-time exposure – as occurred for a vast number of workers in the production and use of DDT – and cancer speaks against any such risk to mankind. However, in 2001 Suzanne Snedeker PhD, Research Project Leader of the Breast Cancer and Environmental Risk Factors Program (BCERF) at Cornell University, USA, concluded that more studies are needed to evaluate the cancer risk of those persons who were exposed to DDT through their occupations.

Stability, fate and environmental effects of organochlorine pesticides

At the beginning of the 1960s Dennis Puleston, an American amateur ornithologist, reported that the number of big birds of prey around Long Island was greatly reduced. During the same period Rachel Carson published her book *Silent Spring* about the reduction in the number of songbirds. This led to scientific investigations which showed deformities and broken (thin-shelled) eggs within the population of fish eagles at Long Island. Further investigations showed the occurrence of DDT and its metabolites in the eggs. By 1970 DDT was abandoned in the State of New York and by 1972 in the whole of the USA. Europe gradually followed.

Follow-up investigations to these incidents disclosed that DDT, some of its impurities and metabolites (DDD and DDE, the latter formed – among other pathways – in the soil both by pure chemical and microbiologically facilitated reactions) and other polychlorinated insecticides show relative low volatilities, are chemically very stable and are lipophilic at the same time. These characteristics lead to their bioaccumulation in animals through bioconcentration (uptake from surrounding medium) and/or biomagnification (uptake from food) as well as to their ecological magnification, i.e. an increase in their concentration through a food chain or food web by transfer from a lower to a higher trophic level.

During the last few decades DDT, methoxychlor and some of the other organochlorine insecticides such as dieldrin have been demonstrated to possess hormone-like activities, which have been associated with the feminization of male alligators in the aquatic US environment among other effects. This has led to discussions of whether these compounds have a role in the decline of sperm counts in man, a decline that most scientists today seem to accept as a fact demonstrated in various environments around the world.

Subsequent studies have revealed that not only most of the organochlorine insecticides but also other highly chlorinated/halogenated compounds, such as the dioxins, are very stable and therefore persistent in the environment.

This knowledge, together with negative experiences with early non-biodegradable sulfonates used as anionic surfactants (detergents) in the household, is the part of the background for our present rules concerning the approval of new pesticides as well as chemicals for other uses. These include compulsory tests for biodegradability and lipophilicity, the latter among others by measuring the octanol–water partition coefficient.

Organochlorine pesticides and food

Nowadays most organochlorine insecticides are banned worldwide. This is due to their persistence in the environment as discussed above. However, DDT still is seen by WHO and other experts as a non-displaceable factor in the combat against certain vector-borne diseases such as malaria in certain regions of the world. Thus, a very restricted use is still occurring.

Despite the ban several decades ago, we still find DDT, DDT impurities, DDT degradation products and other organochlorine pesticides in a number of different food commodities worldwide. This is due to the earlier very intensive use, their already discussed persistence and the fact that at least some of these compounds, among others DDT, undergo a global transfer. That is, DDT shows partitioning into the atmosphere from land and water by being volatized in hot climate zones; the compound vapour is then moved by the wind to low-temperature zones where it condenses and is deposited on to water and soil, even if never used before in the region.

National and international environmental and food authorities still analyse for the occurrence of organochlorine pesticides. Intensive survey programmes are still ongoing worldwide for the concentrations of these compounds in human breast milk. An example of developments in the levels of organochlorines in fish products is seen in Fig. 20.4, which shows a significant decline in the total content of DDT in cod liver from 1988 to the mid-1990s and then almost steady-state conditions. Within the region investigated, i.e. waters around the Scandinavian and Baltic countries, the highest concentrations were found in cod liver from the Baltic Sea and the lowest in cod liver from Skagerrak.

Organophosphate and carbamate insecticides

As the organochlorines were gradually phased out as insecticides and acaricides, new compounds were sought. The first mass-produced agents belonged to the group of so-called *organophosphates* (OPs), i.e. insecticides derived from esters of phosphoric acid. These agents produce their biological action by blocking the nervous tissue enzyme acetylcholinesterase (AChE) in ganglia and in the parasympathetic nervous system. Under normal physiological conditions AChE hydrolyses the neurotransmitter acetylcholine (ACh). However, when this activity is inhibited, ACh accumulates at nerve endings in the synaptic cleft and at effector organs such as glands

and muscle endplates (Fig. 20.5), causing persistent and uncoordinated ACh stimulation.

This kills insects. In man, husbandry and wildlife it causes toxic symptoms such as increased glandular secretions with salivation, excessive bronchial secretion, lacrimation and sweating, increased tonicity of smooth muscles with bronchospasms, miosis, abdominal cramps, and involuntary defecation and urination, supplemented with cardiac effects including bradycardia. All of these symptoms are due to stimulation of muscarinic ACh receptors and are sometimes referred to as the SLUD syndrome (salivation, lacrimation, urination, defecation). The simultaneously occurring stimulation of nicotinic receptors is targeted to the muscle endplate, the sympathetic ganglia and the adrenal medulla, resulting in muscle fasciculations (twitching) and cramps leading to flaccid paralysis with reduced tendinous reflexes. The latter is life-threatening when the diaphragm and respiratory muscles are affected.

While the number of acute fatal intoxications among humans and higher animals was indeed low during the period when the organochlorines were used, this cannot be said for the still very intensively used OPs. The estimated total number of human intoxications with OPs worldwide was 300,000 per annum, and the number of deaths was 30,000 per annum, according to WHO statistics published in 1990. These include accidental poisonings in a work situation and ingested compounds used in committing suicide. Also poisonings did and do occur among wildlife (Fig. 20.6).

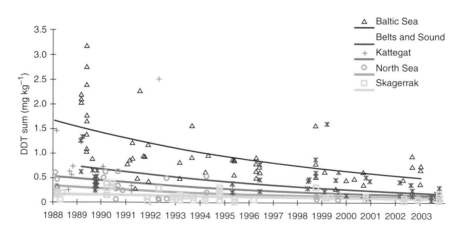

Fig. 20.4. DDT in cod liver from Danish waters, 1988–2003. With permission from the Ministry of Food, Agriculture and Fisheries, Danish Veterinary and Food Administration. Adapted from Fromberg *et al.* (2003).[2]

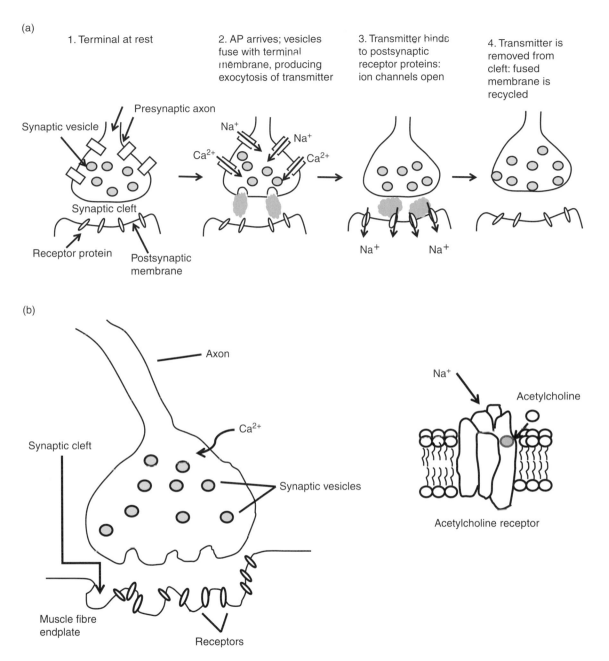

(a)

1. Terminal at rest

2. AP arrives; vesicles fuse with terminal membrane, producing exocytosis of transmitter

3. Transmitter binds to postsynaptic receptor proteins: ion channels open

4. Transmitter is removed from cleft: fused membrane is recycled

Presynaptic axon

Synaptic vesicle

Na$^+$

Na$^+$

Ca^{2+}

Ca^{2+}

Synaptic cleft

Na$^+$

Na$^+$

Receptor protein

Postsynaptic membrane

(b)

Axon

Synaptic cleft

Ca^{2+}

Synaptic vesicles

Na$^+$

Acetylcholine

Acetylcholine receptor

Muscle fibre endplate

Receptors

Fig. 20.5. (a) The events during a chemical transmission from a pre- to a postsynaptic neuron (AP = activating potential). From Randall *et al.* (1997).[3] (b) Schematic of the neuromuscular junction (left) and the associated acetylcholine receptor channel (right). With permission from Cornell University Press, adapted from Reece (2004).[1]

Let us go back and take a look at the history of development of this group of insecticides (including the carbamates) and the reasons for their intensive use despite their generally high toxicity to man and animals.

Organophosphates and war gases

The first compounds within the group of OPs were synthesized in about 1800 by Lassaigne and

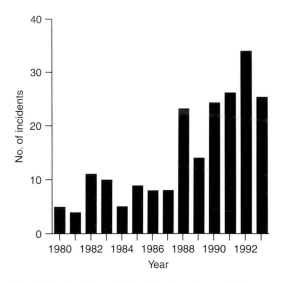

Fig. 20.6. Number of OP and carbamate pesticide-related wildlife mortality incidents; 1980–1993. With permission from the US Geological Survey, adapted from Glacer (1995).[5]

Table 20.2. NATO naming and classification of war gases.

Blood agents	*Vesicants*
Cyanogen chloride: CK	Lewisite: L
Hydrogen cyanide: AC	Sulfur mustard: H, HD, HS, HT
Pulmonary agents	*Incapacitating agents*
Phosgene: CG	Quinuclidinyl benzilate: BZ
Lachrymatory agents	*Nerve agents*
Pepper spray: OC	Sarin: GB
Tear gas: CN, CS, CR	VE, VG, VM

Philip de Clermount. Around 1934 German scientists investigated their potential as insecticides, among them Dr Schrader from the chemical company Bayer AG. He found several to be promising. These findings resulted in the Nazi government abandoning further open research within the field – starting to develop them as war gases instead. Compounds such as tabun, sarin and soman were developed. Sarin is identical to the compound that a Japanese religious sect (Aum Shinrikyo) later used to poison many people in the Tokyo underground. From 1941 the compounds were developed further as insecticides. Following the end of World War II and the founding of the North Atlantic Treaty Organization (NATO) in 1949, most chemical weapons were assigned a one- to three-letter 'NATO weapon designation' in addition to, or in place of, a common name. Some examples including sarin are given in Table 20.2.

TEPP (tetraethylpyrophosphate) developed in 1944 was the first widely used OP insecticide. However, in contrast to the organochlorines, this compound was quite toxic to mammals and had a very short environmental half-life indeed, often being hydrolysed in the presence of water even before it had an opportunity to exert its insecticidal activity. The developmental efforts in the following decades therefore concentrated on two goals: (i) to reduce the acute toxicity to non-target species (keeping the toxicity to insects); and (ii) to make the compounds more stable in the environment.

Parathion (parathion-ethyl) introduced in 1944 soon became a popular insecticide having a somewhat higher environmental stability; however, with a reported LD_{50} in the rat in the range of 3–13 mg kg^{-1} BW, it was (and still is) a problematic compound to work with and to find as a residue in feed and food.

Presently used organophosphates and carbamates

Today more than 100 OPs are used worldwide. Together with the carbamates they make up the group of *AChE inhibitors* developed as insecticides that includes over 200 compounds. OPs are normally esters, thiol esters or anhydride derivatives of phosphoric acid. In TEPP and the war gases the double-bonded atom at the phosphorus is oxygen. However, most of these so-called *oxons* in general are very acutely toxic to mammals since they immediately can inhibit the cholinesterase as a result of the last step in the reaction sequence shown in Fig. 20.7. Parathion-ethyl was the first S-substituted compound (named *phosphorothioates* or earlier *thiophosphates*), where a sulfur atom is double-bonded to phosphorus. These compounds are usually very weak inhibitors and can be compared to pro-drugs that require metabolic activation to the ultimate active compounds, the corresponding oxons. Today, most OPs used as insecticides are S-substituted with the general structure shown in Fig. 20.7 (which also illustrates the activation and enzyme inhibition):

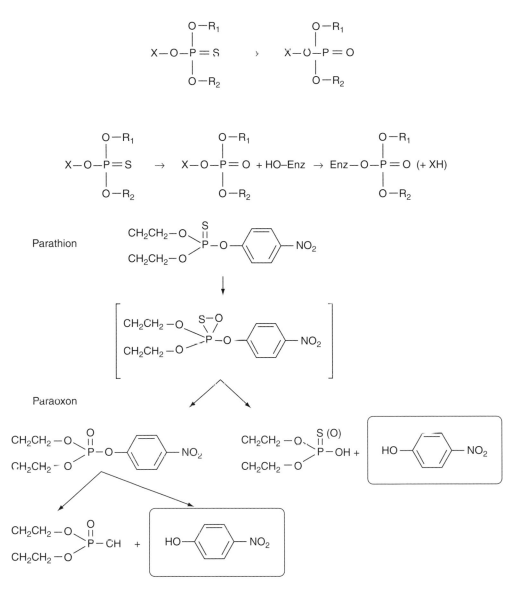

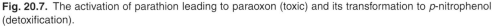

Fig. 20.7. The activation of parathion leading to paraoxon (toxic) and its transformation to *p*-nitrophenol (detoxification).

The activation of the S-substituted compounds is a cytochrome P450-catalysed oxidative desulfuration. This takes place in mammals, e.g. in the liver, as well in insects. However, while mammals can rapidly hydrolyse the newly formed toxic oxon to a non-toxic agent (Fig. 20.7), insects cannot. In this way a certain selectivity of the S-substituted OPs to insects as their target group as opposed to mammals is obtained. For the great majority of the OPs,

R$_1$ and R$_2$ comprise either two methyl groups or two ethyl groups while the leaving group X varies and determines the toxicity to mammals and insects (Table 20.3 and Fig. 20.8).

Further selectivity towards insects thus has been obtained by different means as seen for malathion (Table 20.3 and Fig. 20.9), where the leaving group contains two ethyl ester functions which can be hydrolysed by broad-spectrum esterases

---

present in mammals but not in insects. After hydrolytic cleavage of one (or both) of the ethyl ester functions the compound cannot bind to AChE and hence cannot inhibit this essential enzyme in the nerve synapses.

Table 20.3. Examples of common dimethyl and diethyl OPs and their toxicity to mammals.

Insecticide (type/name)	Toxicity (LD$_{50}$ oral for rat, mg kg^{-1} BW)
Dimethyl	
Dichlorvos[a]	56–108
Parathion-methyl	14–24
Fenthion	190–315
Dimethoate	500–600
Malathion	2800
Diethyl	
Chlorfenvinphos[a]	10–40
Parathion-ethyl	3–13
Triazophos	57–68
Chlorpyrifos	135–165
Diazinon	300–400

[a]Oxons.

The binding of the OPs to AChE that results in its inhibition is to a serine residue at amino acid 203 in the enzyme's active site. The phosphorylated enzyme is spontaneously reactivated, but at a much slower rate than normal after the binding of the natural substrate ACh. Depending on the nature of the two remaining substituents R$_1$ and R$_2$, a so-called *ageing process* with loss of an alkoxy group and formation of a negatively charged phosphorus-containing moiety bound to the enzyme may also occur. The fraction of AChE for which this takes place cannot be reactivated.

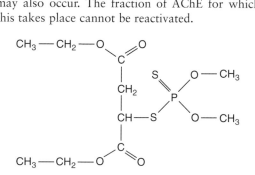

Fig 20.9. Malathion.

OP insectides

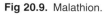

Parathion-ethyl

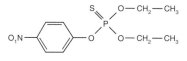

Chlorpyrifos

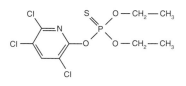

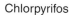
Diazinon

Phenylmethylcarbamate insecticides

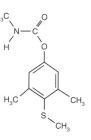

Methiocarb
(= mercaptodimethur)

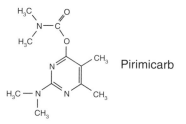
Pirimicarb

Fig. 20.8. Examples of S-substituted OP and carbamate insecticides.

In mammals OPs also inhibit other serine hydrolases, of which a variety exists. Thus, chymotrypsin and trypsin, carboxylesterases (EC 3.1.1.1), plasma pseudocholinesterase (butylcholinesterase (BChE); EC 3.1.1.8) and the so-called neuropathy target esterase (NTE) to some extent are inhibited by covalent binding to a serine residue in the catalytic site. However, OPs exert their acute toxic actions primarily by interfering with cholinergic transmission.

In addition to the acute toxic effects described, some OPs also may give rise to a condition called *intermediate syndrome* and to *organophosphate-induced delayed neurotoxicity* (OPIDN). Intermediate syndrome is a paralytic condition affecting the cranial nerves and caused by such compounds as fenthion and dimethoate among others. OPIDN has been seen after exposure to the insecticide leptophos and reflects damage to the afferent fibres of the peripheral and central nerves, related to inhibition of the aforementioned esterase NTE. The victims face weakness or paralysis and paraesthesia of the legs. The observation of OPIDN has led to the development of special assays to determine whether a compound (an OP) can be expected to cause this syndrome, i.e. the two EU standardized assays 'B.37: Delayed neurotoxicity of organophosphorous substances following acute exposure' and 'B.38: Delayed neurotoxicity of organophosphorous substances 28 day repeated dose study'.

Before we move on to the carbamates it should be mentioned that a commercial preparation of an S-substituted OP insecticide may contain a percentage of the immediately toxic oxon formed by auto-oxidation of the parent compound, thus making the preparation more dangerous in use.

The first commercially available *carbamate* was Sevin® (carbaryl, 1-naphthyl N-methylcarbamate), the structure of which is shown in Fig. 20.10. Carbaryl was discovered and introduced commercially in 1958 by Union Carbide, now a part of Bayer AG.

Comparing this with the structures of two other carbamates, methiocarb and pirimicarb, shown in Fig. 20.8, we can recognize that the carbamate insecticides – another important group that also acts as AChE inhibitors – are carbamate esters with the following general structure:

R–O–C(O)–NHCH$_3$

The plant alkaloid *physostigmine* was the model compound for the synthesis of the carbamate pesticides (Box 20.2). The carbamates also react with serine 203 of AChE, which is then carbamylated instead of being phosphorylated as seen for the OPs. The result

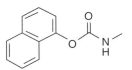

Fig. 20.10. Carbaryl.

is an inhibited enzyme which is, however, subject to rapid hydrolysis and thereby reactivation in mammals. Moreover the carbamylated enzyme is not subject to ageing, the reaction that leads to irreversible inhibition with the OPs. Because of these two differences in the chain of reactions occurring between the carbamates and AChE in the ganglia and at the effector sites it was originally anticipated that carbamates would be less toxic to humans than OP insecticides. Indeed, Sevin showed a relatively low acute toxicity, the LD$_{50}$ being reported as about 250 mg kg^{-1} BW for the rat by the oral route. However, many of the compounds that followed were much more toxic, as shown in Table 20.4 comparing the toxicity of selected carbamates and OPs towards different bird species. Note that large interspecies differences are also seen.

Pyrethrins and synthetic pyrethroids

As already discussed, the natural pyrethrins from the daisy-like flower *T. cinerariifolium* (Trevir.) Schultz-Bip. are non-persistent insecticides of low toxicity to mammals. Chemically the pyrethrins can be divided into two groups (I and II). Both consist of esters of an organic acid containing a 3-carbon ring structure, namely chrysanthemic acid and pyrethric acid, respectively, which in turn are esterified.

Pyrethrin I (and its group members) is the most active ingredient(s) for lethality, while pyrethrin II possesses remarkable knockdown properties for a wide range of household, veterinary and post-harvest storage insects. The natural pyrethrins and early synthetic chrysanthemic acid derivatives are more active as contact poisons than as stomach poisons; this is in contrast to the more recently synthesized agents, which show particular potency when ingested and are less susceptible to biotransformation by insects and mammals.

The genuine plant pyrethrins are still used in sprays indoors for the combat of, for example, houseflies. Here they are normally combined with either piperonyl butoxide or N-octylbicycloheptene dicarboximide. These compounds act as synergists

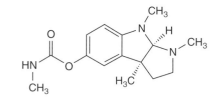
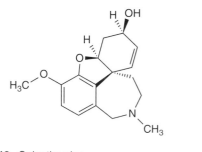
Table 20.4. Toxicity to birds of carbamate and OP pesticides.

Pesticide (class/compound)	Species approximate LD$_{50}$ (mg kg^{-1} BW)		
	Mallard duck	Ring-necked pheasant	Red-winged blackbird
Carbamate			
Aldicarb	3	5	2
Carbaryl	>2000	700	50
Carbofuran	0.5	4	0.5
Methiocarb	15	300	5
OP			
Azinphos-methyl	140	75	10
Dimethoate	40	20	7
Ethion	>2000	1300	50
Phorate	0.5	7	1
Temephos	80	35	40

by inhibiting the mixed-function oxidases of the insects, the enzymes which normally detoxify the pyrethrins in the target organism. The inhibition results in a ten to 20 times increase of the insecticidal activity of the pyrethrins.

Pyrethrins are non-persistent first of all because they are unstable in sunlight. Based on information gained from the isolation and structural elucidation

of the single pyrethrins, a research group led by M. Elliott at the Rothamsted Research in Hertfordshire, UK (Box 20.3) developed the first generation of analogues by synthesis or semi-synthesis, the so-called *pyrethroids*, during the 1960s. This group includes among others allethrin and resmethrin (Fig. 20.13). Resmethrin, as an example, was introduced to the North American market in 1967.

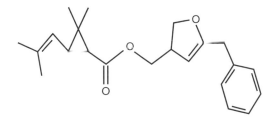

Fig. 20.13. Resmethrin.

Like several other pyrethroids, resmethrin is a mixture of *isomers*. Isomers are molecules made up of the same atoms, joined together in the same sequence, but with different three-dimensional arrangements. One of the isomers of resmethrin is more active insecticidally than the other three. This isomer, called 'bioresmethrin', was introduced separately on the market as an insecticide.

Box 20.3. The history of Rothamsted

Rothamsted is believed to be the oldest agricultural research station in the world. It was founded in 1843 when John Bennet Lawes (Fig. 20.14), the owner of the Rothamsted Estate, appointed Joseph Henry Gilbert, a chemist, as his scientific collaborator. In his youth Lawes had gained an interest in the effect of fertilizers on crop growth. Therefore, he started the first factory for the manufacture of artificial fertilizers in 1842, and in the following year – assisted by Gilbert – he initiated the first of a series of long-term field experiments, some of which continue to this day. The main objective of these experiments is to measure the effect on crop yields of inorganic and organic fertilizers. The collaboration between Lawes and Gilbert lasted 57 years, and it seems fair to say that together they laid the foundations of modern scientific agriculture and established the principles of crop nutrition.

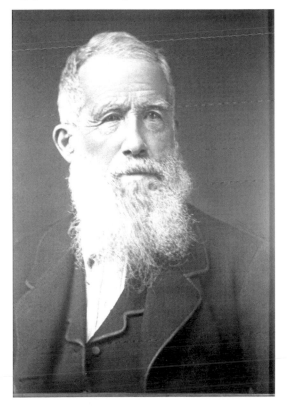

Fig. 20.14. Sir John Lawes. (Copyright Rothamsted Research.)

The introduction of the first pyrethroids was quite timely, considering the persistence problems of the organochlorines and the relatively high toxicity to mammals of the first OP insecticides. This is probably why they quite rapidly increased their market share. Gradually both Rothamsted and a number of industrial players developed new compounds. The aims during the development included higher stability, higher insecticidal effect, and less irritant effect to the skin of man and higher animals than seen for first-generation compounds.

Generally, the pyrethroids evolved from the natural compounds by successive modifications and became a new important class of crop protection chemicals. An example of the structural differences and similarities between the natural and synthetic compounds is shown in Fig. 20.15, where the naturally occurring pyrethrin II is compared with the synthetic permethrin. The pyrethroids really entered the marketplace in 1980 and by 1982 they already accounted for approximately 30% of the worldwide insecticide usage, also within veterinary medicine.

Most of the research to investigate the mechanism(s) by which pyrethroids elicit their effects has been conducted *in vitro* using the cockroach, crayfish or squid giant axon preparations. Pyrethrins and pyrethroids exert their effect primarily by modulating gating kinetics of sodium channels in nerves. This action results in either repetitive discharges or membrane depolarization and subsequent death of the target arthropod. Type I pyrethroid esters affect sodium channels in nerve membranes, causing repetitive (sensory and motor) neuronal discharge and a prolonged negative after-potential, the effects being quite similar to those produced by DDT, i.e. they produce an increase in the time constant for sodium current inactivation. Type II pyrethroids extend the time constant for inactivation by hundreds of milliseconds (to seconds), thereby giving rise to a persistent depolarization.

Pyrethrins and pyrethroids in general are low in toxicity to mammals; the range between the toxicity to insects as compared with mammals is about 1000-fold. This is due among other factors to rapid metabolism by esterases in the mammals. However, they are quite toxic to fish and a number of water-living insects. Also, resmethrin (with added piperonyl butoxide) was shown to kill the red swamp crayfish (*Procambarus clarkii*) – a freshwater crustacean (resembling a small lobster) that is produced in great quantities in the USA – at a concentration of 0.8 ppb, which is only about 7% of the concentration needed to kill mosquitoes. Another characteristic for this group of compounds is that they are more effective towards insects at low temperatures.

The pyrethroids can be divided into at least four generations. The first generation is represented by allethrin and the second by tetramethrin, bioresmethrin, bioallethrin and phenothrin. They are more potent than pyrethrum in knockdown potency but decompose rapidly on exposure to sunlight. The third generation is more potent and even more photostable, as represented by fenvalate and permethrin. The fourth-generation compounds such as cypermethrin, flucythrinate and fluvalinate are up to ten times as potent and *very persistent* in the environment. Unfortunately this makes them favour the development of resistance.

In conclusion, today we have a large number of OPs as well as carbamates in use as insecticides in the different agricultural and horticultural sectors producing commodities for the feed and food industry. While this gives good possibilities for plant protection schemes targeted to the specific conditions, it also results in a need for a very powerful analytical setup (with regard to selectivity as well as sensitivity) at the regulatory authorities to analyse for residues. When adding the group of pyrethroids just discussed, the pallet of compounds becomes even wider.

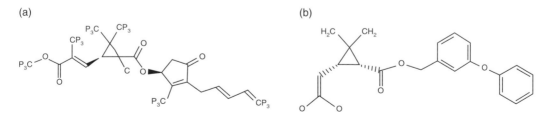

Fig. 20.15. Pyrethrins and pyrethroids: (a) pyrethrin II; (b) permethrin.

20.3 Herbicides and Fungicides

To produce an insecticide that is non-toxic to man is difficult since basically we are not that different from the insects, mites and ticks that we want to kill. This was clearly demonstrated in the previous section. When it comes to killing plants and fungi, however, things look different. Both types of organism possess a number of characteristics with respect to anatomy (overall and cellular), physiology and biochemistry that differ from the animal organism and hence can be used as targets for the development of pesticidal compounds that kill plants or fungi specifically. This also means that, at least with regard to acute toxicity, we must expect the groups of herbicides and fungicides to be less problematic for man, his husbandry and wildlife. When it come to adverse effects of chronic exposure or to possible carcinogenicity things can be different, however.

Herbicides

A *herbicide* is a chemical compound that kills weeds. *Non-selective herbicides* may be used to kill all vegetation before cultivation and planting begin. Once the crop has emerged, *selective herbicides* must be used. These should target the troublesome weeds and leave other weeds and the growing crop unharmed. Some have a residual action in the soil – allowing, for example, weed seedlings to be exposed to the chemicals as they emerge, which then kills them.

Contact herbicides destroy only the plant tissue in contact with the chemical. Generally, these are the fastest-acting herbicides. *Systemic herbicides*, on the other hand, are translocated through the plant from foliar application down to the roots, or from soil application up to the leaves. They can destroy a greater amount of plant tissue. Soil-applied herbicides are applied to the soil and are taken up by the roots of the target plant.

The first herbicide to be used was not only effective, it was even selective in its mode of action, i.e. it could (can) distinguish between monocotyledonous plants (monocots) and dicotyledonous plants (dicots). The agent was sulfuric acid and the reasons for its selectivity can be found in two factors:

- The monocots include among others the grasses, and as such all of the grains. Normally these plants have relatively highly waxed leaves. The dicots include all of the so-called broadleaved plants, whether herbs, bushes or trees. The leaves of these plants normally have a less developed wax layer but most often a leaf-covering hair layer.
- While the sulfuric acid runs off the wax layer of the monocot leaves thereby doing no harm, it sticks to the hairs of the dicot leaves, ultimately causing corrosion of the leaves and killing the plant.

Sulfuric acid never became a widely used herbicide for many reasons, so let us turn to the earliest synthetic organic compounds used as herbicides. These were the so-called *yellow agents*, such as DNOC (4,6-dinitro-o-cresol; Fig. 20.16).

Although these compounds could be used to kill broadleaved weeds in cereals, their overall selectivity was still very limited indeed. Thus, they could be used not only as herbicides, but also as insecticides, acaricides and fungicides. This also meant that the toxicity towards warm-blooded animals was very high (oral LD_{50} in the rat):

- DNOC, 25–40 mg kg^{-1} BW; and
- dinoseb (2,4-dinitro-6-sec-butylphenol; DNBP), 50 mg kg^{-1} BW.

For ruminants the oral doses leading to poisoning with methaemoglobinaemia and intravascular haemolysis for both compounds were to be found in the interval of 2–50 mg kg^{-1} BW.

The compounds inhibit oxidative phosphorylation in the mitochondria of cells. As a contact herbicide, DNOC was used to control broadleaved weeds in cereals and to desiccate potato and leguminous seed crops before harvesting. Since it is strongly phytotoxic for broadleaved plants its use as an insecticide has been limited to dormant sprays, especially for such fruit trees as apples or peaches. In the USA, EPA cancelled the registration of DNOC as a pesticide agent starting in 1991. DNBP, which was a less expensive and more effective herbicide, had already begun to replace DNOC by the late 1980s. Today none of these compounds is registered in the USA or in Europe.

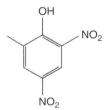

Fig. 20.16. The structure of DNOC.

The second generation of herbicides (after yellow agents) comprised the *chlorophenoxy herbicides*, also termed *hormone agents*. These synthetic organic compounds exert the same effect on the plant cells as the natural plant hormone auxin (= indole-3-acetic acid; IAA). These so-called *auxin herbicides* are more stable in plants than the main natural auxin and show systemic mobility and selective action, preferentially against dicot weeds in cereal crops. Hence, dicots can be eradicated in a field of monocots such as a grain field. Although the finer details of the mechanism behind the phytotoxicity (with selectivity for dicots) have been investigated for decades, it is only recently that we have begun to get some understanding (which, however, will not be dealt with here). The first compound within this group was 2,4,5-T (2,4,5-trichlorophenoxyacetic acid). Developed in the late 1940s the compound was found to be effective in defoliating broadleaved plants. The compound seemed to be more or less an ideal herbicide since the acute toxicity to mammals (including man) was low, with an oral LD_{50} of about 400 mg kg^{-1} BW in mice and 500 mg kg^{-1} BW in rats. Soon 2,4,5-T was used extensively in the USA. New compounds within the same group were gradually marketed such as 2,4-dichlorophenoxyacetic acid (2,4-D), 2-methyl-4-chlorophenoxyacetic acid (MCPA) and dichlorprop (Fig. 20.17). The latter, which possesses an asymmetric carbon and is therefore a chiral molecule, appeared on the market in 1960s. Initially it was sold as a racemic mixture of

stereoisomers, but since then advances in asymmetric synthesis have made possible production of the enantiopure compound. Today, only the active *R*-dichlorprop (also called dichlorprop-p or 2,4-DP-p) and its derivatives are sold as pesticides.

The chlorophenoxy compounds soon became very popular around the world. However, in 1961 the US military took to using 2,4,5-T in the Vietnam war. A product called *agent orange* (a mixture of equal amounts of 2,4,5-T and 2,4-D) was sprayed from aircrafts over the jungle in order to remove the leaves of the trees to better be able to identify Vietnamese Vietcong partisans and possibly North Vietnamese soldiers from the air. The US military herbicide programme in South Vietnam took place between 1961 and 1971. Herbicides were sprayed in all four military zones of Vietnam. More than 19 million gallons of various herbicide combinations were used.

After some years it was recognized that synthetic 2,4,5-T contained a number of impurities from the syntheses, compounds that gradually were revealed to be very toxic indeed to certain animal species such as the guinea pig. We are talking here about the so-called *dioxins*. The dioxins are a group of compounds with a basic skeleton structure of dibenzo-*p*-dioxin (two benzene rings joined by two oxygen bridges). The most toxic members of this family of chemical compounds are those with a high degree of chlorination, such as TCDD (2,3,7,8-tetrachlorodibenzodioxin). Also compounds from

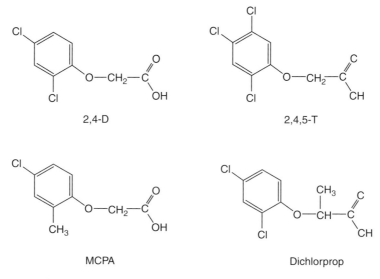

Fig. 20.17. The structures of selected chlorophenoxy herbicides.

the group of *dibenzofurans* (which contain two benzene rings fused to one furan ring in the middle) are counted when we talk about dioxins generally in a toxicological context.

Gradually the chemical companies learnt to control the syntheses in such a way that the formation of dioxins and dibenzofurans was minimized. Also a shift to some different members of the synthetic auxins (other than 2,4,5-T) meant a reduction in the toxic risk, since impurities other than TCDD were formed. In a number of European countries 2,4,5-T was never approved. However, huge amounts of, for example, 2,4-D were used in the 1980s and 1990s. After having solved the problems with the dioxin impurities these herbicides were regarded as just about perfect.

Nevertheless, at the end of the 1990s these compounds were found more and more frequently in groundwater, e.g. in European countries such as Denmark. Prior to this a number of evaluations based on models of soil composition and structure had denied that this could happen. In many countries most of the compounds were now required to go through a new process of approval, resulting in several of the compounds being abandoned. However, MCPA stayed in common use.

In 1970 USDA halted the use of 2,4,5-T on all food crops except rice, and in 1985 EPA terminated all remaining uses of this herbicide in the USA. The international trade of 2,4,5-T is restricted by the Rotterdam Convention, which covers pesticides and industrial chemicals that have been banned or severely restricted for health or environmental reasons.

Examples of herbicides taking over after a reduction in use of the chlorophenoxy herbicides include dicamba, triclopyr, prosulfocarb and glyphosate (Fig. 20.18). As an example from Europe, the Danish registered use of herbicides in 2006 amounted to 2500 t of which 42% was glyphosate followed by prosulfocarb (22%) and MCPA (12%).

Dicamba, a benzoic acid herbicide which can be applied to leaves or soil, controls annual and perennial broadleaved weeds in grain crops and grasslands, and brush and bracken in pastures. It will kill broadleaved weeds before and after they sprout. Legumes are also killed by dicamba. In combination with a phenoxyalkanoic acid or other herbicide, dicamba is used in pastures, rangeland and non-crop areas (fence-rows, roadways and wastage) to control weeds. The reported oral LD_{50} for dicamba in the rat ranges from about 750 to 1700 mg kg^{-1} BW. However, dicamba is very irritating and corrosive and can cause severe and permanent damage to the eyes.

Triclopyr is a systemic, foliar herbicide. It is used to control broadleaved weeds while leaving grasses and conifers unaffected. The oral LD_{50} of triclopyr in rats is about 700 mg kg^{-1} BW.

Prosulfocarb has low acute oral toxicity in the rat (LD_{50} = 1820 mg kg^{-1} BW in males and 1958 mg kg^{-1} BW in females). The compound was re-evaluated in the EU in 2007, which resulted in the approval of an ADI of 0.005 mg kg^{-1} BW.

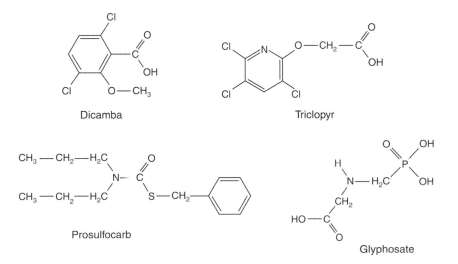

Fig. 20.18. The structures of selected modern herbicides.

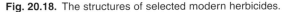

Pesticides and Persistent Organic Pollutants

Glyphosate, N-(phosphonomethyl)glycine, is a broad-spectrum systemic herbicide used to kill weeds, especially perennials. It is absorbed through the leaves, but may also be injected into the trunk, or applied to the stump of a tree. It was patented initially by Monsanto Company in the 1970s under the trade name Roundup®. The US patent expired in 2000. Glyphosate is currently the most used herbicide in the USA, where some 2270–3630 t are used on lawns and yards and 38,500–40,800 t are used in US agriculture annually. The mode of action is to inhibit an enzyme involved in the synthesis of the amino acids tyrosine, tryptophan and phenylalanine. It is absorbed through foliage and translocated to growing points. Because of this mode of action, it is effective only on actively growing plants; it is not effective as a pre-emergence herbicide. The toxicity to mammals is very low indeed with an acute oral LD_{50} for the rat of 5600 mg kg^{-1} BW.

In conclusion, the herbicides we use in our food production have changed from compounds showing an oral LD_{50} to mammals of about 30 mg kg^{-1} BW to compounds which in practice we classify as acutely non-toxic with LD_{50} values ranging from approximately 1000 mg kg^{-1} BW and upwards, to several grams per kilogram of body weight. In most cases relatively few compounds dominate the use.

Fungicides

The presently known fungicidal compounds that have or have had a use as fungicides can be broadly divided into the following four classes when it comes to their mode of action: (i) inhibitors of the electron transport chain; (ii) inhibitors of enzymes; (iii) inhibitors of nucleic acid metabolism and protein synthesis; and (iv) inhibitors of sterol synthesis.

The oldest fungicide in use – sulfur – disrupts electron transport along the cytochromes and has been used as a non-systemic contact and protective fungicide (and acaricide) from long back in time, normally applied as sprays or a dust. It is relatively non-toxic to mammals, but can cause irritation of the skin and mucous membranes. Copper (i.e. Cu^{2+} ions) in the form of the so-called *Bordeaux mixture* (a mixture of copper sulfate with calcium hydroxide) has been used for more 150 years, originally especially in vineyards to control downy mildew. Later it was also used to control fungal diseases in potatoes, apples and hops. Copper acts by causing a non-specific denaturation of proteins and enzymes necessary for the fungus. Both of these fungicidal agents had to be applied to the plant leaves before the attack of the fungus, i.e. they protect the plant by killing the attacking fungus before it has penetrated the plant.

The mercury fungicides – starting with the inorganic salts such as the mercuric and the mercurous chlorides together with mercuric oxide, followed by the metallo-organic compounds such as methylmercury – also acted this way. All mercury compounds have been phased out of use today due to the extreme toxicity of this metal.

Although the fungicides used nowadays in the production of different food commodities in general show low acute as well as chronic toxicity, historically some of the most tragic epidemics of pesticide poisoning were due to fungicides. Mostly they occurred because of mistaken consumption of seed grain treated with such fungicidal compounds as organic mercury or hexachlorobenzene (HCB). For example, close to 4000 people in south-east Anatolia (Turkey) developed porphyria during 1955–1959 due to long-term ingestion of HCB, a fungicide added to wheat seeds. The exposures led to the development of bullae on sun-exposed areas, hyperpigmentation, hypertrichosis and porphyrinuria. The condition was called *kara yara* or *black sore*. Several breast-fed children under the age of 2 years whose mothers had ingested HCB-treated grain died from a disease known as *pembe yara* or *pink sore*. In a follow-up study of 252 patients some 20–30 years after exposure, many had dermatological, neurological and orthopaedic symptoms and signs. In Iraq an outbreak of poisoning happened in the winter of 1971/72 in a rural region where farmers consumed home-made bread made from seed wheat treated with a methylmercury fungicide. Analysis of the flour used gave an estimated amount of 1–4 mg of mercury per loaf of bread. The bread was eaten over a period from 2 weeks to 2 months depending on the family in question. Out of 49 children investigated clinically 2 years after the incident, 40 still had symptoms relating to the nervous system.

Indeed, fungicides that had to be applied prior the attack and that were effective only when present on the plant surface represented the sole means of protecting plants from fungal diseases until the emergence of the first systemic fungicides. These finally started to appear in 1960 as a result of many attempts to develop compounds that were able to enter the plant and consequently could prevent penetration of the fungus from within or kill fungus which had already penetrated. The first systemic fungicide for use in horticulture was the compound triamiphos (Wepsyn®). Within the next approximately 10–15 years this was followed by others such as pyrazophos (Curamil®), dimethirimol (Milcarb®), oxycarboxin (Plant wax®), benomyl (Benlate®) and thiabendazole (Tecto 60®).

The present-day fungicide market is characterized by being very diverse not only with regard to the number of compounds, but also the variation of their basic chemical structures. Major groups include benzimidazoles, dicarboximides, dithiocarbamates, OPs, strobilurins and (tri)azoles. Most fungicides approved today have very low acute toxicity indeed, whether surface active or systemic, and whether belonging to one or the other chemical group:

- Benzimidazoles (e.g. thiophanate-methyl): rat oral LD_{50} = 6640 mg kg^{-1} BW.
- Dicarboximides (e.g. vinclozolin): rat oral LD_{50} > 10,000 mg kg^{-1} BW.
- Dithiocarbamates (e.g. maneb): rat oral LD_{50} = 3000–8000 mg kg^{-1} BW.
- OPs (e.g. fosetyl-Al): rat oral LD_{50} = 5400 mg kg^{-1} BW.

- Strobilurins (e.g. azoxystrobin): rat oral LD_{50} > 5000 mg kg^{-1} BW.
- (Tri)azoles (e.g. tebuconazole): rat oral LD_{50} = 1700 mg kg^{-1} BW.

Now let us look into the possible chemical food safety problems with fungicides in today's production of food commodities. In general fungicides are cytotoxic and many show positive results in one or more *in vitro* mutagenicity tests, a characteristic inherent to this group of biocides. Several chemical classes of fungicide – the imidazoles (imazalil), the triazoles (propiconazole, myclobutanil, tebuconazole, triflumazole) and the morpholines (dimethomorph) – inhibit sterol (ergosterol) production and affect membrane synthesis by inhibiting cytochrome P450 enzymes in the sterol pathways. The process of steroidogenesis seems to be highly conserved throughout living organisms, and indeed several fungicides (fenarimol and prochloraz) inhibit aromatase (converts C19 androgens to aromatic C18 oestrogens) activity in mammals and affect mating behaviour. This being said, most fungicides still seem to pose few problems, the only exception possibly being the *dithiocarbamates* (Fig. 20.19).

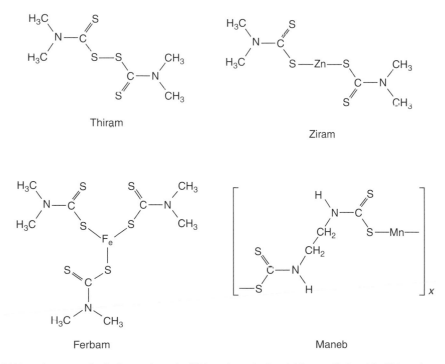

Thiram

Ziram

Ferbam

Maneb

Fig. 20.19. Dithiocarbamates (including polymeric dithiocarbamate fungicides = ethylenebisdithiocarbamates).

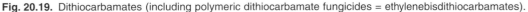

Within the group of dithiocarbamates we find some polymeric fungicides, i.e. the *ethylenebis-dithiocarbamates* (EBDCs), a group of non-systemic (surface-acting) fungicides that includes maneb, mancozeb and metiram. EBCDs are used on a wide range of crops worldwide including potatoes, cereals, apples, pears and leafy vegetables. They control many fungal diseases such as blight, leaf spot, rust, downy mildew and scab. Mancozeb is also used for seed treatment of cotton, potatoes, maize, safflower, sorghum, groundnuts, tomatoes, flax and cereal grains. Degradation of these compounds will, on the plant at the field as well as during processing, give rise to the formation of the metabolite ethylenethiourea (ETU). According to a report from the US EPA from 2002, there is sufficient evidence that three dithiocarbamates – maneb, mancozeb and metiram – can induce a common effect (thyroid cancer) by the formation of the common metabolite, ETU. These three chemicals should be grouped, as in the past, when conducting a risk assessment. When measuring actual residues most authorities today also analyse for ETU.

The industrial development of new fungicides has resulted in a wide range of structural classes being used, representing both surface-active compounds and systemically acting agents which are taken up by the plant.

20.4 Persistent Organic Pollutants and Synthetic Environmental Endocrine Disrupters

Chemical contaminants in food may consist of elements (e.g. metals) or different organic molecules. The latter can be present as a result of, for example, fungal activity (mycotoxins), application of pesticides or use of veterinary drugs directly in production of the food commodity, or they may come from the environment. In the latter case especially compounds that are not easily degraded and maybe even (in addition) possess characteristics that favour their accumulation in living organisms, such as being easily absorbed after ingestion or being lipophilic and hence stored in metabolically less active tissues, are of major concern. Overall we often group such compounds under the designation POPs (*persistent organic pollutants*).

POPs thus are organic compounds that are resistant to environmental degradation through chemical, biological and photolytic processes. Therefore, they also are capable of long-range transport, and hence can bioaccumulate in animal and human tissues and biomagnify in food chains to be found in high concentrations even far away from their place of origin.

We have already touched upon some POPs. Thus, several of the earlier used chlorinated pesticides including DDT belong to this group. In 1995, the United Nations Environment Programme Governing Council (GC) began an investigation into POPs, starting with a shortlist comprising the following 12 compounds, known as the 'dirty dozen': aldrin, chlordane, DDT, dieldrin, endrin, heptachlor, hexachlorobenzene, mirex, polychlorinated biphenyls, polychlorinated dibenzo-*p*-dioxins, polychlorinated dibenzofurans and toxaphene.

Of these 12 compounds two should be defined further, i.e. mirex and toxaphene (Fig. 20.20). Mirex is a chlorinated hydrocarbon commercialized as an insecticide and later banned because of its impact on the environment. It was popularized to control fire ants but by virtue of its chemical robustness and lipophilicity it was soon recognized as a bioaccumulative pollutant. The US EPA prohibited its use in 1976. Also, toxaphene is an insecticide which, from 1947 to 1980, was used primarily in the southern USA on cotton crops. Today widespread use of toxaphene has been banned in the USA.

Separately from the emerging focus on POPs, interest was additionally aroused in the so-called *environmental oestrogens* (and *anti-androgens*) – also grouped together as endocrine disrupters. To some extent the two groups proved to overlap, which is why here we treat them together as 'POPs and synthetic environmental endocrine disrupters'. As our focus is on food safety, in the following we concentrate only on POPs, i.e. polychlorinated dibenzo-*p*-dioxins (dioxins) and polychlorinated

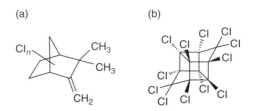

Fig. 20.20. The structures of mirex (a) and toxaphene (b).

dibenzofurans together with PCBs (polychlorinated biphenyls), and supplement with information on nonylphenol.

Dioxins, furans and dioxin-like polychlorinated biphenyls

As already mentioned in the previous section when discussing the chlorophenoxy herbicides, members from the group of dioxins were formed as by-products (synthesis impurities) when synthesizing, for example, the herbicide 2,4,5-T. However, today we know that dioxins are formed in many reactions where organic and chlorine-containing substances (e.g. PVC) are heated (burnt) together, such as in incinerators. This is why many communities presently have strict rules about the temperature at which incinerators should operate, in order to minimize the formation of dioxins.

Strictly taken, dioxins are polychlorinated dibenzo-*p*-dioxins (PCDDs). In the PCDDs, the chlorine atoms are bound at one or more of the eight free places on the molecule, i.e. at positions 1–4 and 6–9. In this way 75 different types of PCDD congener come into existence (Fig. 20.21).

The toxicity of PCDDs depends on the number and positions of the chlorine atoms. Congeners that have chlorines at positions 2, 3, 7 and 8 have been found to possess significant toxicity in a number of contexts. However, in today's risk assessment activities focusing on the toxic potential of these compounds we most often merge them with relevant members of two other groups of chemical, namely the polychlorinated dibenzo-furans (PCDFs) and the so-called dioxin-like PCBs. This is due to the assumption that all 2,3,7,8-substituted PCDDs and PCDFs (Fig. 20.21), as well as the dioxin-like PCBs (Fig. 20.22), have the same mode of action, elicited by binding to the same receptor – the Ah receptor – and show comparable qualitative effects, but with different potencies.

The dioxin-like PCBs include those where chlorines occupy: (i) usually no more than one of the ortho positions; (ii) both *para* positions; (iii) at least two *meta* positions; and where (iv) the structure is not hindered from assuming the preferred planar configuration.

While the PCDFs – like the dioxins – are formed during heating/burning of different organochlorines (including PCBs) and mixed materials with a content of chlorine, the PCBs themselves have quite another origin. The first mixture of PCBs was synthesized in 1881 and later different such mixtures with physical characteristics ranging from light oily substances to greasy and waxy substances were marketed and widely incorporated in a number of products, being used for a range of technical applications. These included the direct use as insulating fluids in the electrical industry, and the use as components in materials and products such as plasticizers, paints, lubricants, insulating tapes, fireproofing materials and hydraulic fluids. PCB production in general was terminated around 1980; however, at that time, more than half a billion kilograms had been produced in the USA alone.

Dioxins

The toxicity of the dioxins has been investigated over several decades with quite astonishing observations gradually being made. First of all, these compounds show a very different acute toxicity depending on the actual number and placement of chlorine atoms. That is, we see a great variation between the 75 different congeners, of which actually only the following seven are classified today as being toxic: 2,3,7,8-TCDD, 1,2,3,7, 8-PeCDD, 1,2,3,4,7,8-HxCDD, 1,2,3,6,7,8-Hx-CDD, 1,2,3,7,8,9-HxCDD, 1,2,3,4,6,7,8-HpCDD and 1,2,3,4,6,7,8,9-OCDD (where T = tetra, Pe = penta, Hx = hexa and O = octa).

Second, it soon became clear that for the most acutely toxic compound (TCDD) the species

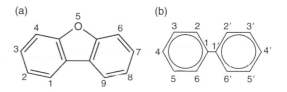

Fig. 20.22. Basic structure of (a) dibenzofuran (the skeleton of the PCDFs) and (b) biphenyl (the skeleton of the PCBs).

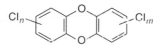

Fig. 20.21. General structure of PCDDs where *n* and *m* can range from 0 to 4.

difference is indeed enormous. Thus, the oral LD_{50} values (Table 20.5) reported for a number of species vary from approximately $0.5\,\mu g\,kg^{-1}$ BW for the guinea pig to about $1\,mg\,kg^{-1}$ BW for the frog and hamster. This corresponds to a factor of 2000 between the most and the least sensitive species. Compared with the default factor of 10 normally used in risk assessment to reflect species differences, this clearly is exceptional.

The high acute toxicity of TCDD and some other dioxins to a number of animal species prompted a great fear of these compounds, which of course led to much research as well as prompting attempts to regulate this area. Then the Seveso accident happened.

The 10th of July 1976 became a fatal day for the Italian town of Seveso, 15 miles from Milan. On that day the local chemical company Icmesa was struck by an accident. The alkaline hydrolysis of 1,2,3,4-tetrachlorobenzene to produce 2,4,5-T, to be used in the manufacture of herbicides, ran out of control. Overheating resulted in the formation of dioxins and when a valve broke a little after noon that Saturday, close to 3000 kg of the reaction mixture was released into the air and spread over an area of about 1800 ha. The amount of dioxins involved is still not known, but has been estimated to be anywhere from about 100 g to 20 kg, or even more according to some sources. Three days afterwards dead animals were found among the wild fauna and soon approximately 5% of local farm animals also died. The rest, about 80,000 animals, were killed to prevent contamination of the food chain.

The authorities divided the area around the chemical plant into three zones depending on the concentration of dioxins in the topsoil. In zone A (87 ha) the average concentration was

Table 20.5. The acute toxicity measured as LD_{50} of TCDD for different species.

Species	LD_{50}
Chicken	$25\,\mu g\,kg^{-1}$ BW ($0.025\,mg\,kg^{-1}$ BW)
Dog	$1\,\mu g\,kg^{-1}$ BW ($0.001\,mg\,kg^{-1}$ BW)
Frog	$1\,mg\,kg^{-1}$ BW
Guinea pig	$500\,ng\,kg^{-1}$ BW ($0.0005\,mg\,kg^{-1}$ BW)
Hamster	$1157\,\mu g\,kg^{-1}$ BW ($1.157\,mg\,kg^{-1}$ BW)
Mouse	$114\,\mu g\,kg^{-1}$ BW ($0.114\,mg\,kg^{-1}$ BW)
Rabbit	$115\,\mu g\,kg^{-1}$ BW ($0.115\,mg\,kg^{-1}$ BW)
Rat	$20\,\mu g\,kg^{-1}$ BW ($0.02\,mg\,kg^{-1}$ BW)

$235\,mg\,m^{-2}$ with a maximum of approximately $5500\,mg\,m^{-2}$. In this zone a quarter of the animals died immediately. Zone B (269 ha) showed an average of $3\,mg\,m^{-2}$ with a maximum of $50\,mg\,m^{-2}$. Zone C had sporadic contamination of up to about $5\,mg\,m^{-2}$. A total of 36,000 inhabitants were evacuated from the area 2 weeks after the incident. Strikingly, no people died, only animals. The only symptom that was seen was chloracne, a severe skin rash. Out of 1300 exposed children, 1046 were hit by this effect. The blood dioxin concentration in the exposed victims as measured in 1976 ranged from 200 to 10,000 times higher than that of normal unexposed Italians. No strict correlation was found between blood dioxin concentrations and the occurrence/severity of chloracne.

The fact that no people died in Seveso and that only chloracne was observed as an acute effect, together with similar observations from exposures involving hundreds of workers at different industrial plants worldwide, led to the conclusion that man is less sensitive to the acute toxicity of dioxins than most animals. It also prompted discussions about whether dioxins actually represented a threat to humans at all in the longer perspective.

Today we know that dioxins are a threat. But let us start by going back to the people exposed in Seveso and look at their dioxin burden 20 years after the disaster. From the Seveso exposure scenario (together with other analysed scenarios) we learnt that the half-life for dioxins in man is high: on average 7.5 years, but with a sixfold variation between individuals for TCDD. Thus, it cannot be a surprise that the average blood dioxin concentration in the Seveso victims was still elevated 20 years after the exposure, with the highest concentrations found in: (i) women; (ii) persons who had been eating locally grown vegetables; and (iii) obese persons. Twenty-five years after the exposure a large study was published that demonstrated a significant increase in breast cancer frequency and found individual serum TCDD concentration to be significantly related to breast cancer incidence among women in the Seveso Women's Health Study Cohort.

Today IARC has concluded that 2,3,7,8-TCDD is carcinogenic to humans, based on being an unequivocal animal carcinogen, limited human information (epidemiological/other) and mechanistic plausibility; furthermore, that other dioxin-like compounds are likely to be carcinogenic and that complex environmental mixtures of such compounds therefore also are likely to be carcinogenic to man. On 25 March 2010, the US Department of Veterans Affairs published a proposed regulation that will establish B-cell leukaemias (such as hairy cell leukaemia), Parkinson's disease and ischaemic heart disease to be associated with exposure to agent orange. Eligible Vietnam veterans may thus receive disability compensation for these diseases when the regulation becomes final.

The mechanism behind the carcinogenesis is not yet totally clear; however, it seems certain that it is elicited by binding to the Ah receptor.

The Ah receptor

The Ah (aryl hydrocarbon) receptor or AhR is a member of the so-called basic helix–loop–helix (bHLH)-Per-ARNT-Sim (PAS) family of transcriptional regulators controlling a number of developmental and physiological events, including neurogenesis, tracheal and salivary duct formation, toxin metabolism, circadian rhythms, response to hypoxia, and hormone receptor function. AhR is a cytosolic factor responsive to both natural and man-made environmental compounds that is normally inactive, bound to several co-chaperones. Upon ligand binding (TCDD) the chaperones dissociate, resulting in AhR translocating into the nucleus and dimerizing with ARNT (AhR nuclear translocator), leading to changes in gene transcription. Much of our knowledge of AhR function stems from analyses of the mechanisms by which the ligand TCDD induces the transcription of *CYP1A1*. This gene encodes the microsomal enzyme cytochrome P4501A1, which oxygenates various xenobiotics as part of their stepwise detoxification. Additional routes of AhR-mediated actions have been proposed. Thus, it was demonstrated that TCDD induces changes in protein phosphorylation through the activation of protein tyrosine kinases within 10 min. This effect was shown to be AhR-dependent and occurred under cell-free conditions in the absence of a nucleus. Based on these results the TCDD-induced protein phosphorylation pathway may be considered a separate route of AhR signalling from the well-established nuclear translocation-dependent pathway. Figure 20.23 shows the two different signalling pathways of AhR upon ligand binding.

In the rat the liver is the main target organ for carcinogenesis, which seems not to be the case for humans. This might be explained by the fact that dioxins induce transcription of both *CYP1A1* and *CYP1A2* in rats, whereas *CYP1A1* transcription is not induced in human liver.

Dioxins and dioxin-like compounds and food

Food in general accounts for about 95% of human exposure to dioxins (and dioxin-like compounds including dioxin-like PCBs). Since the compounds accumulate in the fat of animals, the highest sources in the human diet are beef, pork, lamb, fish, shellfish, butter, cheese, processed meats, eggs, poultry and milk. Dioxins can also be taken up by plants; usually the concentrations are considerably lower, though. Dioxin levels tend to be highest in fatty fish from contaminated areas near industries that produce dioxin. Generally, old, high-fat-content bottom fish, collected close to the contaminant source, have the highest levels, whereas lower-fat, non-stationary fish have much lower concentrations, even in the vicinity of the contaminant source.

In the Annex to Commission Regulation (EC) No. 1881/2006, Section 5, we find that the EU defines and regulates dioxins and PCBs in the following way. For each group of commodities the maximum level is set for the content of 'dioxins' as the sum of PCDDs and PCDFs (PCDD/F), expressed as WHO toxic equivalents (TEQ) using the WHO toxic equivalency factors (WHO-TEFs). In addition, another maximum level is set for the total sum of 'dioxins and dioxin-like PCBs' (sum of PCDDs, PCDFs and PCBs; PCDD/F-PCB), again expressed as WHO-TEQ using the WHO-TEFs. A few examples are given below.

- Meat and meat products (excluding edible offal) of bovine animals and sheep (sum of dioxins (in PCDD/F-TEQ)/sum of dioxins and dioxin-like PCBs (in PCDD/F-PCB-TEQ)): 3.0 pg g^{-1} fat/4.5 pg g^{-1} fat.
- The corresponding maximum levels for muscle meat of eel (*Anguilla anguilla*) and products thereof are 4.0 pg g^{-1} wet weight/12.0 pg g^{-1} wet weight.

Nonylphenol

Nonylphenol originates principally from the degradation of nonylphenol ethoxylates, which are

---

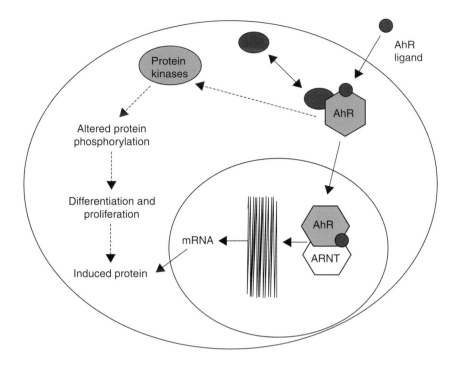

Fig. 20.23. Binding of the ligand (e.g. TCDD) to the AhR results in the release of associated proteins (chaperones, e.g. HSP90, heat shock protein 90) and translocation to the nucleus followed by dimerization with ARNT. The AhR–ARNT complex binds the xenobiotic response element (XRE) promoting target gene transcription. Ligands can also exert their effects in the cytoplasm through AhR-associated protein kinases to alter the function of a variety of proteins through a cascade of protein phosphorylation. From Pocar *et al.* (2005).[6]

widely used as industrial surfactants. It is classified as an endocrine disrupter capable of interfering with the hormonal system of numerous organisms. Nonylphenol ethoxylates reach sewage treatment works in substantial quantities where they biodegrade into several by-products including nonylphenol. Due to its physico-chemical characteristics, such as low solubility and high hydrophobicity, nonylphenol accumulates in environmental compartments that are characterized by high organic content, typically sewage sludge and river sediments, where it persists. The occurrence of nonylphenol in the environment is clearly correlated with anthropogenic activities such as wastewater treatment, landfilling and sewage sludge recycling. Nonylphenol is found often in matrices such as sewage sludge, effluents from sewage treatment works, river water and sediments, soil and groundwater. The impacts of nonylphenol in the environment include feminization of aquatic organisms, a decrease in male fertility and the survival of juveniles at concentrations as low as $8.2 \, \mu g \, l^{-1}$. Owing to the harmful effects

of the degradation products of nonylphenol ethoxylates in the environment, the use and production of such compounds have been strictly monitored in many countries such as Canada and Japan and banned in EU countries. In July 2003 the EU passed Directive 2003/53/EC, which restricts the marketing and use in Europe of certain products and product formulations that contain more than 0.1% of nonylphenol ethoxylates or nonylphenol by weight. This applies to many industries, including the textile and leather industries among others.

Although it has been shown that the concentration of nonylphenol in the environment is decreasing, it is still found at concentrations of $4.1 \, \mu g \, l^{-1}$ in river waters and $1 \, mg \, kg^{-1}$ in sediments. Nonylphenol has been referred to in the list of priority substances in the Water Frame Directive and in the third draft Working Document on Sludge of the EU. Consequently there is currently a concern within some industries about the possibility of future regulations that may impose the removal of trace contaminants from contaminated effluents.

The significance of upgrading sewage treatment works with advanced treatment technologies for removal of trace contaminants is discussed.

What are endocrine disrupters?

We have now discussed a number of pesticides used in food production, a number of POPs which are harmful due to their carcinogenicity and nonylphenol, which has been regulated due to being an endocrine disrupter. But what is an endocrine disrupter and which compounds fall under this designation?

An *endocrine disrupter* is an exogenous substance or mixture that alters function(s) of the endocrine system and consequently causes adverse health effects in an intact organism, or its progeny, or (sub)populations. Some chemicals can act on the endocrine system to disturb the homeostatic mechanisms of the body or to initiate processes at abnormal times in the life cycle. The chemicals can exert their effects through a number of different mechanisms:

- They may mimic the biological activity of a hormone by binding to a cellular receptor, leading to an unwarranted response by initiating the cell's normal response to the naturally occurring hormone at the wrong time or to an excessive extent (*agonistic effect*).
- They may bind to the receptor but not activate it. Instead the presence of the chemical on the receptor will prevent binding of the natural hormone (*antagonistic effect*).
- They may bind to transport proteins in the blood, thus altering the amounts of natural hormones that are present in the circulation.
- They may interfere with metabolic processes in the body, affecting the synthesis or breakdown rates of the natural hormones.

Up to now, because of a series of observations in both humans and wildlife, the spotlight has focused on disruption to those hormones that play a major part in the control of reproduction and development. The main area of concern has been the steroid hormones produced by the gonads, which, in conjunction with some other hormones (particularly those produced by the pituitary), control processes such as reproduction and sexual behaviour, fetal differentiation and development, and maturation. They also influence the immune system and general metabolism. The main sex steroids fall into two groups.

- Oestrogens: a group of chemicals of similar structure mainly responsible for female sexual development and reproduction. They are produced mainly by the ovaries but also by the adrenal glands and adipose (fat) tissue. The principal human oestrogen is 17-β-oestradiol.
- Androgens: chemicals responsible for the development and maintenance of male sexual characteristics. They are structurally similar to oestrogens; indeed, oestrogens are produced in the body from androgenic precursors. Testosterone, produced mainly by the testes, is the principal human androgen.

More recently research has indicated that some chemicals may disrupt thyroid function, with concerns focusing particularly on the role of the thyroid in the developmental process.

The main evidence suggesting that exposure to environmental chemicals can lead to disruption of endocrine function comes from changes seen in a number of wildlife species. Effects suggested as being related to endocrine disruption have been reported in molluscs, crustaceans, fish, reptiles, birds and mammals in various parts of the world.

There is also some limited evidence in humans that adverse endocrine-mediated effects have followed either intentional or accidental exposure to high levels of particular chemicals. The clearest example of an endocrine disrupter in humans is diethylstilbestrol (DES), a synthetic oestrogen prescribed in the 1950s and 1960s to 5 million pregnant women for the prevention of spontaneous abortion. It was found that some of the children who had been exposed *in utero* had developmental abnormalities, and that some of the girls developed an unusual form of vaginal cancer when they reached puberty. As a consequence, DES was banned in the 1970s. In addition, a number of adverse changes have been suggested to have occurred in the population living near a chemical plant in Seveso, Italy, as a result of the accidental release of the chemical dioxin, a suspected endocrine disrupter.

Chemicals with hormonal activity, i.e. potential endocrine disrupters, include the following:

- Natural hormones from any animal released into the environment and chemicals produced by one species that exert hormonal actions on other animals, e.g. human hormones unintentionally reactivated during the processing of human waste in sewage effluent, may result in changes to fish.

- Natural chemicals including toxins produced by the components of plants (the so-called phyto-oestrogens, such as genistein or coumestrol) and certain fungi.
- Synthetically produced pharmaceuticals that are intended to be highly hormonally active, e.g. the contraceptive pill and treatments for hormone-responsive cancers, may also be detected in sewage effluent.
- Man-made chemicals and by-products released into the environment. Laboratory experiments have suggested that some man-made chemicals might be able to cause endocrine changes. These include some pesticides (e.g. DDT and other chlorinated compounds), chemicals in some consumer and medical products (e.g. some plastic additives) and a number of industrial chemicals (e.g. PCBs, dioxins). The hormonal activity of these chemicals is many times weaker than the body's own naturally present hormones. For example, nonylphenol (a breakdown product of alkylphenol ethoxylate surfactants), found as a low-level contaminant in some rivers in Europe, has an oestrogenic activity that is only about 1/10,000th of that of the natural hormone, oestrogen.

20.5   Conclusion

There are several reasons accounting for why we try worldwide today to reduce the exposure – through food and other sources – to chemicals such as pesticides and other POPs, reasons that include risks for the development of cancer as well as our present observations on the possible adverse effects of compounds with endocrine-disrupting potential.

Notes

[1] US NLM (2009) TOXNET Toxicology Data Network, ChemIDplus Dictionary. US National Library of Medicine; Rockville, MD; available at http://toxnet.nlm.nih.gov/cgi-bin/sis/htmlgen?CHEM

[2] Fromberg, A., Larsen, E., Hartkopp H., Larsen, J., Granby, K., Jørgensen, K., Rasmussen, P., Cederberg, T. and Christensen, T. (2003) *Chemical Contaminants 1998–2003. Part I.* Danish Veterinary and Food Administration, Søborg, Denmark; available at http://www.food.dtu.dk/Default.aspx?ID=8338

[3] Randall, D., Burggren, W. and French, K. (1997) *Eckert Animal Physiology – Mechanisms and Adaptations*, 4th edn. W.H. Freeman and Company, New York, New York.

[4] Reece, W.O. (ed.) (2004) *Dukes Physiology of Domestic Animals*, 12th edn. Cornell University Press, Ithaca, New York.

[5] Glacer, L.C. (1995) Wildlife mortality attributed to organophosphorus and carbamate pesticides. In: LaRoe, E.T. *et al.* (eds) *Our Living Resources. A Report to the Nation on the Distribution, Abundance, and Health of US Plants, Animals, and Ecosystems.* US Department of the Interior, National Biological Services, Reston, Virginia, pp. 416–418; available at http://biology.usgs.gov/

[6] Pocar, P., Fisher, B., Klonisch, T. and Homback-Klonisch, S. (2005) Molecular interactions of the aryl hydrocarbon receptor and its biological and toxicological relevance for reproduction. *Reproduction* 129, 274–389.

Further Reading

Committee on the Implications of Dioxin in the Food Supply, National Research Council (2003) *Dioxins and Dioxin-like Compounds in the Food Supply; Strategies to Decrease Exposure.* National Academies Press, Washington, DC.

EFSA (2004) *Dioxins – Methodologies and Principles and Setting Tolerable Intake Levels for Dioxins, Furans and Dioxin-like PCBs. EFSA Scientific Colloquium Summary Report.* European Food Safety Authority, Parma, Italy.

EFSA (2007) *Dioxins – Cumulative Risk Assessment of Pesticides to Human Health: The Way Forward. EFSA Scientific Colloquium Summary Report.* European Food Safety Authority, Parma, Italy.

Marrs, T.C. and Ballantyne, B. (eds) (2004) *Pesticide Toxicology and International Regulation (Current Toxicology Series).* John Wiley & Sons, Hoboken, New Jersey.

Ware, G.W. and Whitacre, D.M. (2004) *The Pesticide Book*, 6th edn. Meister Media, Willoughby, Ohio.

21 Contaminants From Processing Machinery and Food Contact Materials

- We discuss the compounds that may contaminate foods as a result of different types of physical contact.
- Contact with mechanical machinery may lead to contamination with lubricants.
- Contact with machinery as well as with storage/packaging materials may lead to contamination with a number of elements (metals) and organic compounds.

21.1 Lubricants

Processing machinery in the food industry, like all machinery, needs lubrication. Examples can be pumps, filling equipment and conveyer belts. In the case of a leakage at, for example, a gear, contamination of the food product under production may occur. While no official (state) agencies to date have any programmes for approval of lubricants for the food industry in place, the US-based independent organization National Sanitation Foundation (NSF) – which since 1944 has developed and offered tests and certification of a number of products within the area of water, food and consumer goods – has developed a three-stage certification system for lubricants. Today many food industries that work internationally use only NSF-certified lubricants. Lubricants for food producing industries fall into one of the following three categories:

- NSF H1: the lubricant can be accepted to be in limited contact with a food product (an example could be a lubricant for gears and hydraulic equipment).
- NSF 3H: the lubricant is approved by NSF for direct contact with a food product (an example could be a 'food grade mould release' product to be used as a slip-agent on grills, frying pans, etc.).
- NSF H2: the lubricant is approved for storage together with food products but not for contact with such.

A number of commercially available products of this kind are added antibacterial substances.

21.2 Food Contact Materials

Food has always been prepared, stored and ingested using a number of storage and processing pots, pans and containers as well as packaging materials for wrapping around food. Back in time (and presently still to a limited extent in some cultures) jars/vessels were made of hollowed fruits (e.g. 'calabash', a bowl-shaped vessel manufactured from different types of gourd from members of the gourd plant family). Later copper, tin and ceramics were used intensively. Today in modern (industrial) food production the materials that food mostly comes into contact with are metal tanks with or without epoxy coating and tubes of plastic or rubber, while materials used in large volumes for retail packaging include glass, paper, lacquered metal and plastics.

Glass and ceramics have been used for food storage and transport purposes for hundreds (or actually thousands) of years. This gave rise to a number of problems with leakage of lead and later also of cadmium into the stored products. Often this was due to the use of colourings containing these toxic heavy metals applied in the fabrication of the glass or ceramic. For this reason a number of countries in Europe had national legislation concerning the maximum level of leakage of these two compounds into food. However, gradually plastic materials took over in a number of cases, and these problems with migration of toxic compounds into food seemed to be solved. Or were they?

Plastics

A plastic material is made up primarily of one or more polymers, the chains of the polymer(s) forming a more (crystalline) or less (amorphous) organized network. In addition, all plastic materials typically contain a small percentage of so-called *additives*, used in order to ensure that:

- the mixture can polymerize and be cast (residues of catalysing substances and additives to ensure that the product loosens from the mould); and
- the plastic is protected against degradation (antioxidants, stabilizers against UV irradiation and heat degradation):

Depending on conditions during production, the material may further contain:

- residues of monomers; and
- oligomers.

During the 1960s and 1970s it became apparent that finished plastic materials most often are not just inert polymers. Of special importance, it was found that many products made from PVC in fact contained – and could leak – quite high concentrations of the monomer (vinyl chloride), as shown in the following examples:

- In 1973 it was found that alcoholic beverages in PVC bottles could contain up to 0.2–0.5 mg of vinyl chloride per litre.
- Later, butter/margarine holding up to 50 mg kg^{-1} and vegetable oils with concentrations of 15 mg kg^{-1} were reported to be found on the commercial market.
- A 13-week study on rats clearly showed that vinyl chloride at a dose of 30 mg kg^{-1} BW was toxic. The compound was subsequently shown also to be carcinogenic.

Despite this our present-day plastics usage is not restricted to just hard/brittle materials: a lot of different plastics are made soft by the addition of so-called *plasticizers* (softeners), although PVC – the first plastic material to be made soft by this process – remains the most prominent material in this respect. Soft PVC may contain up to 50% of plasticizers by weight. Examples of additives used or formerly used in plastics include: (i) anti-oxidants such as butylated hydroxyanisole (BHA) and butylated hydroxytoluene (BHT); (ii) anti-static additives such as quarternary ammonium compounds (e.g. cetylmethylammonium bromide – teratogenic); (iii) flame-retarding compounds (halogenated – chlorinated and brominated – hydrocarbons, organophosphate esters); and (iv) plasticizers such as esters of dicarboxylic acids, polyesters of adipic acid and glycols (polymeric softeners), and epoxidated soybean oil (ESBO; acts as softener, heat stabilizer and lubricating mould substances).

Gradually national legislation together with industrial efforts meant that limits were set for residues of monomers, and the problems were also gradually solved from the technical point of view.

But that was not the end. In 1987 the UK Ministry of Agriculture, Fisheries and Food (MAFF) reported that a number of food products contained the two plastic softeners DEHA (= di-(2-ethylhexyl)adipate) and DEHP (= di-(2-ethylhexyl)phthalate). Of these, DEHA was used mainly to soften PVC film to wrap, for example, food products. DEHP (and other phthalates) were used also for many non-food purposes (in other kinds of products), which is why they are found spread in the environment to a much larger degree. From the environment they may enter the food chain in different ways and

---

Box 21.1. DEHP and milk from cow to mouth

Among the measures taken to solve these new problems in Denmark, one can find:

- legislation against the use of tubes softened with DEHP in milking machines, put into action by 1989;
- following this legislation the Danish Food Agency monitored the content of DEHP in milk marketed for consumption up to 1997; and

- for the whole of the period the content was shown to be very low, giving rise to a human exposure far below the level found tolerable.

By 1997 the first limit for migration was set – as a substitute for a ban. Today a Specific Migration Limit (SML) of 1.5 mg kg^{-1} food simulant is approved in the EU for DEHP on the basis of a risk assessment (Commission Directive 2007/19/EC).

expose humans and animals even more directly. However, DEHP has also been used in plastic for food containers and to soften tubes, for example, used for milking machines (Box 21.1).

Migration of low-molecular-weight additives may also occur from rubber products. The compound 2-mercaptobenzothiazol (MBT) is used in the production of latex (natural rubber). Accordingly residues of MBT have been found in teats/nipples from feeding-bottles and in dummies made of rubber. MBT is thought to play a major role in the development of allergy to products made from latex. The European Committee for Standardization (CEN) has set a limit for the migration of MBT from rubber products. The limit is 8 mg kg^{-1} rubber product as determined by a CEN developed test. A Danish investigation in 1999 showed that several dummies on the market did not pass the test. Conclusion: there is nearly always something that migrates!

The migration of DEHA (and to a certain extent DFHP) from packaging materials to food products – the 'new' problem faced as a result of the use of softened plastic containers and wrappings – clearly also had to be 'solved'. For this the EU now sets limits for migration while industry makes attempts to find new technical solutions. The latter include the use of so-called *polymeric softeners* such as polyesters of adipic acid and glycols and the earlier mentioned ESBO. However, ESBO also migrates. Thus, elastic wrappings meant for food products may contain up to about 11% ESBO by weight while PVC seals in bottle closures have been shown to contain up to 34% ESBO by weight; moreover, weaning food from bottles with such closures was found to contain ESBO in the range from 0.5 and up to 51 mg kg^{-1} food product!

Ready-cooked foods and microwave ovens

As our dependency on convenience and ready-cooked foods has increased, the plastic and packaging industry gradually has developed quite complex materials. Nowadays we expect to be able to enter a shop, buy a full dish which we can transport to our home in our shopping bag without any problems, put it in the oven or the microwave oven and heat for consumption. This actually means that the package, which weighs only a few grams, must stand a hot fill packing under aseptic conditions and maintain an efficient barrier for 6 months in a freezer at −18°C and withstand a short heating

period to about 100°C in the microwave oven or in boiling water. The materials developed for such purposes often consist of multilayered structures built up of several types of polymers, adhesives, lacquers and printing inks. At the same time this structure should not leak its constituents to the food. Indeed, this is not a simple thing.

Legislation

After these historical examples, let us turn to the current legislation. In the EU, the general legislative requirements concerning materials in contact with food are found in Regulation (EC) No. 1935/2004 of the European Parliament and of the Council of 27 October 2004 on materials and articles intended to come into contact with food. Later this regulation was followed by a GMP Regulation (EC) No. 2023/2006 of 22 December 2006 on good manufacturing practice for materials and articles intended to come into contact with food. The following fundamental principles are stated in Regulation 1935/2004:

- general 'inertness' of materials; and
- no transfer of substances to the foodstuffs in quantities which could bring an unacceptable change in the composition of the foodstuffs or endanger human health or give rise to deterioration in the organoleptic properties.

The regulation foresees separate legislation for each of the following classes of material: (i) active and intelligent materials and articles; (ii) adhesives; (iii) ceramics; (iv) cork; (v) rubbers; (vi) glass; (vii) ion-exchange resins; (viii) metals and alloys; (ix) paper and board; (x) plastics; (xi) printing inks; (xii) regenerated cellulose; (xiii) silicones; (xiv) textiles; (xv) varnishes and coatings; (xvi) waxes; and (xvii) wood.

So far only the plastics have been thoroughly treated in a 'full' piece of legislation, i.e. in the Directive 2002/72/EC of 6 August 2002 relating to plastic materials and articles intended to come into contact with foodstuffs, as amended several times.

The Directive contains a 'List of monomers and other starting substances which may be used in the manufacture of plastic materials and articles' and a 'List of additives which may be used in the manufacture of plastic materials and articles'.

The Directive further sets the limits for migration into foods. This is done by a multi-tiered set of rules. Thus, an overall maximum limit for total migration to the food is set at 60 mg unspecified plastic ingredients per kilogram (or maximum 10 mg dm^{-2}). In addition, many monomers/starting materials as well as additives have a Specific Migration Limit (SML) or a Maximum Residual Quantity in the material (Qm) prescribed. As an example we can take the additive 2-aminoethanol, for which an SML of 0.05 mg kg^{-1} has been set and for which we further find a more detailed specification saying: 'Not for use in polymers contacting foods for which simulant D is laid down in Directive 85/572/EEC and for indirect food contact only, behind the PET layer'.

This immediately brings us to wonder what simulant D means. The simulants are used when testing a material for its compliance with the legislation. Thus, a test must be performed where the material is brought into contact with one or more of the four food stimulants, i.e. (food simulants from Directive 85/572/EEC):

- distilled water (simulant A);
- 3% w/v acetic acid (simulant B);
- 10% (15%) v/v ethanol (simulant C); and
- rectified olive oil (simulant D).

The test conditions must be chosen as based on the expected/approved use of the plastic material.

1. Materials without any restriction in their use (examples):

- for general use at all conditions, e.g. 2 h at 175°C in oil or 4 h at 100°C in aqueous simulants;
- for use at ambient temperature, e.g. 10 days at 40°C, all food simulants.

2. Materials labelled with restrictions in their use:

- select specific test conditions accordingly with respect to food simulant(s), temperature and exposure period.

After the test(s) have been performed the total migration into the simulant is determined by weight, while specific migrations are determined by analysing for the specific compound in the simulant.

Bisphenol A

Before we leave the subject of migration into foods we just have to mention bisphenol A (BPA), not because it is more interesting than many other compounds that one could look into further, but because it is one of those compounds that has been discussed in scientific circles as well as the public arena for decades (and indeed is still being discussed). BPA (Fig. 21.1) is a key monomer in the production of the most common form of polycarbonate plastic, which is clear and nearly shatter-proof and which is used to make a variety of common products including baby and water bottles, sports equipment, medical and dental devices, dental fillings and sealants, and eyeglass lenses.

BPA-based plastics have been in commerce for more than 50 years and it has been known since the 1930s that the compound can mimic the female sex hormone, oestrogen. Therefore, the effects on fertility and reproduction have been subject to intense scientific debate, linked to reports of low-dose effects of BPA in rodents. In short, BPA is one of several chemicals also having the potential to interact with hormone systems in the human body, i.e. an endocrine disrupter.

Especially from 2006 onwards this fact has prompted a lot of risk assessment and review activities around the exposure to and risk (if any) from BPA. In Europe EFSA carried out a new review of BPA in 2006, since around 200 scientific papers had been published on BPA after the previous review by SCF in 2002. Furthermore, a consensus statement by 38 experts on BPA was published in 2007 in the scientific journal *Reproductive Toxicology* as a result of a conference sponsored by among others the US EPA and the Commonwealth and held in Chapel Hill, North Carolina, USA. In April 2008 the US National Toxicology Program (NTP) published a draft brief in which it concluded that there was some concern for neural and behavioural effects in the fetus, infant and child at current levels of exposure. At the same time reports from Health Canada and Environment Canada also raised concerns over possible adverse effects on newborns and infants, and in particular on the elimination of the substance from the bodies of newborns and infants.

The last-mentioned concerns prompted the European Commission to ask EFSA to further assess the differences between infants and adults in the elimination of BPA from the body, taking into

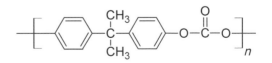

Fig. 21.1. The repeating sequence in a polycarbonate plastic, showing the bisphenol A moiety.

account the most recent information and data available. As a result EFSA published another new opinion on BPA in July 2008. The current status in Europe is that the EFSA Panel on Food Additives, Flavourings, Processing Aids and Materials in contact with Food (AFC) has now established a TDI of 0.05 mg kg^{-1} BW, using the usual 100-fold uncertainty factor. According to calculations made by EFSA a 3-month-old bottle-fed baby who weighs around 6 kg would need to consume more than four times the usual number of bottles of baby formula per day before he/she would reach the TDI.

21.3 Conclusion

Migration of compounds from materials in contact with food is one of several means by which a food commodity may be contaminated. No matter which material we choose migration will occur depending on the material, the characteristics of the food item (fat content, pH, alcohol content, etc.) and the storage/processing conditions (temperature and time).

Further Reading

Barnes, K., Sinclair, R. and Watson, D. (eds) (2006) *Chemical Migration and Food Contact Materials. Woodhead Food Series No. 136*. Woodhead Publishing Limited, Cambridge, UK.

Forest, M. (2009) *Food Contact Materials – Rubbers, Silicones, Coatings and Inks. Rapra Review Reports No. 186*. Smithers Rapra Press, Shrewsbury, UK.

22 Toxic Compounds Formed During Processing or Improper Storage

- A large number of toxic compounds may be formed as a result of processing or improper storage – and of very different chemical structure.
- Some are mutagenic and/or carcinogenic.
- Some are acutely toxic.
- Some are single compounds while others consist of groups of compounds.

22.1 Introduction

A number of very different new organic compounds are formed when we process our food. Heat treatments in particular, and among these the high-temperature processing methods, have proved to result in numerous different classes of new compounds of which several include very toxic and/or carcinogenic agents. The first result of food heat processing that was recognized by chemists was browning. When we toast our bread we initiate a highly complex reaction (actually a high number of parallel reaction chains) today named the Maillard reaction. This leads to the formation of the toxic acrylamide, the toxic water-soluble premelanoidins and the insoluble dark-brown polymeric pigments called melanoidins. So, before we discuss the many different groups of process toxins, let us take a look at the Maillard reaction.

The first step of the famous Maillard reaction is the reaction of a reducing sugar, such as glucose, with an amino acid. The reaction is named after Louis Camille Maillard (1878–1936), a French scientist, who studied the reactions of amino acids and carbohydrates in 1912 as part of his PhD thesis. Pentoses such as ribose react faster than hexoses (glucose, fructose) and disaccharides (sugar/sucrose, lactose). Sugar alcohols or polyols (sorbitol, xylitol) do not participate in the Maillard reaction. The first reaction product is a so-called *Amadori compound*, which differs depending on the amino acid and the sugar, which means that the first step (theoretically)

already results in over 100 different reaction products. The Amadori compounds easily isomerize into three different structures (Fig. 22.1), each of which may react differently in the next steps. The amino acid may for example be removed, which results in reactive compounds that are further degraded to the flavour components furfural and hydroxymethylfurfural (HMF), or the so-called *Amadori rearrangement* (the starting point of the main browning reactions) may take place (Fig. 22.2).

After the Amadori rearrangement three different main pathways can be distinguished leading to a very large number of compounds including, in the early stages, the water-soluble premelanoidins and at later stages a mixture of insoluble dark-brown polymeric pigments called melanoidins, i.e. the dark pigments of the browning reaction when toasting, etc.

22.2 Acrylamide

In the year 2002 Swedish scientists detected the compound acrylamide (acrylic amide) in a number of starch-rich food products. Further analysis confirmed that, while heating commodities rich in protein but low in carbohydrates gives rise to acrylamide formation up to a level of about 5–50 µg kg^{-1}, much higher levels from 150 to 4000 µg kg^{-1} result when heating the carbohydrate-rich potato and beetroot. No acrylamide could be found in commodities that were not heated.

The finding of acrylamide in food products was most unexpected. Until then this compound, with

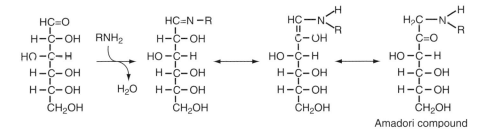

Fig. 22.1. The initial step of the Maillard reaction between glucose and an amino acid (RNH₂), in which R is the amino acid side group.

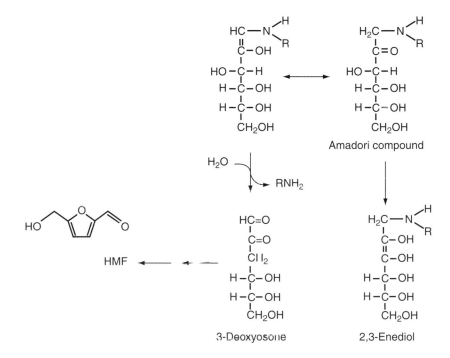

Fig. 22.2. Formation of HMF and Amadori rearrangement.

chemical formula C₃H₅NO and IUPAC name 2-propenamide, had mostly been known as a white crystalline solid used extensively in industry for the production of polyacrylamide. Industrial exposure of workers had proved it to be neurotoxic, the toxicity being manifested by paraesthesias, numbness, peeling and sloughing of skin, and muscle weakness. If nerve fibres of victims are biopsied, there is a loss of myelinated fibres, and axons are noted to be swollen with masses of neurofilaments. Like two other compounds, i.e. 2,5-hexanedione and carbon disulfide, acrylamide also inhibits some glycolytic enzymes directly by reacting with

proteins to form pyrrole adducts. This is believed to be part of the mechanism behind the damage to the nervous system seen for acrylamide.

However, when acrylamide was found in food commodities the neurotoxicity was not the major concern that prompted both JECFA and EFSA soon after to start a risk evaluation on the basis of the findings reported from Sweden (and quickly after from a number of other countries). IARC already by then had classified acrylamide as being 'probably carcinogenic to man', and this was the reason for looking in more detail at acrylamide and its occurrence in foods.

Several theories have been presented as to the mechanism of formation of acrylamide in heat-processed foods. Since a number of deep-fried products were shown to contain the compound, the early focus was on a role of the lipids in the frying fat. Hydrolysis of triacylglycerols can lead to the formation of acrolein. This compound can be oxidized to acrylic acid among others, which in turn may react with an amino group to form acrylamide. Even though possible, this mechanism is not currently regarded as being of any real significance, however. Instead most experts agree that acrylamide is formed via a Maillard reaction including as

reactants the amino acid asparagine and a reducing sugar (glucose) (Fig. 22.3).

In conclusion, acrylamide is formed upon heat processing of carbohydrate-rich foods at temperatures from 120°C upwards. Several experiments have confirmed that higher temperatures lead to a higher content and that in general a significantly higher acrylamide level is found near to the surface than in the core of the product.

From the point of view of the neurotoxicity of acrylamide, the concentrations found so far in foodstuffs give no cause for concern. Whether the carcinogenic potential established through a number

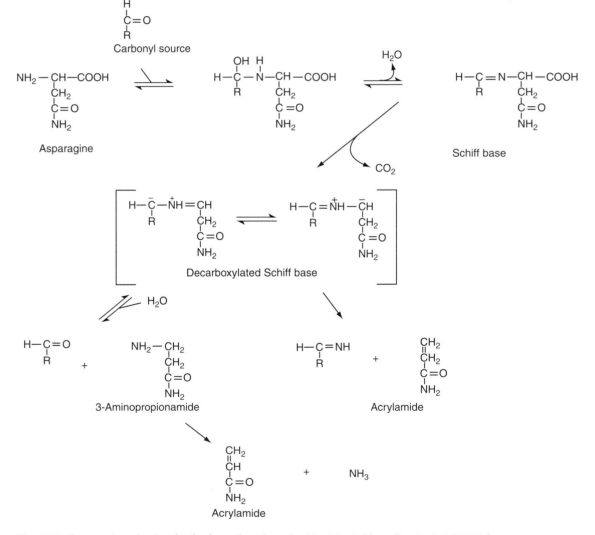

Fig. 22.3. Proposed mechanism for the formation of acrylamide. Adapted from Zyzak *et al.* (2003).[1]

of animal experiments gives reasons for further risk management initiatives is another question, however. This was discussed by the Codex Committee on Food Additives and Contaminants (JECFA) in 2004. JECFA concluded that measures to further reduce the content of acrylamide in food products should be developed and advised, a point of view supported by the Scientific Panel on Contaminants in the Food Chain (CONTAM) under EFSA in its statement of April 2005 and as repeated in 2008.

22.3 Nitrite and Nitrosamines

Nitrite (NO_2^-) is toxic and can serve as a substrate necessary for the formation of carcinogenic so-called *nitrosamines*. Nitrite, and nitrate (NO_3^-), commonly used as a fertilizer, are both part of the natural nitrogen cycle, prevalently taking place in matrices such as aerobic soils, sediments and wastewater treatment plants. Nitrite thus can be formed by either microbial nitrification of ammonia or by chemical and microbial reduction of nitrate. A microbial reduction of nitrate to nitrite can also occur in the oral cavity. Because of their high solubility in water, nitrite and nitrate ions may occur naturally in groundwater, and thereby in drinking water, as well as in various types of food, especially plant foods. However, both nitrate and nitrite also may be used as food additives in the so-called *meat curing process*. We now look at the ways that nitrite and nitrate (as a source of nitrite formation) enter our food and the possible consequences.

Nitrite in meat

Curing is a method of processing for conservation that includes the use of different chemicals. The curing of meat, like other methods of preserving meat at ambient temperatures, developed from drying. First salt (NaCl) was used to assist the drying process. It is believed that the deliberate introduction of nitrate resulted from an original use of crude salt with a content of nitrate and subsequent observation of the benefits that this change in the chemistry of the process brought about. Sodium chloride in itself has an inhibitory effect on microorganisms due to lowering of the water activity level and a specific inhibitory effect of the Na^+ ion. Nitrate later was found to be a reservoir for the continuous formation of nitrite, the true curing agent in addition to the salt. In 1899, German scientists thus showed that nitrite is the active agent in formation of the characteristic (red) curing

colour of meat, while it had to wait until the 1920s for the antimicrobial action of nitrite to be demonstrated. The most significant is the action against *Clostridium botulinum*, which causes the potentially deadly disease botulism.

The origin of the process of meat curing is unknown; however, the industrialization of this process for mass production took place in the south-western county of Wiltshire in the UK. While the original methods relied on packing the meat in a dry mixture of NaCl and other curing agents, the 'Wiltshire cure' used tank curing in concentrated brines. Nowadays Wiltshire bacon is produced in many countries.

Today, nitrite (or in some cases nitrate) is used in cured meat products for a number of reasons:

1. It prompts the red curing colour.
2. It plays a part in the formation of the characteristic curing flavour.
3. It has an important antimicrobial effect.
4. It acts as an antioxidant.

Nitrate is only used for slow curing in a few special products requiring a long-term reservoir of nitrite, which can be released throughout the curing process with the aid of a starter culture containing nitrate-reducing bacteria.

The formation of the curing colour is indeed very complex and has been clarified only relatively recently. In brief, nitrite is reduced to nitric oxide (NO). Parallel with this MbFe(II) (Mb = myoglobin) present in the fresh meat is oxidized by the added NO_2^- to form MbFe(III), which then reacts with NO to form an intermediary meat pigment. This is reduced into the red pigment nitrosylmyoglobin, MbFe(II)NO, by either endogenous or exogenous reductants. Upon heating, MbFe(II)NO turns into the final heat-stable pink pigment nitrosylhaemochrome (Fig. 22.4).

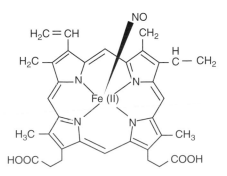

Fig. 22.4. The structure of nitrosylhaemochrome.

A strong and stable curing colour in cooked, cured meat products is obtained with a nitrite level of 25–50 mg kg^{-1} meat, but often about 150–300 mg NaNO$_2$ (corresponding to 100–200 mg NO$_2^-$ ion) is added per kilogram of meat in whole-muscle brine-injected products.

An estimated 30–50 mg NO$_2^-$ kg^{-1} meat is necessary for the development of cured meat flavour. The chemistry behind this is not yet fully understood, however.

As already mentioned the main antimicrobial effect of nitrite in cured meat products is that against *C. botulinum* through inhibition of the outgrowth of the germinated spore and thereby toxin production. This is particularly important when the cured meat is vacuum packed, since *C. botulinum* is an anaerobic bacterium. The effect of nitrite is favoured by reduced pH and is furthermore enhanced by the occurrence of other curing factors such as salt. To create a microbiological hurdle, reportedly initial nitrite levels of the order of at least 100 mg kg^{-1} cured meat are necessary.

Table 22.1 shows examples of the maximum limits for nitrite and nitrate as curing agents in the EU. For comparison it can be mentioned that the USA allows about 100 mg NaNO$_2$ kg^{-1} meat for curing, whereas Russia does not allow nitrite at all.

Nitrate – a source of nitrite – in the diet

As mentioned, nitrate can be reduced to nitrite by microorganisms present in the oral cavity and this happens to up to 8% of ingested nitrate. The dietary intake of nitrate is therefore of great significance for the total human exposure to nitrite. It is estimated that only about 10% of this nitrite stems from cured meat and other nitrate/nitrite-containing foods and the remaining 90% originates from the conversion of nitrate in vegetables and other sources including water.

Nitrate from plant foods

Overall, vegetables are the major sources of nitrate in the human diet. It is estimated that they account for 60–80% of the total nitrate intake, whereas water contributes about 20%.

The level of nitrate in a certain plant raw material depends on the plant species, the tissue, the amount of fertilizer used, the humidity and temperature, and the exposure to sunlight (more sunlight giving rise to less nitrate in the plant). In general nitrate levels therefore will be higher in raw materials from temperate regions such as Northern Europe than from subtropical or tropical regions such as Mediterranean countries. As a result of the intensive use of synthetic nitrogen fertilizers as well as livestock manure in agriculture today, food and drinking water may in general contain higher amounts of nitrate than in the past.

A number of food plants are especially well known for having the potential to accumulate nitrate at rather high concentrations. These include vegetables such as iceberg type lettuce, other types of fresh head lettuce (*Lactuca sativa*) and spinach (*Spinacea oleracea*). A survey from Germany showed that these, along with other vegetables including cress, radish, fennel and beetroot, may have nitrate levels of the order of 1500–2300 mg kg^{-1} FW. The EU has legal maximum levels for nitrate in spinach, head lettuce and iceberg lettuce as well as baby foods; some examples are shown in Table 22.2.

According to a 2003 report on the findings by the Danish Institute for Food and Veterinary

Table 22.1. Curing agents in meat products in the EU (extracted from Directive 2006/52/EC of the European Parliament and of the Council of 5 July 2006 amending Directive 95/2/EC on food additives other than colours and sweeteners and Directive 94/35/EC on sweeteners for use in foodstuffs).

E-number	Name	Foodstuff	Maximum amount added during manufacturing (expressed as NaNO$_2$) (mg kg^{-1})	MRL (expressed as NaNO$_2$) (mg kg^{-1})
E249	Potassium nitrite	Meat products	150	–
E250	Sodium nitrite	Sterilized meat products	100	–
	–	Traditional immersion-cured meat	100	50–175
	–	Other traditional cured meat products	180	50
E251	Potassium nitrate	Non-heat-treated products	300	50
E252	Sodium nitrate	Traditional immersion-cured meat	300	10–250

Chapter 22

Table 22.2. Maximum levels of nitrate in spinach, head lettuce, iceberg lettuce and baby foods (extracted from Commission Regulation (EC) No. 1881/2006 of 19 December 2006 setting maximum levels for certain contaminants in foodstuffs).

Product		Maximum level (mg NO_3^- kg^{-1} FW)
Fresh spinach	Harvested 1 October to 31 March	3000
	Harvested 1 April to 30 September	2500
Preserved, deep-frozen or frozen spinach		2000
Fresh lettuce	Harvested 1 October to 31 March	
	• Grown under cover	4500
	• Grown in the open air	4500
	Harvested 1 April to 3 September	
	• Grown under cover	3500
	• Grown in the open air	2500
Baby foods and processed cereal-based foods for infants and young children		200

Research concerning the nitrate content in vegetables, selected crops showed levels within the following ranges (mg kg^{-1} FW): (i) head lettuce (greenhouse – Danish), 520–3900; (ii) head lettuce (foreign), 1100–1800; (iii) iceberg (Danish), 290–1000; (iv) iceberg (foreign), 480–1400; (v) fennel (Danish), 905–1100; (vi) fennel (foreign), 140–1300. In general these levels are not especially high compared with the tabulated maximum levels. However, it becomes interesting when one turns to the results for rucola lettuce, analysed to have by far the highest mean content of nitrate of 5399 mg kg^{-1} FW. Values from the years 2000 and 2002 showed a similar trend for rucola.

Nitrate from water

Water also may be a significant source of nitrate and nitrite, as mentioned above. Therefore, most countries have set maximum levels for the content of these two chemical entities. Often these follow the WHO guideline value for nitrate in drinking water of 50 mg l^{-1}. This value is set so that even the highest-risk group (refer to below under toxicity), bottle-fed infants, are not at risk for acute intoxication when consuming the water. Because both nitrate and nitrite can be present in the water concurrently, the sum of the ratios of the concentration of each substituent to its guideline value should not be greater than one. In 2007 WHO published a valuable document that provides further background information in this respect, entitled *Nitrate and Nitrite in Drinking-water – Background Document for Development of WHO Guidelines for Drinking-water Quality* (WHO/SDE/ WSH/07.01/16), which can be consulted online (http://www.who.int/water_sanitation_health/dwq/ chemicals/nitratenitrite2ndadd.pdf).

Depending on the most common source(s) of drinking water different situations are seen in different countries and regions. However, at least one important lesson learnt during recent decades is worthwhile mentioning. Until recently nitrate was not usually found in deep drillings in countries such as Denmark. While this still is true in clay soils, because of the use of fertilizers nitrate is now found even in rather deep drillings in sandy soils. One mg NH_4^+ eventually gives 3.4 mg NO_3^-. This transformation of ammonia to nitrate via nitrite can often account for 5–10 mg NO_3^- l^{-1} drinking water as reported by the local government of Vallensbæk in 2008.

Furthermore, nitrification in the water distribution system can potentially more than double the content of nitrite in drinking water up to more than 3 mg l^{-1}. This is the background for the two different maximum limits for nitrite seen in Table 22.3.

The toxicology of nitrite

While nitrate is virtually non-toxic by the oral route this is by no means the case for nitrite. The ADI of

Table 22.3. Maximum legal limits of nitrate and nitrite in drinking water in Denmark (Danish Environmental Protection Agency, 2006).

	Maximum limit (mg l^{-1})
Nitrate	50
Nitrite, at exit from waterworks	0.01
Nitrite, in distribution pipes	0.10

nitrate set by JECFA is 5 mg kg⁻¹ BW expressed as sodium nitrate, corresponding to $3.7\,mg\,NO_3^-\,kg^{-1}$ BW (the ADI does not apply to infants below the age of 3 months). This value originates from risk assessments taking into account the connection between intake of nitrate and possible exposure to nitrite and its carcinogenic products of reaction (nitrosamines) as discussed below. The JECFA ADI for nitrite established at the same JECFA meeting is 0.07 mg kg⁻¹ BW. Recent studies show mean nitrate intake for adults of 50–140 mg day⁻¹ in Europe and 40–100 mg day⁻¹ in the USA.

Acute nitrite toxicity – methaemoglobinaemia

Acute nitrite toxicity occurs because nitrite can oxidize haemoglobin (oxyHb), which has iron in the Fe^{2+} state, to methaemoglobin (metHb) where iron is in the Fe^{3+} state:

$$oxyHb(Fe^{2+}) + NO_2^- \rightarrow metHb(Fe^{3+}) + NO_3^-$$

Oxygen binds poorly to methaemoglobin, which therefore cannot transport oxygen to the tissues, leading to a state of anoxia. This condition can be life-threatening, especially to infants who are more sensitive to nitrite toxicity due the following four factors:

1. A temporary deficiency of NADH-methaemoglobin reductase, which is the major enzyme responsible for the reduction of methaemoglobin.
2. Young infants may still have a significant amount of the easily oxidized fetal haemoglobin present in the blood.
3. Young infants have a higher gastric pH than older children and adults. This means that nitrite is less rapidly degraded in the stomach and more is left to be absorbed in the small intestine and released into the bloodstream.
4. Young infants have a high energy intake relative to body weight (a general consideration).

Methaemoglobinaemia is often referred to as *blue baby syndrome*. The clinical features are oxygen deprivation with cyanosis, cardiac arrhythmias and circulatory failure, and progressive CNS effects ranging from mild dizziness and lethargy to coma, convulsions and even death in the most severe cases. Normal methaemoglobin levels are around 1% of total haemoglobin. Cyanosis occurs at levels of 10–20%, whereas levels of 30–50% will lead to severe symptoms of methaemoglobinaemia including respiratory distress, dizziness, headache and fatigue. Lethargy and stupor develop at methaemoglobin levels above 50%, while levels above 70% can cause death if not treated immediately.

The first reported incident of an infant with methaemoglobinaemia is from 1941. The first fatality was described in 1945, the cause being contaminated well water. From 1945 to 1971, a total of 2000 cases were reported in North America and Europe. Approximately 8% of the cases resulted in death. In contrast to this, only one infant death by methaemoglobinaemia was reported in the period from 1972 to 1979. A few fatalities and some sporadically occurring non-fatal cases were then again reported during the 1980s and 1990s. For many other geographical and political regions such statistics do not exist. Consumption of infant formula mixed with nitrate-contaminated well water was the most common cause. Nitrite can originate from water contaminated with both nitrate and bacteria with a nitrate reductase.

According to WHO, doses of $33–250\,mg\,NO_2^-$ kg⁻¹ BW (corresponding to 50–375 mg NaNO₂) may give rise to lethal methaemoglobinaemia, the higher amounts referring to healthy adults. Toxic doses resulting in non-lethal methaemoglobinaemia are stated to be found in the range of $0.4–200\,mg\,NO_2^-$ kg⁻¹ BW (0.6–300 mg NaNO₂).

Long-term nitrite toxicity: *N*-nitroso compound (nitrosamine) formation

This section is mainly about nitrosamines as representatives of the bigger group of so-called *N*-nitroso compounds, which are still discussed concerning the risk for the development of cancer due to human exposure from different sources. In the rich part of the Western world the human exposure to nitrosamines is now estimated to be down to about 0.1 mg day⁻¹ due to a drastic reduction in contents in foods and beverages that has taken place over the past 30 years or so. In comparison, the exposure to nitrosamines for a cigarette smoker from inhalation may be around 100 times greater.

Nitrosamines have been described in the chemical literature for over 100 years. In 1956, nitrosodimethylamine (NDMA) was first discovered to cause liver tumours in rats. This started an interest in the carcinogenesis of *N*-nitroso compounds, especially after NDMA later caused a large outbreak of liver disease in sheep in Norway.

By the year 2000, approximately 300 N-nitroso compounds had been tested. About 90% of these were found to cause cancer in an array of experimental animals. NDMA has been found to be carcinogenic in the more than 40 of the species tested so far. Most other nitrosamines are also carcinogens, and some are even transplacental carcinogens. Representatives of several other groups of N-nitroso compounds have also been proved to be carcinogenic in a number of experimental animals, although many differences exist as to which organs are affected. Humans are exposed to both preformed N-nitroso compounds and N-nitroso compounds formed *in vivo*. The main exposure is to nitrosamines, but also a few nitrosamides – which are generally more toxic to the nervous system – are met.

Preformed *N*-nitroso compounds

Preformed N-nitroso compounds may occur in foods such as cured meats and fish, cheeses and in alcoholic beverages. In most instances beer is no longer a principal source of nitrosamines, since the process of drying the barley malt has been converted from direct-fire drying to indirect-fire drying. It has been shown that the group of volatile nitrosamines include the main carcinogenic nitrosamines. Common volatile nitrosamines in a Western diet include NDMA, nitrosodiethylamine, nitrosopiperidine from spices, and nitrosopyrrolidine from, for example, fried bacon. Among these, nitrosopyrrolidine is one of the more carcinogenic nitrosamines that may be found at levels of about 100 ppb in fried bacon.

Cured meats may contain nitrosamines due to the meats' natural content of amines combined with the addition of a curing agent, most often $NaNO_2$ as already discussed. Fresh meats do not contain high levels of amines, but the level is increased during fermentation. Only secondary amines can form stable nitrosamines. Furthermore, the pH must be low enough or metal ions must be present to form NO^+, a key intermediate in the overall reaction scheme:

(a) $NaNO_2 + H^+ \rightarrow HNO_2 + Na^+$

$HNO_2 + H^+ \rightarrow NO^+ + H_2O$

(b) $2HNO_2 \rightarrow N_2O_3 + H_2O$

$N_2O_3 \rightarrow NO + NO_2$

$NO + M^+ \rightarrow NO^+ + M$

RNH_2 (primary amine) $+ NO^+ \rightarrow RNH-N=O + H^+ \rightarrow$ unstable

R_2NH (secondary amine) $+ NO^+ \rightarrow R_2N-N=O + H^+$

R_3N (tertiary amine) $+ NO^+ \rightarrow$ no nitrosamine formation

In the above, M/M^+ represents a transition metal like Fe^{2+}/Fe^{3+}.

When cured meats are heat processed at temperatures >130°C, the amount of nitrosamines will increase greatly, since these conditions are very conductive to nitrosamine formation.

N-nitroso compounds formed *in vivo*

N-nitroso compounds can also be formed endogenously in the human body. This *in vivo* formation can take place via either acid-catalysed or bacterial nitrosation or by NO formation during inflammation. The process takes place in the gastric juice in the stomach and is increased during inflammation. Ingested or endogenous nitrate and nitrite can form nitrosating agents as previously described for meat curing. The nitrosating agents react with amines, which are present in a wide range of foods, for example meat, and form nitrosamines.

Nitrosamines and human cancer

With the clear carcinogenic effect of many N-nitroso compounds in experimental animals in mind, it may seem surprising that a variety of human epidemiological investigations have not shown an indisputable relationship between nitrate/nitrite intake and the risk of cancer in man. However, one has to understand how difficult it is to compare the results from epidemiological studies on the connection between dietary intake and risk, especially when it comes to the effects of long-time exposure.

An example can be presented by looking at the Iowa Women's Health Study, which examined cancer incidences among 21,977 women who had used the same water supply for more than 10 years. For all types of cancer taken as one disease group there was no association with increasing nitrate content in the drinking water. However, positive relationships between both bladder cancer and ovarian cancer and the nitrate content in drinking water were shown. On the other hand, there were inverse associations between nitrate and both uterine and rectal cancer.

The most significant problems in such analyses are the methods used to assess intake, the definition of meat, the addition of prepared or raw meat, covariance, confounding and the representativeness of the study population. It has been shown that ascorbic acid and other antioxidants in the diet will reduce the amount of nitrosamine formation. This could perhaps be an important factor explaining why no clear association between the total intake of dietary nitrate/nitrite and cancer has been made: most dietary nitrate originates from vegetables, which in turn also have a relatively high content of vitamin C, i.e. the degree of nitrosamine formation will be diminished.

22.4 *Trans* Fatty Acids

Lipids in our diet

Lipids (fats and oils) are triacylglycerol esters with different carboxylic acids (often termed *fatty acids*). The acid composition with regard to chain length and number (but not placement) of double bonds is shown in Table 22.4 for a number of generally important sources of fat.

No matter what our diet, fats and oils represent an important component providing us with energy as well as essential fatty acids and being the bearer of a number of different fat-soluble vitamins, the concentration and selection depending on the source of the fat.

We need a number of unsaturated essential fatty acids which we as animals cannot biosynthesize ourselves. These include acids containing double bonds in either the *n*-3 (omega-3) or the *n*-6 (omega-6) position. Both linoleic acid (18:2*n*-6) and linolenic acid (18:3*n*-3) are usually consumed with plant products. Linoleic acid is converted by animals to arachidonic acid (20:4*n*-6) and linolenic acid to eicosapentaenoic acid (EPA, 20:5*n*-3). Arachidonic acid and EPA are subsequently converted into a number of compounds essential for our physiological regulation such as prostaglandins, prostacyclins and thromboxanes.

We consume fats in meat, milk and from plant sources, the latter especially as oils present in seeds (energy storage) or exceptionally in fruit pericarps (olive oil). In general the physical properties of a fat/oil depend on the chain average length of the acids as well as on the overall degree of unsaturation (number of double bonds) in these. The higher the degree of unsaturation, the more liquid the oil will be. Likewise the occurrence of double bonds makes oil vulnerable to oxidation and maybe polymerization, especially upon heating as occurs during pan-frying and deep-frying.

Table 22.4. Fatty acid composition of selected fats and oils from different sources.

	Content (g per 100 g)					
	Canola	Coconut	Maize	Cottonseed	'Fish'	Lard
C6:0	–	0.6	–	–	–	–
C8:0	–	7.5	–	–	–	–
C10:0	–	6.0	–	–	–	0.1
C12:0	–	44.6	–	–	–	0.2
C14:0	–	16.8	–	0.8	9.3	1.3
C16:0	4.8	8.2	10.9	22.7	17.1	23.8
C18:0	1.6	2.8	1.8	2.3	2.8	13.5
C16:1	–	–	–	0.8	12.5	2.7
C18:1	53.8	5.8	24.2	17.0	11.4	13.5
C18:2	22.1	1.8	58.0	51.5	1.5	41.2
C18:3	11.1	1.8	0.7	0.2	1.6	10.2
C20:1	–	–	–	–	1.6	–
C20:4	–	–	–	–	2.0	–
C20:5	–	–	–	–	15.5	–
C22:5	–	–	–	–	2.4	–
C22:6	–	–	–	–	9.1	–

Different oils and fats dominate in different parts of the world, although the industrialization of the world food market has levelled out the disparities to a great extent. As illustrated in Fig. 22.5, the overall degree of unsaturation is high for a considerable number of the important genuine plant-derived oils, which thus provide us with the essential fatty acids needed. However, solid and chemically stable fats which without addition of high concentrations of antioxidants can be stored at room temperature have some technical advantages in food processing, and have a longer shelf-life.

Industrial processing of oils and formation of *trans* fatty acids

Oils can be transformed industrially by transesterification, fractionation and hydrogenation. In order to produce more solid fats with a long shelf-life for the industrial plant, oils are hardened by hydrogenation (Fig. 22.6).

Compared with naturally occurring highly saturated plant fats (e.g. coconut oil) and unhydrogenated liquid plant oils, industrially hardened fats contain acids with one or more double bonds in a *trans* configuration formed as a by-product of the hydrogenation process, as opposed to the *cis* configuration normally found in fats and oils. Such industrially produced (IP) *trans fatty acids* (TFAs) often occur in concentrations of up to about 30%

by weight and in special cases IP-TFAs can constitute up to 60% by weight of the fat in certain foods. TFAs are also produced in microbiological processes in the rumen of ruminants, which is why so-called ruminant TFAs (R-TFAs) can constitute up to about 6% of a diet by weight.

Trans fatty acids and health risks

Intake of TFAs is associated with increased risk of coronary heart disease (CHD). An article in the well-known scientific journal *Atherosclerosis* in 2006 stated there was at that time definitive evidence from multiple randomized trials that TFAs have adverse effects on blood lipids, near-definitive evidence that TFAs increase inflammatory markers in blood, and strong evidence from prospective epidemiological studies that high TFA intake is associated with elevated risks of CHD. Shortly after, a meta-analysis of four large prospective studies found that an intake of TFAs corresponding to 2% of energy intake – approximately 5g day^{-1} – is associated with a 25% increased risk of CHD. CHD refers to the failure of coronary circulation to supply adequate circulation to cardiac muscle and surrounding tissue.

Restaurant-produced deep-fried foods and industrial fried and baked products are the most important sources of TFAs worldwide. A survey concerning the possible consumption of TFAs and the health risks conducted in 26 countries during

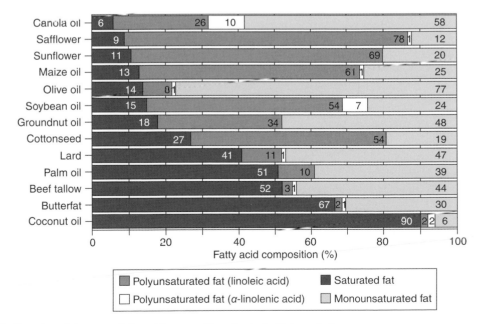

Fig. 22.5. Overview of the gross fatty acid composition of selected fats and oils.

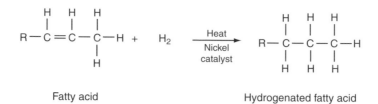

Fatty acid   Hydrogenated fatty acid

Fig. 22.6. Hydrogenation with nickel as the catalyst.

the period 2004–2006 defined a 'high trans menu' as a large serving of French fries and nuggets, 100 g of microwave popcorn and 100 g of biscuits/wafers/cakes. The investigation showed that such a 'high trans menu' provided more than 20 g of IP-TFA in 17 of the countries surveyed, with Hungary, Czech Republic, Poland, Bulgaria and the USA ranking highest with 42, 40, 38, 36 and 36 g, respectively.

In Denmark the content of TFAs was less than 1 g; however, a similar analysis performed earlier in the country had shown a content of 30 g TFAs in a similar menu. The reason for this great difference is clear: in 2004 Denmark – as the only country worldwide – limited the IP-TFAs in foods to a maximum of 2% of fat content by legislation. In this context it is interesting to note that the first-mentioned investigation found that the IP-TFA content of the McDonalds servings (French fries) varied from less than 1 g in Copenhagen (Denmark) and Beijing (China) to 10 g in New York City (USA), while another chain, KFC (Kentucky Fried Chicken), showed even bigger differences ranging from below 1 g in Germany to 24 g in Hungary. A considerable part of these differences could be ascribed to differences in the content of TFAs in the frying oils used.

The TFA content of hardened oils varies according to the hardening process used. The level can be reduced by using a low temperature (105–120°C), effective stirring and copper as the catalyst. Yet nothing is without drawbacks; even a small residual content of copper catalyst in deep-frying oil will cause a higher rate of hydrolysis of the lipids during the frying.

22.5 Cooking and Frying Mutagens (Browning Products)

Polycyclic aromatic hydrocarbons

Formation and occurrence

In 1775 Percivall Pott in England observed that chimney sweeps showed a high frequency of scrotal cancer.

(a)   (b)   (c)

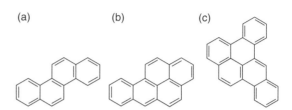

Fig. 22.7. Examples of PAHs: (a) chrysene (MW 228); (b) benzo[*a*]pyrene (MW 252); (c) dibenzo[*a,e*]pyrene (MW 302).

He related this to the fact that it is difficult to wash off the tar components from the surface of the scrotum. Later a number of studies related professions with close contact to coal tar and soot to different forms of cancer. In 1925 Kennaway produced in the laboratory some high-boiling tar fractions that proved to provoke cancer, and by 1930 he isolated the compound benzo[*a*]pyrene (3,4-benzpyrene) which was shown to be carcinogenic in laboratory animals. Benzo[*a*]pyrene belongs to the group of so-called *polycyclic aromatic hydrocarbons* (PAHs), which includes more than 100 compounds of which several are carcinogenic. The most feared have molecular weights between 226 and 302 and consist of from four to six fused rings (Fig. 22.7).

PAHs are formed by pyrolytic decomposition of various organic compounds at high temperatures (typically 300–400°C) and thus are found in the combustion from cars, in smoke from chimneys, and in tobacco smoke. PAHs can also be formed when preparing meals, especially when using cooking methods that involve intense heat with limited availability of oxygen such as roasting and grilling. High-fat food products are especially prone to the formation of PAHs. Thus, charcoal-broiled meats may contain up to 200 ppb of benzo[*a*] pyrene and comparison of a high-fat hamburger with lean beef typically reveals differences of about 50 ppb as compared with 5 ppb of total PAHs, respectively. Also charred crusts of bread products, broiled fish and roasted coffee have been shown to contain elevated concentrations of total PAHs. A special example of PAHs entering the food chain is that of deliberate production of smoke-cured products (see later).

Owing to the many sources of PAHs human exposure varies to a great extent, processed food products being only one source. Studies in towns in Europe, the USA, Australia and South Africa (highly industrialized regions) showed a huge variation in summer versus winter levels of PAHs (expressed as benzo[a]pyrene) in the air: 0.03–4 µg per 1000 m^3 as opposed to 0.6–104 µg per 1000 m^3, respectively. Airborne particulate PAHs will be inhaled and deposited on the surface of plant commodities. Food commodities produced in regions with a high level of PAHs in the air thus normally will have a much higher PAH content. As an example let us look at apples produced in an industrial area as opposed to a village suburb. Contents reported in the literature were: industrial area 30–60 (peel)/0.2–0.5 (inner part) and in the village suburb 5–6/0.1–0.4 µg benzo[a]pyrene kg^{-1} DW, respectively. According to the investigation about 20% of the benzo[a]pyrene could be removed from the peel by rinsing with water.

Another important source of PAHs is tobacco smoke. Active smokers may have a death rate from lung cancer about 15 times that of non-smokers. Furthermore, a meta-analysis of passive smoking showed that the excess risk of lung cancer was approximately 25% among lifelong never smokers who lived with a smoker. The principal carcinogens responsible are PAHs, together with nitrosamines and aromatic amines.

In conclusion, human exposure to PAHs varies depending on place of living, lifestyle (smoker/non-smoker), and awareness of how to treat and process food.

Mechanism of action

As already mentioned a number of PAHs are carcinogenic. Parental administration of benzo[a]pyrene thus has resulted in tumour formation in a number of organs in mice and rats, i.e. lungs and skin, as well as in the development of mamma cancer. Moreover, oral administration resulted in the formation of tumours in the lung, liver and blood vessels of mice and in the mammae of mice and rats, as well as reproductive and haematopoietic disturbances.

The compounds are genotoxic carcinogens after enzymatic activation. One of the most studied compounds, benzo[a]pyrene, is first oxidized by cytochrome P4501A1 to form a variety of products, including (+)-benzo[a]pyrene-7,8-epoxide. This product is metabolized by epoxide hydrolase, opening the epoxide ring to yield (–)-benzo[a]pyrene-7,8-dihydrodiol. The ultimate carcinogen is formed after still another reaction with cytochrome P4501A1, to yield (+)-benzo[a]pyrene-7,8-dihydrodiol-9,10-epoxide. This diol epoxide binds covalently to DNA, causing mutations (initiation of carcinogenesis) which can eventually result in tumour formation.

Smoke-curing and smoke flavourings

Among the multiple methods used to improve the shelf-life of food products (refrigeration and freezing, canning, irradiation, drying/dehydration, freeze-drying, salting, pickling, pasteurizing, fermentation, carbonation, chemical preservation and smoke-curing), smoke-curing deserves special attention when it comes to chemical food safety.

Smoke-curing (or simply smoking) is the process whereby the material is placed in/passed by freshly generated smoke. According to many sources of information the method has been used for preserving foods for thousands of years. The process, which is traditionally applied to certain perishable foods such as fish and meat, also imparts colour and flavour to food.

Smoking is applied among other foods to meat products such as pork products (ham, bacon), beef products (pastrami), lamb (e.g. in Iceland; 'hangikjöt' is smoked lamb leg or shoulder), various sausages, fish such as herrings (when salted and cold-smoked called 'kippers' or 'bloaters'), eel and farmed Atlantic salmon (*Salmo salar*) – a product exported worldwide, especially from Norway, and produced in very large amounts. However, also cheeses, certain vegetables such as garlic, ingredients used to make beverages such as whisky, and the Chinese 'lapsang souchong' tea are smoked.

Most often smoking does not stand alone as a method of food preservation. Salting, drying and smoking have been widely used in combination as a means to preserve fish such as herring and salmon, and the fundamental principles of this hurdle technique are still utilized by the commercial smoking industry. However, due to the development of sophisticated refrigeration and packaging technologies, the preservative action of the unit operations involved has become less important.

Thus, the extent of salting, drying and smoking of products has been significantly reduced, and so-called cold-smoked salmon nowadays appears as a lightly preserved product with a salt content in the range 2.0–3.9%, water activity in the range 0.93–0.98, pH in the range 5.4–6.2 and total phenol content in the range 3–14 mg kg^{-1}.

In Europe traditionally the smoke was generated by burning wood such as alder (or oak and beech) – restricting the air delivery – directly under the food products, which were hanging above. In North America hickory and mesquite and several other wood types are commonly used for smoking. Modern forced-convection industrial ovens for smoking of food, such as the 'Torry kiln' with a capacity of up to 750 kg of fish, have separate smoke generators. These may work in either a rather traditional way, by causing pyrolysis of wood dust (with a water content of 20–40%) by heating it on a hot plate, or in other ways such as by friction between a wood stick and a carborundum drum or by the heating of fluidized wood dust in a very hot inert gas. In general one subdivides the food smoking process into *cold smoking* (product temperature during the process from 18 to 30°C), *medium-temperature smoking* (about 40°C) and *warm smoking* (70–90°C). Together with the smoking temperature and time, both the source(s) of wood and the method of smoke generation are of importance for the chemical safety of the final food product, the latter determining the composition of the smoke.

Major wood smoke components include acetic acid (and higher acid homologues), methanol and 'soluble tar substances' such as different phenolic compounds. All together more than 450 compounds have been identified in different wood smokes analysed. The preservative action of the smoking process depends on: (i) the product drying during the smoking; (ii) the lowering of the pH as caused by the acids; and (iii) an antimicrobial effect of many of the phenolic substances. The surface colour formation depends mostly on Maillard reactions as initiated by reactions between formaldehyde (about 1%) in the smoke and amino groups in the product's proteins. The flavour is very complex in that a high number of different compounds each gives its own contribution: esters, aromatic ketones and phenolic aldehydes (sweet), pentadione (caramel-like), diacetyl (bread-like), vinyl guaiacol (smoke-like), etc.

While most of the compounds we have mentioned so far do not give rise to great concerns, one

group does. This is the group of PAHs. CAC recommends the combustion temperature in the smoke generator to be in the range of 250–350°C to minimize formation of compounds with adverse health effects such as PAHs.

With the development of other methods of food preservation and of effective chains of cold storage from producer to consumer, gradually the preservative effect obtained by traditional smoking has become less important. However, the flavour is still wanted by the consumer, which is why *liquid smoke flavouring products* have gained increasing popularity and importance. These products are not new. In their impressive two-volume encyclopaedia entitled *Handbuch der Drogisten-Praxis; ein Lehr- und Nachschlagebuch für Drogisten, Farbwarenhändler und so weiter* from 1919, the German authors Buchheister and Ottersbach describe the production of so-called 'holz säure' (wood acid) as a by-product of the production of wood tars, which were and still are used in dermatological practice. They do not stop there, however; they also describe the use of the wood acid as a means of preserving especially fish while at the same time obtaining the smoked flavour.

The modern commercially available smoke flavours still are produced on the basis of wood which is thermally degraded in a limited supply of oxygen (pyrolysis). The smoke (vapours) is condensed to give a liquid product which by physical means is separated into two to three phases: an aqueous phase, an oily phase and a water-insoluble high-density tar phase. The aqueous phase (more or less identical to the traditional wood acid) perhaps as supplemented with components from the tar phase is the basis for the production of the smoke flavour by means of further refinement steps such as extraction, distillation, concentration, absorption or membrane separation. Naturally, the basic condensates used for this further refinement also contain PAHs, which is why the EU nowadays sets maximum limits for these substances, among others, in smoked foods as well as in liquid smoke flavouring products.

Regulations and maximum limits

In 2006 the European Commission implemented a maximum limit of 5 μg benzo[a]pyrene per kilogram of smoked food product, a limit which applies to the whole of the EU. A subsequent survey made in Denmark in collaboration between professional societies of the Danish fish producers and the Danish meat producers showed the following results:

- A great variety of smoke ovens from small manually controlled table-top types to huge electronically controlled industrial ovens were used for the production of smoked foods marketed in Denmark.
- Technically, the pallet of ovens included both the ones that generate the smoke directly in the smoking chamber (direct smoking) and the ones having a separate smoke generator (indirect smoking).
- Analysis of close to 180 samples showed that a majority had a content of benzo[a]pyrene below $1\,\mu g\,kg^{-1}$.
- Analysis also showed that the total sum of 25 PAHs analysed was less than half in the indirectly smoked products compared with the directly smoked foods.
- Warm-smoked salmon compared with cold-smoked showed more than double the content of PAHs (total of 25 PAHs analysed).

At the end of 2003 the EU also implemented a new piece of legislation regulating the area of smoke flavourings used or intended for use in or on foods (Regulation (EC) No. 2065/2003). According to this each producer shall have his 'smoke flavouring primary product' (from which the different specific flavour products are produced) approved. Approval will be based on an application, which must describe the production process in details and report on the quantitative content of 15 specified PAHs and on the results of the following toxicological tests performed according to international protocols such as the OECD *Guidelines for the Testing of Chemicals*: (i) subchronic toxicity, a 90-day feeding study in rodents; (ii) a test for the induction of gene mutations in bacteria; (iii) a test for induction of gene mutations in mammalian cells *in vitro*; and (iv) a test for induction of chromosomal aberrations in mammalian cells *in vitro* (or *in vivo*) (Guidance from the Scientific Panel of food additives, flavourings, processing aids and materials in contact with food; Guidance on submission of a dossier on a Smoke Flavouring Primary Product for evaluation by EFSA).

Interestingly, among eight products risk-assessed by EFSA one was not approved as communicated to the public by an EFSA press release of 21 June 2007. The reasons for the Panel not being able to

establish its safety in use when added to food was that the product was weakly genotoxic *in vivo*.

Heterocyclic aromatic amines

Just as acrylamide and PAHs are formed upon heat processing of foods, so too are the *heterocyclic aromatic amines* (HAAs; also called HAs or HCAs = frying mutagens). While acrylamide mostly is formed in starch-rich products and PAHs are formed on the surface of fatty meat and fish, the amines discussed here are formed primarily from creatinine and/or amino acids. The HAAs thus may be divided into two classes:

1. The so-called *IQ compounds* (imidazo quinolines and imidazole quinoxalines), formed by reaction between a Maillard reaction product (pyridines and pyrazines) and creatinine (Fig. 22.8). Optimum temperatures for their formation were found to be about 200°C. The compounds are not formed in non-muscular tissues (e.g. liver) since these do not contain creatine/creatinine.

2. The *aminopyridines*, which seem to be formed directly as products of protein pyrolysis at temperatures higher than 300°C. For example, tryptophan has been shown to be the precursor of the mutagen 3-amino-1-methyl-5*H*-pyrido[4,3-*b*] indole.

When looking at the minimum/optimum temperatures for the formation of the two compound classes it is evident that pan-frying or broiling enhances formation of the HAAs compared with

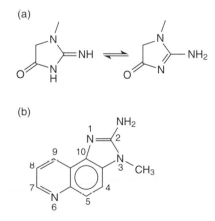

Fig. 22.8. (a) Creatinine (a degradation product of creatine phosphate in muscle); (b) the mutagenic HAA 2-amino-3-methylimidazo(4,5-*f*)quinoline.

deep-frying or stewing. Actually a rare to medium-rare (beef) steak fried at up to about 150°C will contain much fewer mutagens of these two types than will a well-done steak.

Members from both classes of compound were shown in the 1980s to be mutagenic (especially frameshift) after activation by liver enzymes (S9 mix) when investigated in bacteria (Ames test and related tests). This is in agreement with later findings that they are activated through N-hydroxylation by cytochrome P450. The N-hydroxyl compound formed requires further activation by O-acetylation or O-sulfonation to be able to react with DNA. The compounds are in general absorbed rapidly in the gastrointestinal tract, and many have been shown to be carcinogenic in rodents.

Glucose-derived advanced glycation end-products

The already discussed Maillard reaction between a reducing sugar (pentoses and hexoses) and aliphatic primary or secondary amines of amino acids is the starting point for the formation of the mixture of insoluble dark-brown polymeric pigments called *melanoidins*, i.e. the dark pigments of the browning reaction when toasting, etc. During the early stages of this process a large number of water-soluble compounds are formed, which as a group are termed *premelanoidins*. Some of these mixtures and individual compounds were demonstrated to inhibit growth, cause liver damage and interrupt reproduction in laboratory animals. However, of even greater interest nowadays is the discussion on whether an Amadori modification of a protein, which typically will mean a reaction between a dissolved reducing saccharide such as glucose or lactose with a free amino group at a lysine residue in a protein (remembering that lysine possesses two amino groups), can lead to health-impairing effects. Such products are also called *advanced glycation end-products* (AGEs). The reason for this discussion is the fact that glucose-derived AGEs are associated with, and according to some scientists may be a causal factor, in the development of vascular complications of diabetes. Thus, AGEs, a heterogeneous group of molecules that form spontaneously *in vivo* via non-enzymatic glycoxidative reactions between reducing sugars and proteins (and lipids), accumulate slowly in vascular and renal tissues with ageing and at a significantly higher rate in diabetes.

22.6   Urethane

The New York Times reported on 29 December 1987 that the US distilling industry had proposed voluntary guidelines for reducing levels of a contaminant in whisky and other alcoholic beverages. The reason for this action was that studies conducted in Canada in 1985 had shown the presence of urethane (ethyl carbamate) in wines and distilled beverages and that Canada had established a maximum value in distilled beverages of $150\,\mu g\,l^{-1}$, based on consumption patterns and an ADI of $0.3\,mg\,kg^{-1}$ BW. The contaminant as we can understand was urethane and the risks were malignant tumours and leukaemia found with greater frequency in rats injected with up to $0.1\,mg\,kg^{-1}$ BW.

In the USA, FDA sampled the market in 1987 and found that imported brandies contained the highest levels of urethane averaging about $1200\,\mu g\,l^{-1}$, followed by sake with $\sim300\,\mu g\,l^{-1}$ and then bourbon (whisky) with levels averaging $150\,\mu g\,l^{-1}$. Table wines had levels of $\sim15\,\mu g\,l^{-1}$, but dessert wines, such as sherries and liqueurs, averaged $\sim115\,\mu g\,l^{-1}$.

The voluntary guideline accepted as its target by the industry in 1987 was $125\,\mu g\,l^{-1}$ for urethane levels in all new whisky produced as of 1 January 1989. As a follow-up on the first sampling and the agreement with US industry, a new sampling of domestic and foreign products was done in 1991 by FDA and the US Bureau of Alcohol. The results shown in Table 22.5 indicate that urethane levels in most instances had decreased.

Today the USA imposes the value of $125\,\mu g\,l^{-1}$ as the maximum limit for all imported distilled beverages.

Urethane occurs naturally in many (especially fermented) foods and beverages. In table wines, the levels are usually in the range of $10-50\,\mu g\,l^{-1}$ as a result of the enzymatic degradation of arginine into urea, which reacts with ethanol to produce urethane. For this reason the US Wine Institute in the 1990s recommended grape growers to minimize fertilization, since heavily fertilized vineyards tend to produce grapes that contain high levels of arginine, thus leading to higher urea and urethane levels. The levels further increase with product overheating during the distillation of spirits. This is particularly true in the distillation of some beverages made from stone fruits rich in cyanogenic glycosides, such as amygdalin. For such fruit

Table 22.5. Urethane levels as found in different products.

Product	Average urethane level (ppb)		
	1987	1991	
		Domestic	Imported
Brandy (grape)	40	10	45
Brandy (fruit)	1200	5	255
Bourbon (retail)	150	70	55
Rum	20	2	5
Liqueur	100	10	25
Scotch	50	a	55
Sherry	130	10	40
Port	60	23	26
Grape wine	13	10	15
Sake	300	55	60

a Scotch is not manufactured in the USA.

brandies urethane concentrations higher than $1500 \mu g \, l^{-1}$ have been reported. One chemical pathway proposed for this latter formation of urethane involves the oxidation of cyanide (CN^-) formed from the cyanogenic glycoside(s):

$$2Cu(II) + 4CN^- \rightarrow 2Cu(CN)_2$$

$$2Cu(CN)_2 \rightarrow 2CuCN + C_2N_2$$

$$C_2N_2 + 2OH^- \rightarrow NCO^- + CN^- + H_2O$$

$$NCO^- + C_2H_5OH + H^+ \rightarrow C_2H_5OCONH_2$$
$$\text{(urethane)}$$

There is still a focus on urethane, which is classified in Group 2B by IARC: the agent (mixture) is possibly carcinogenic to humans, i.e. it is reasonably anticipated to be a human carcinogen based on sufficient evidence of carcinogenicity in experimental animals. When administered in the drinking water to rats among others, the compound induced lung adenomas, lymphomas (mainly lymphosarcomas), liver angiomas and haemangiomas, papillomas and sebaceous carcinomas of the skin. Also various tumours were seen in experiments using hamsters.

Entering the 21st century, the level of urethane therefore has gradually become the main obstacle for the exportation of different distilled beverages from certain producer countries – as has happened for Brazil, for example, concerning its sugarcane spirits. Therefore, Brazil established a 5-year limit for

sugarcane distilleries to attain the same maximum acceptable level as Canada. A survey published in 2007 subsequently showed that about 45% of products sampled from Rio de Janeiro contained urethane above the level of $150 \mu g \, l^{-1}$, with an average of $160 \mu g \, l^{-1}$. The lower values were from samples from alembics (distilling apparatuses) using low-temperature and high-reflux-rate distillation.

As already mentioned in Chapter 18 in the introduction to contaminants, in 2009 EFSA began collecting data on the presence of ethyl carbamate in foods and beverages within Europe. However, having talked about the risk of cancer from the exposure to urethane in alcoholic beverages, it should not be overlooked that the consumption of alcohol (ethyl alcohol) in itself is a significant risk factor when it comes to the development of a number of cancer forms. This is also pointed to by IARC, which classifies alcoholic beverages as carcinogenic to humans (Group 1).

Many people will know 'polyurethane' as a type of white rigid foam used for many different purposes. However, as described in Box 22.1, this has little direct connection with what we have just discussed.

22.7 Biogenic Amines

All animal organisms produce a number of amines, each of which plays an important role for the normal function of the species in question. In higher animals these include among others neurotransmitters such as noradrenaline (norepinephrine), dopamine, serotonin (5-hydroxytryptamine, 5 HT) and histamine, as well as adrenaline (epinephrine). Histamine also plays an important role in the immune system in that it is present in a high concentration in mast cells from where it is released upon their degradation. The specific actions of histamine include constriction of bronchial smooth muscle, venous constriction and increase in capillary permeability, effects that are the result of the interaction of histamine with histamine receptors (types H1 and H2).

Plants also biosynthesize a number of amines essential for their general function. Examples are the diamine putrescine and the polyamines spermidine and spermine with different roles in the processes of cell division and flowering. Moreover, some plants store large amounts of tyramine together with the *N*-methylated compounds *N*-methyl tyramine and *N*-methyl-β-phenylethylamine. These

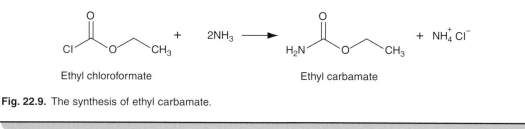
compounds are thought to be the causative agents of intoxications in husbandry when eating leaves of plants such as *Acacia berlandieri*.

The amines can be aliphatic, aromatic or heterocyclic depending on their origin, which in general is by enzymatic decarboxylation of amino acids such as lysine, ornithine, phenylalanine, tyrosine, histidine or tryptophan. Amines formed this way are often called *biogenic amines*.

Biogenic amines can also be formed by decarboxylation of amino acids released upon hydrolytic degradation of proteins, both processes being facilitated by microorganisms. Such formation of especially the amines histamine (together with putrescine and cadaverine) and tyramine are well described as leading to food poisonings.

Scombroid poisoning

Scombroid is a moderately common technical term in zoology, deriving ultimately from the Greek *scombros* = tuna, which also led via Latin to *scomber* as an uncommon English word for mackerel, but which is now only used as the formal name for this genus of fish. The scombroid fish is a group of about 100 species that include mackerel, tuna, marlin and swordfish. Many of us

are most likely to encounter the word in the phrase *scombroid poisoning*, a poisoning which is caused by eating fish that contains histamine produced by bacterial activity as a result of poor storage.

Low levels of biogenic amines normally represent no risk to humans; however, eating food with a high content may lead to symptoms of food poisoning. The adverse effects of these compounds can be potentiated by the simultaneous intake of alcohol or certain kinds of medicine. If food products (especially scombroid fish) are stored incorrectly, e.g. at too high a temperature for a long period, bacteria naturally occurring in the product can form histamine and other biogenic amines by hydrolysis of the fish proteins and subsequent decarboxylation of the formed amino acids. This may lead to toxic reactions when eating the food products.

Fish species described to be involved in this kind of food intoxication include tuna, kahawai, mackerel, bonito and butterfly kingfish, as well as certain non-scombroid fish including Western Australian salmon, sardines, 'mahi-mahi' (dolphin-fish) and blue marlin.

The most important bacterium with respect to the protein degradation and the formation of the amines in fish is *Morganella morganii*. However, several other species are also found to be implicated: *Klebsiella pneumoniae*, *Proteus* spp., *Enterobacter aerogenes*, *Hafnia alvei* and *Vibrio algenolyticus*. In fermented fish products, several *Lactobacillus* spp. have also been implicated in histamine production.

It is important to note that cooking, canning and/or freezing do not reduce the toxicity. The distribution of the toxin within an individual fish fillet or between cans in a case lot can be very uneven, with some sections of a product causing illness and others not.

Food products with a high concentration of histamine may give a burning sensation on the tongue as well as on the lips and in the throat. Blisters may occur on the tongue and the lips. If one encounters these symptoms the food should immediately be spat out and the rest should not be eaten. Other symptoms of histamine intoxication include reddishness in the face and on the chest (urticaria), headache, vomiting, stomach pains and swollen lips. Sometimes itching is also seen, together with dizziness and low blood pressure. In the case of severe intoxication pain from the lungs and shock may also occur. The onset of the symptoms can occur immediately up to about 30 min to 2 h and diminish within about 3 h to 1 day. Histamine (scombroid) poisoning is often misdiagnosed as fish allergy (Box 22.2).

Investigations in guinea pigs have shown a potentiating effect of the two biogenic amines putrescine and cadaverine on the symptoms of histamine toxicity when the substances are administered orally. Also, it has been demonstrated that spermine and spermidine can enhance the absorption of histamine in the gastrointestinal tract.

In places such as the USA and certain European countries where statistics on the occurrence of food poisonings are relatively well established, scombroid poisoning has proved to be quite common. Some examples from Denmark are given in Box 22.3.

Biogenic amines in other food products

A number of other food products and beverages can contain biogenic amines in concentrations that may result in adverse health symptoms. These include cheese, wines and different soy products. Cheese is the type of food product next most often associated with biogenic amine poisonings after fish. Outbreaks have been described for Gouda, Cheddar, Gruyère, Cheshire and different Swiss types of cheese. The relative occurrence of the different protein amino acids in milk, coupled with the enzymatic activities of the involved bacteria, means that in cheese normally one will see a formation of all four biogenic amines: histamine, tyramine, cadaverine and putrescine. This was demonstrated in an investigation on the effect of using bactofugated milk on the formation of biogenic amines when producing Emmental cheese.

In cheese, species of *Lactobacillus* plays an important role in the formation of histamine, tyramine and putrescine; however, certain coli forms and species of *Enterococcus* are also described as being important especially concerning the formation of tyramine. If the raw milk used for the cheese production is pasteurized, coli forms are inactivated while some enterococci may survive. *Enterococcus faecalis* and *Enterococcus faecium* have been implicated in the formation of biogenic amines in cheese.

In 1985 a Swiss cheese was identified as the food source causing an outbreak of histamine poisoning. A subsequent investigation resulted in the isolation of a strain of *Lactobacillus buchneri* able to produce 42 mg of histamine per 100 g of medium, a very high production. The high histidine decarboxylase activity found was shown to be both species- and strain-specific. Subsequent investigations using such strains of *L. buchneri* in the production of Gouda cheese has provided detailed knowledge about the factors influencing the histamine formation. In conclusion, the resulting histamine level

---

Box 22.2. Allergy to fish proteins

Allergy to fish is an immune reaction to a fish-specific protein present in most fish species. Thus, most people allergic to fish are allergic to all fish. However, tuna is special in this respect, so if a person has an allergy to tuna it is possible that he/she is allergic only to this species. The allergens of fish are in general very heat-stable, which means that it is not possible to remove the problem by boiling or frying. Very sensitive individuals may react with allergic reactions just by breathing in the steam from boiling fish.

---

was higher in cheeses produced using a high storage temperature, a high pH and/or a high salt concentration, as compared with cheeses stored at low temperature, low pH and/or salt concentration, respectively.

22.8   3-MCPD and 1,3-DCP

The traditional soy sauce from Japan and surrounding countries is normally produced by fermentation of soybeans; it takes about 4–5 months to make the traditional product. However, in order to speed up the process, hydrolysis of the protein using a relatively strong acid (HCl) and elevated temperature has been introduced by a number of producers.

In 2001, FSA in the UK warned against unacceptable levels of two potentially carcinogenic compounds found in soy sauce products from China, Taiwan and Thailand. These are the compounds 3-MCPD (3-monochloropropane-1, 2-diol) and 1,3-DCP (1,3-dichloro-2-propanol). Of these, 3-MCPD is in the pipeline for new formal evaluations by IARC. The compounds are formed as a result of a hydrolysis of the lipids also present in the soybeans. The hydrolysis leads to the release of glycerol, which by reaction with HCl forms the two compounds. Japanese soy sauce products investigated showed no such contents.

The conclusions of risk assessments made for especially 3-MCPD have changed through time. Within the EU, SCF evaluated 3-MCPD in 1994 and concluded as follows, based on the results reported for a carcinogenicity study and the fact that the compound in the Ames test causes base-pair substitutions:

A safe threshold dose cannot be determined and 3-MCPD should be considered as an undesirable contaminant in food. Therefore residues of 3-MCPD in food products should be undetectable by the most sensitive analytical method.

SCF again looked at 3-MCPD in 1997 but stated there was no reason to change the conclusion drawn in 1994. However, in the year 2001 yet another new opinion was published by SCF on 3-MCPD. This time things had changed. Three new studies published in 1997 and 2000 had shown that 3-MCPD did not induce unscheduled DNA synthesis in the liver of male rats, was found to be negative in the bone marrow micronucleus test in male rats and showed no evidence of gentoxicity in an assay using *Drosophila melanogaster* (generally called the 'common fruit fly' or the 'vinegar fly'). On this basis SCF now concluded that:

taking into account the lack of genotoxicity *in vivo* and the likely secondary mechanisms of the tumorigenic affects seen in the chronic toxicity study in rats a threshold-based approach for deriving a Tolerable Daily Intake (TDI) would be appropriate.

Using an overall uncertainty factor of 500, SCF established a TDI of $2 \mu g \, kg^{-1}$ BW. Perhaps we have not heard the last about this compound; only time will tell.

22.9 Conclusion

Processing food is an ever ongoing activity around the world; every second millions of people are preparing meals in their home, at restaurants and institutions, or in an industrial setting. These activities ensure that we get delicious and easily digestible food which – if prepared according to the normal procedures developed locally over time – most often also is safe from a microbiological point of view. This chapter has demonstrated that simultaneous formation of new chemical entities that can result in adverse effects acutely or chronically may accompany our food processing activities. However, the chapter also has described the current knowledge that allows us to minimize these consequences of (especially heat) processing.

Note

[1] Zyzak, D., Sanders, R.A., Stojanovic, M., Tallmadge, D.H., Ebehart, L., Ewald, D.K., Gruber, D.C., Morsch, T.R., Strothers, M.A., Rizzi, G.P. and Villagram, M.D. (2003) Acrylamide formation mechanism in heated foods. *Journal of Agricultural and Food Chemistry* 51, 4782–4787.

Further Reading

Dabrowski, W.M., Zdzislaw, E. and Sikorski, Z.E. (eds) (2004) *Toxins in Food*. CRC Press, Boca Raton, Florida.

Seal, C.J., de Mul, A., Eisenbrand, G., Haverkort, A.J., Franke, K., Lalljie, S.P.D., Mykkänen, H., Reimerdes, E., Scholz, G., Somoza, V., Tuijtelaars, S., van Boekel, M., van Klaveren, J., Wilcockson, S.J. and Wilms, L. (2008) Risk–benefit considerations of mitigation measures on acrylamide content of foods – a case study on potatoes, cereals and coffee. *British Journal of Nutrition* 99, S1–S46.

23 Veterinary Drugs and Contaminant Overall Conclusion

- Veterinary drugs may give rise to residues – the problem is discussed.
- An overall conclusion concerning contaminants is presented.

23.1 Veterinary Drugs

In the more industrialized parts of the world animal production has become more and more intensive with production units containing a large number of animals. Veterinary drugs play a vital role as effective therapeutic and preventive (prophylactic) means for controlling animal diseases and in the control of transmission of disease from animals to humans (*zoonoses*). Also the use of growth promoters in order to obtain the most optimal production economy is part of this consideration. The use of veterinary drugs in the production of food-producing animals – like the use of pesticides to protect our food crops – means that we risk consuming residues of these compounds, residues that may be present in edible tissues and products such as milk and eggs.

In order to prevent the occurrence of health-threatening drug residues pharmaceutical companies wishing to register new products must submit a dossier of data to the relevant authorities for approval. This must contain toxicological data for the compound including an NOAEL determined through animal studies. Furthermore, the results of measurements of concentrations found in different edible tissues and other products such as milk/eggs after different periods of time following treatments of relevant production animals must be reported. Based on the toxicological data an ADI value is calculated for the compound using the normal procedures (see Chapter 27). Thereafter, an MRL is set for different tissues and products so that in general the ADI will not be exceeded. In order to ensure that these MRLs are not exceeded in tissues and products from treated and later slaughtered animals, the farmer

must follow the advised treatment regimes (doses, etc.) and obey the withdrawal periods. A *withdrawal period* is set as the time for residues to fall to a concentration below the MRL in each tissue where an MRL has been set for the animal species in question.

One way of classifying the veterinary drugs of relevance is as:

- *therapeutic agents* used to control infectious diseases in farm animals;
- *prophylactic agents* used to prevent outbreaks of diseases and control parasitic infections, e.g. at certain times of the year;
- *growth promoters* belonging to either the class of antimicrobial promoters or the group of anabolic agents; and
- *hormonal drugs* used to control reproduction in farm animals.

However, as we see below, several compounds may be used in more than one of these situations.

Therapeutic agents used in production animals include:

1. *Antimicrobial compounds* such as sulfonamides, β-lactams (penicillins and cephalosporins), tetracyclines, aminoglycosides (e.g. streptomycin), macrolides (e.g. tylosin) and quinolones/fluoroquinolones.
2. Four groups of *anthelmintic agents*, i.e. benzimidazoles, tetrahydroimidathiazoles (e.g. levamisole) and the related compounds, avermectines and anilides.
3. *Coccidiostats*, which include a broad number of compounds with the so-called *ionophores* (monensin and related compounds) as the most important.

Several of these compounds are also used in prophylactic regimes and certainly as growth promoters.

Anabolic growth promoters include the stilbene compounds (e.g. DES) and a number of naturally occurring steroids as well as derivatives of such steroids. While a number of anabolic growth promoters are allowed and used in cattle production in the USA, this is not the case in the EU. The group of synthetic anabolic agents with oestrogenic activity, the stilbene compounds, was prohibited in 1982 because of fears about adverse health effects from residues. Later on, the use of anabolic growth promoters was totally prohibited in the EU.

Today many countries worldwide have implemented a surveillance programme for veterinary drug residues in food products of animal origin. The EU Directive 96/23/EEC sets out the sampling regime and the veterinary drugs that must be monitored. If we use the results of surveillance in the UK as an example we can get an idea about the frequencies of occurrence and the levels of residues found for the different types of drug. During 1998 some 25,028 samples of red meat were tested for residues of veterinary drugs. Only 13 (0.05%) of the samples contained residues above the MRL, while a further 17 (0.07%) samples contained residues at a level below the MRL for the compound in question. For the poultry meat samples analysed, 1.2% (96 samples) was found to contain a drug residue above the MRL. Muscle samples from farmed fish were also analysed, in this case four out of 814 samples contained residues above the MRL. The compound in all four cases was a tetracycline. Analysis of eggs showed an occurrence of drug residues above the MRL level at a frequency of 2.5%; nicarbazin was the drug most often found in this case.

From the above it seems safe to conclude that in well-controlled societies the occurrence of veterinary drug residues does not represent a general problem.

23.2 Contaminants – Overall Conclusion

Especially when we talk about the old very lipophilic pesticides such as DDT and its fellow chlorinated insecticides, the methylmercury occurring in fatty fish, the PCBs used earlier in transformers, etc. and the dioxins as well as other persistent man-made compounds such as the brominated flame retardants used in computers and televisions, we will always have to think about the possible consequences of accumulation in the body for different age groups including the unborn child. Thus, different national food agencies have had different but still restrictive recommendations for pregnant women concerning the intake of fatty fish. The reason for this is that a cost–benefit analysis has to be made between the risk of a damaging effect on the development of the fetal CNS and the high nutritional value of these fish with respect to for instance fat-soluble vitamins and important unsaturated fatty acids.

Likewise, at the time of writing this text, experts are discussing which recommendations to give concerning the optimal duration of breast-feeding. At present WHO recommends 6 months of breast-feeding followed by a further 6-month period with a gradual shift to solid foods. However, given that after 4–6 months of breast-feeding the concentration of several of the above-mentioned compounds in the baby's body has in general reached a level similar to that in the mother, some experts have suggested that breast-feeding should be terminated in the period between 4 and 6 months of age. Again it is a question of balance, since many different factors must be taken into account when making such a recommendation. Examples of such factors are the availability and quality of alternative food resources for the baby, the economic feasibility of the family purchasing the good alternatives, and the quality (chemical and microbiological) of the water available for the preparation of, for example, breast-milk substitutes.

Taking a final example of the difficulties faced in risk assessment, management and communication concerning food contaminants, we should recapitulate the great difference in the risk of developing liver cancer as a result of exposure to aflatoxins found between individuals with HBV as opposed to non-infected individuals. In this case unfortunately most HBV-positive individuals live in regions of the world where the likelihood of encountering high exposure to aflatoxins also is the greatest, such as Africa south of Sahel and South-east Asia.

23.3 Conclusion

A high number of compounds of very different origin and chemical structures can be found as contaminants in our food products. Good food production practices combined with legislative regulations and effective control systems can, however, ensure that with our current scientifically based knowledge we avoid both most acute and most chronic adverse effects.

Further Reading

Botsoglou, N.A. and Fletouris, D.J. (2001) *Drug Residues in Foods: Pharmacology, Food Safety and Analysis*. Marcel Dekker, New York, New York.

Cannavan, A. (ed.) (2005) *Development of Strategies for the Effective Monitoring of Veterinary Drug Residues in Livestock and Livestock Products in Developing Countries. Book of Abstracts of the 2nd International Symposium on Recent Advances in Food Analysis, Prague, Czech Republic, 2–4 November 2005*. Food and Agriculture Organization of the United Nations, Rome.

Schmidt, R.H. and Rodrick, G.E. (eds) (2003) *Food Safety Handbook*. John Wiley & Sons, Hoboken, New Jersey.

24 Food Additives and Flavourings, Etc.

- We define food additives and list the different major groups and their uses.
- We look at the safety of food additives through history up until today.
- We define flavourings and describe the different ways of production together with their safety.

24.1 Introduction to Food Additives

Food additives may be defined in a number of ways; thus, different national and regional pieces of legislation have different wording. However, the actual meaning of the different texts is more or less identical. For simplicity in this chapter we refer to the EU legislation and its definitions.

According to the EU, *food additives* are substances added intentionally to foodstuffs to perform certain technological functions, such as to colour, to sweeten or to help preserve foods, or said in more complicated legal text:

> any substance not normally consumed as a food in itself and not normally used as a characteristic ingredient of food, whether or not it has nutritive value, the intentional addition of which to food for a technological purpose results in it or its by-products becoming directly or indirectly a component of such foods. (Council Directive 89/107/EEC)

Under European legislation, additives must be explicitly authorized at European level before they can be used in foods. Upon authorization an additive is given an identity number, a so-called *E-number*, which together with its function in the finished food (e.g. preservative, colour, emulsifier, gelling agent) must always be stated in the ingredient list of the product. All authorized additives must comply with approved purity criteria, which are laid down in other directives.

The EU legislation was originally structured with three individual directives; namely, Directive 94/35/EC on sweeteners for use in foodstuffs and Directive 94/36/EC on colours for use in foodstuffs, both launched in 1994, and Directive 95/2/EC implemented the following year covering food additives other than colours and sweeteners.

In 2008 a new regulation, Regulation (EC) No. 1333/2008 of the European Parliament and of the Council of 16 December 2008 on food additives, was put into force. Gradually – as annexes are produced – this will replace the three aforementioned directives. The new regulation further constitutes part of a whole new regulatory package on Food Improvement Agents which further includes food enzymes (Regulation (EC) No. 1332/2008) and flavourings and certain food ingredients with flavouring properties (Regulation (EC) No. 1334/2008), as well as an additional fourth regulation establishing a common authorization procedure for these (Regulation (EC) No. 1331/2008).

Before authorization all additives as well as food enzymes and flavouring must undergo a safety evaluation for use of the agent as intended. For additives, those permitted before 20 January 2009 are foreseen to all be re-evaluated by December 2020 by EFSA. A guidance document exists on how to prepare such an application (http://ec. europa.eu/food/food/chemicalsafety/additives/ flav16_en.pdf).

The application dossier must include a toxicological section, which normally must describe the results obtained from such core studies as:

- metabolism/toxicokinetics;
- subchronic toxicity;
- genotoxicity;
- chronic toxicity and carcinogenicity; and
- reproduction and developmental toxicity.

In addition the application dossier must include information on, among other things, chemical name and structure, specifications and methods for analysing the substance, production procedures, technological requirement and levels intended for use in food.

So far we have mostly been describing food additives from a legislation point of view, and therefore also to a certain extent in legislative terms. Now let us take a more descriptive look at food additives and their main functions.

Food additives (including nutritional fortifications) serve five main functions:

1. *Maintain the wholesomeness of foods.* Contamination from bacteria can allow food-borne illnesses to occur. Preservatives and antioxidants reduce the spoilage that air, fungi, bacteria or yeast can cause. Preservatives and antioxidants help baked goods preserve their flavour by preventing the fats and oils from becoming rancid. They also keep fresh fruits from turning brown when exposed to air.

2. *Provide colour and enhance flavour.* Certain colours improve the appearance of foods. Similarly artificial sweeteners, many spices, natural and synthetic flavours and flavour enhancers (e.g. monosodium glutamate) may constitute or bring out the best in the flavour of food.

3. *Control the acidity and alkalinity, and provide leavening.* Specific additives help change the acidity or alkalinity of foods to obtain a desired taste, colour or flavour. Leavening agents that release acids when they are heated react with baking soda to help biscuits, cakes and other baked goods rise.

4. *Maintain product consistency.* Emulsifiers provide a consistent texture and prevent products from separating. Stabilizers and thickeners provide a uniform texture. Anticaking agents enable substances to flow freely.

5. *Improve or preserve the nutrient value.* Fortification and enrichment of foods have made it possible to improve the nutritional status of populations worldwide. For example, vitamins and minerals (e.g. iodine) may be added to many foods including flour, cereal, margarine and milk. What is allowed to be added depends on national/regional legislation. Such additions help to make up for vitamins or minerals that may be low or completely lacking in a person's diet. In most countries/regions all products that contain added nutrients (fortifications) must be labelled.

24.2 Origin, Identity and Purity

Food additives as well as flavourings may have very different origins. Some are more or less purified extracts of plants, animals or microorganisms, examples being the additives carnauba wax and cassia gum mentioned previously (Chapter 11 and Chapter 2, respectively) in other contexts; others are semi-synthetic compounds such as glycerol ester of wood rosin (E445) used to keep oils in suspension in water and therefore common in soft drinks and lemonades; and some are purely synthetic products.

For each additive or flavouring that a company wants approved, the origin, identity and purity (discussed above as specifications and production procedures) must be described. The purity includes the total amount of impurities in percentages and the identity of the impurities. Obviously, the latter will be a function of both origin and the detailed production method. Look for example at the description of the identity, production and resulting purity of cassia gum in Chapter 2.

24.3 Single Groups of Additives

In this chapter we do not comprehensively treat all the different groups of additives and not even those groups we look into further with some degree of detail. Rather we describe some examples in order to point to key issues, historically as well as for the current situation worldwide.

Artificial sweeteners

Sweeteners are compounds that are added to food to sweeten them instead of sucrose, especially in light products and products for diabetics. Very often at least two different sweeteners are added because they act synergistically.

The history behind the development of the different artificial sweeteners that we have on the market today began with saccharine, which was discovered in 1878 when a chemist named Constantin Fahlberg spilled a working product on his hands in a lab at Johns Hopkins University. During World War I, sugar shortages made it very popular. The discovery of cyclamate dates back to 1937, when Michael Sveda, a graduate student at the University of Illinois, was working on the synthesis of anti-pyretic (anti-fever) drugs. He put his cigarette down on the lab bench. When he put it back in his mouth, he discovered the sweet taste of cyclamate. Aspartame, marketed as Equal® and NutraSweet®, was discovered in much the same way. In 1965, Jim Schlatter, a chemist at G.D. Searle, was working on ulcer treatments. He claimed to lick his finger as he reached for a paper and tasted something sweet. The name aspartame comes from aspartyl-phenylalanine methyl ester, the compound Schlatter was working on.

Saccharin (E954)

Saccharin (Fig. 24.1) is a non-nutritive sweetener, 500 times sweeter than sucrose.

- ADI = 2.5 mg kg^{-1} BW;
- LD$_{50}$ = 17 g kg^{-1} BW oral for rats and mice.

It is used for soft drinks, ice cream, chocolates, light products and instead of sugar in coffee and tea. The daily intake is 54–173 mg for diabetics and 25–155 mg for non-diabetics based on food consumption surveys. These are older figures; they may be higher today because of the increased intake of light soft drinks in particular.

Toxicity testing using animals has shown that saccharin is not teratogenic, mutagenic or genotoxic. No carcinogenic effect was seen in mice, guinea pig or apes even after high dosing. An increased incidence of bladder tumours was seen in male rats in the second generation when the dose of saccharin in the feed was higher than 1% by weight. Saccharin was dosed to the parents during their full lifetime; the offspring were exposed to saccharin during the fetal stage, nursing stage and for the rest of their lifetime. The effect was not seen when the dose was less than 1% by weight of feed. In other experiments it has been shown that saccharin can promote the growth of bladder tumours if the cells have been initiated by nitroso compounds.

Several retrospective epidemiological investigations of the relationship between human bladder cancer and saccharin consumption have been conducted. These studies could not establish a significant difference in bladder tumour incidence between the control group and the groups using saccharin. These investigations are, however, difficult to analyse as it is very difficult to estimate the exposure to agonists/antagonists, which could be smoking, drinking coffee, medications and exposure to environmental contamination.

Saccharin is absorbed well from the gastrointestinal tract and excreted unchanged in the urine; 90% of the dose will be excreted within 24 h. Saccharin has an anticariogenic effect further promoted by the low intake of sugar.

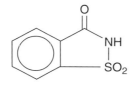

Fig. 24.1. Saccharin.

Aspartame (E951)

The synthetic sweetener aspartame (Fig 24.2) is 150–200 times sweeter than sucrose, being a dipeptide consisting of aspartic acid and phenylalanine.

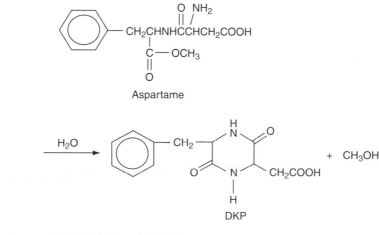

Fig. 24.2. Aspartame and its hydrolysis to yield DKP.

Food Additives and Flavourings

- ADI = 40 mg kg^{-1} BW;
- LD$_{50}$ = 17 g kg^{-1} BW oral for rats.

A typical content, for example, in some Danish food products is marmalade, 1 g kg^{-1}; ice cream and marinade for fish, 200–300 mg kg^{-1}; chocolates, 2 g kg^{-1}; and chewing gum, 5.5 g kg^{-1}. It is used mostly in products with low pH and products which are stored for a short time at low temperature. Long-time storage at high temperature and high pH will initiate hydrolysis of the compound to diketopiperazine (DKP) and methanol, giving a bitter taste (see Fig 24.2).

As the compound contains two secondary amines that may form nitrosamines, the compound was suspected to be carcinogenic, but several chronic toxicity studies using rats, mice and dogs did not show any carcinogenic, teratogenic or reproductive toxicity. Very high doses (3–4 g kg^{-1} BW) given to monkeys can cause spasms like an epileptic attack. This might be due to aspartic acid as this compound gives the same symptoms at high concentration. Aspartic acid is a decomposition product of aspartame, which decomposes in the gastrointestinal tract to aspartic acid, phenylalanine and methanol. No toxic effect has been seen in man but people with phenylketonuria should not eat too much food with aspartame (Box 24.1).

The safe intake of aspartame (often described as 'the most tested compound in the world') has been questioned a number of times by different 'alternative consumer groups'. For this reason, among others, it has been re-evaluated again and again by different authorities. By 2009 EFSA had on several occasions reviewed the safety of the sweetener aspartame. In 2008 EFSA felt forced to re-evaluate aspartame due to the occurrence of a new Italian study. The EFSA's Panel on Food Additives and Nutrient Sources added to Food (ANS) concluded that, on the basis of all the evidence currently available including the Italian study by the European Ramazzini Foundation published in 2007, there was no indication of any genotoxic or carcinogenic potential of aspartame and no reason to revise the previously established ADI for aspartame of 40 mg kg^{-1} BW.

Box 24.1. Definition of phenylketonuria

Phenylketonuria (PKU) is a genetic disorder characterized by an inability of the body to utilize the essential amino acid phenylalanine. In 'classic PKU' the enzyme that metabolizes phenylalanine, phenylalanine hydroxylase, is completely or nearly completely deficient. This enzyme normally converts phenylalanine to tyrosine. Without this enzyme, phenylalanine accumulates in the blood and body tissues. A normal blood phenylalanine level is about 1 mg dl^{-1}, whereas in classic PKU levels may range from 6 to 80 mg dl^{-1}, usually greater than 30 mg dl^{-1}. Chronically high levels of phenylalanine and some of its breakdown products can cause significant brain problems. Classic PKU is the most common cause of high levels of phenylalanine in the blood. Classic PKU affects about one of every 10,000–20,000 Caucasian or Oriental births. The incidence in African Americans is far less. These disorders are equally frequent in males and females.

Infants with PKU appear normal at birth. Today, in many countries most symptoms of untreated PKU are avoided by newborn screening, early identification and management. Untreated PKU symptoms – currently a rarity – include the following. About 50% of untreated infants have early symptoms, such as vomiting, irritability, an eczema-like rash and a mousy odour to the urine. Some may also have subtle signs of nervous system function problems, such as increased muscle tone and more active muscle tendon reflexes. Later, severe brain problems occur, such as mental retardation and seizures. Other commonly noted features in untreated children include microcephaly (small head), prominent cheek and upper jaw bones with widely spaced teeth, poor development of tooth enamel and decreased body growth.

For the screening of newborns a few drops of blood are obtained by a small prick on the heel, placed on a card and then sent for measurement. If the screening test is abnormal, other tests are needed to confirm or exclude PKU. The goal of PKU treatment is to maintain the blood level of phenylalanine between 2 and 10 mg dl^{-1}. Some phenylalanine is needed for normal growth. For PKU sufferers this means a diet that has some phenylalanine but in much lower amounts than normal. High-protein foods, such as meat, fish, poultry, eggs, cheese, milk, dried beans and peas, are avoided. Instead, measured amounts of cereals, starches, fruits and vegetables, along with a milk substitute, are usually recommended. Phenylalanine-free formulas are available for all age groups.

Cyclamate sodium salt (E952)

Cyclamate sodium salt (Fig. 24.3) is a synthetic sweetener that is 150–200 times sweeter than sugar, and is used daily in households as well as commercially.

- ADI = 11 mg kg^{-1} BW (established by JECFA and used in the EU before 2005), now 7 mg kg^{-1} BW (established later by EFSA and used in the EU today);
- LD$_{50}$ = 10 g kg^{-1} BW oral for rats and mice.

It is used for soft drinks, marmalade (1 g kg^{-1}) and ice cream (250 mg kg^{-1}).

Part of the ingested cyclamate is converted in the intestine to cyclohexylamine and oxidative products thereof. Cyclohexylamine and cyclamate have very different toxicological properties. Cyclohexylamine may cause the release of catecholamine, which increases blood pressure. Cyclamate does not show any teratogenic or reproductive toxicity in toxicity tests with several generations; it may, however, cause testis atrophy in rats after long-time exposure. Chronic toxicity studies using rats, mice and guinea pigs could not detect any carcinogenicity for either cyclamate or cyclohexylamine, but some experiments indicate that cyclamate can induce bladder tumour growth if the cells have been initiated by a mutagen. Results of epidemiological studies do not give any indication of a higher frequency of bladder cancer in exposed people compared with controls.

Cyclamate is very well absorbed and is a laxative at high doses (more than 70 mg kg^{-1} BW). It is excreted through the liver and kidneys after 1–2 days.

The ADI for cyclamate was decreased recently (2005) after a safety evaluation had taken place. The use of cyclamate in ice cream and some other sweets is no longer allowed in the EU.

Acesulfame K (potassium; E950)

Acesulfame K (Fig. 24.4) is a synthetic compound about 150 times sweeter than sucrose.

- ADI = 9 mg kg^{-1} BW;
- LD$_{50}$ = 7430 mg kg^{-1} BW oral and 2240 mg kg^{-1} BW intraperitoneal for rats.

It is added to milk products (300 mg kg^{-1}), ice cream (800 mg kg^{-1}), marmalade (1 g kg^{-1}) and soft drinks (350 mg l^{-1}).

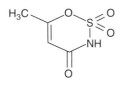

Fig. 24.3. Cyclamate as sodium salt (left) and calcium salt (right).

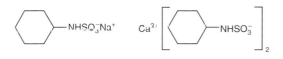

Fig. 24.4. Acesulfame.

In toxicity studies, acute toxicity tests using rats dosed for 90 days with 0, 1, 3 and 10% acesulfame by weight of feed showed only a very weak toxic response at the high concentration. A slight increase of liver and kidney size was seen together with diarrhoea. The NOAEL of 900 mg kg^{-1} BW day^{-1} was determined from an experiment using dogs. No chronic toxicity and carcinogenicity was found during a 120–123-week period in experiments using rats given doses of 0, 0.3, 1 and 3% acesulfame by weight of feed.

Acesulfame is absorbed rapidly from the gastrointestinal tract and excreted in the urine; 98% of the dose is excreted within 24 h. The compound is not metabolized and it does not bioaccumulate.

Sugar alcohols (mannitol (E421), sorbitol (E420) and xylitol (E667))

The sugar alcohols are polyhydroxy compounds used as naturally occurring sugar substitutes.

- ADI = 0–160 mg kg^{-1} BW for mannitol (none for the others);
- LD$_{50}$ = 14–22 mg kg^{-1} BW oral for rats (same as for sucrose).

They are used in many products such as candy, chewing gum and soft drinks.

Toxicity studies have shown that these compounds are absorbed slowly and metabolized by gastrointestinal bacteria. The effects seen after ingestion of high doses are an enlarged appendix, diarrhoea, increased calcium uptake and changes in the kidney. Adrenal tumour growth may be observed, but it may be caused by the increased uptake of calcium, which can cause increased content of adrenaline and noradrenaline in the adrenal cortex. This effect has not, however, been seen in humans. The sugar alcohols do not cause teratogenicity or changes in reproduction. A Finnish epidemiological study in which 50 people consumed 60–70 g xylitol daily for 2 years did not give rise to any effects.

Sucralose (E955)

Sucralose (Fig. 24.5) is a new artificial sweetener, 500–600 times sweeter than sucrose:

- $LD_{50} > 16$ g kg^{-1} BW oral for mice.

Sucralose was first approved for use in Canada in 1991, after it had undergone a risk assessment by JECFA in 1990. Subsequent approvals came in Australia in 1993, in New Zealand in 1996, in the USA in 1998 and in the EU in 2004. Unlike aspartame, sucralose is stable under heat and over a broad range of pH conditions. Thus, it can be used in baking or in products that require a longer shelf-life. The quick commercial success of sucralose-based products stems from its favourable comparison with other low-calorie sweeteners in terms of taste, stability and safety.

Stevioside

Stevioside (Fig. 24.6) is 250–300 times sweeter than sucrose.

Stevioside is one of several naturally occurring glycosides responsible for the sweet taste of the leaves of the stevia plant (*Stevia rebaudiana, Asteraceae*) found in the Brazilian state of Mato Grosso do Sul and Paraguay. These compounds range in sweetness from 40 to 300 times sweeter than sucrose, are heat-stable and pH-stable, and do not ferment. In 1970 Japan approved stevia extracts and stevioside as sweeteners and flavour enhancers for food use in Japan. In Europe, EFSA (Scientific Panel on Additives) has assessed the safety of steviol glycosides and established an ADI

of 4 mg kg^{-1} BW. The assessment was sent to the European Commission during 2010. The Commission will consider whether or not to authorize the substances in the EU for their proposed use, in particular in sugar-free or reduced-energy foods such as certain flavoured drinks, confectionery with no added sugar and energy-reduced soups. This ADI is consistent with that already established by JECFA.

Food colourants

In the USA, FDA characterizes *food colourants* as 'colour additives', but they are also known as food colourings, food colourants and dyes. To the best of our knowledge colour has been added to food since time immemorial. Archaeologists tell us that food colours most probably emerged around 1500 BC. Saffron is mentioned as a colourant in Homer's *Iliad*, and Pliny the Elder remarks that wines were artificially coloured in 400 BC. In the beginning food colouring mostly relied on what was readily found in nature. For instance, saffron has long been used to give a yellow tint to rice, and squid ink gives pasta a black appearance (Spaghetti al Nero di Seppia). Other popular natural colourants have included paprika, turmeric, beet extract and petals of various flowers.

The only contact with food colour that a peasant of the Middle Ages had was with poisoned bread. As well-refined white flour and bread were preferred by the elite, manufacturers often produced

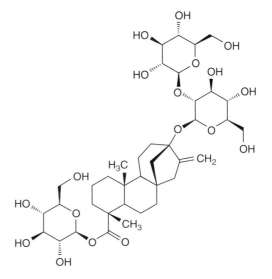

Fig. 24.6. Stevioside.

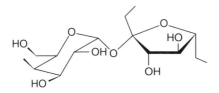

Fig. 24.5. Sucralose (1,6-dichloro-1,6-dideoxy-β-D-fructofuranosyl-α-D-galactopyranoside).

cheap versions for the peasantry that used lime, chalk or even crushed bones to attain the desired effect. The proliferation of bread tainted with deleterious white colourings spawned one of the oldest surviving instances of food adulteration regulations, from the time of King Edward I (1272–1307). We also have knowledge of a few other early pieces of legislation concerning colouring of food. Early colouring laws include a 1396 French edict against the colouring of butter, and a 1574 French law that made it illegal to add colouring to pastries to simulate the presence of eggs.

The English chemist Friedrich Accum was the first to bring a steadily growing problem of food adulterations – including the adding of colours – to the public's attention with his book *A Treatise on Adulterations of Food and Culinary Poisons*, published in 1820. Not only was bread mentioned but also numerous examples of adulterations of beer, wine, spirituous liquors, tea, coffee, cream, confectionery, vinegar, mustard, pepper, cheese, olive oil, pickles and other articles employed in domestic economy. Confections were loaded up with poisonous chemicals, seeking to appeal to children through bright colours. Accum thus documented sweets coloured with vermillion (contains mercury), red lead, white lead, verdigris (a copper salt), blue vitriol (contains copper) and Scheele's green (contains copper and arsenic). According to one publication,[1] 46% of the candy sampled for analysis in Boston in 1880 was found to contain at least one toxic mineral pigment, predominantly lead chromate.

Realizing this situation and its catastrophic effects, in the USA the Federal Government intervened and outlawed coloured metal salts and other injurious pigments with the Wiley Act (Federal Food and Drugs Act of 1906), 28 U.S.C. §1–15, 1934 (repealed 1938).

Since then a number of organic synthetic colourants have been developed, some brought into use and later banned, others still being in use. Constantly, food colourants have been in the focus of both the authorities and the public. This is still so. In Europe EFSA is re-evaluating all food colours which are authorized for use in the EU on a case-by-case basis. The first colour to be re-evaluated was Red 2G in July 2007. Subsequently this agent was withdrawn following concerns expressed by the AFC Panel. Lycopene was re-evaluated in January 2008. For this colour the AFC Panel established an ADI of 0.5 mg kg^{-1} BW from all sources. However, it was also pointed out that some high

consumers of lycopene-containing foods, such as pre-school children and schoolchildren, may exceed this ADI. Lycopene is a bright red carotenoid pigment found in tomatoes and other red fruits and vegetables, such as red carrots, watermelons and papayas (but not strawberries or cherries). It has no vitamin A activity.

In September 2009 the EFSA ANS Panel provided scientific advice on six food colours. As a result of these risks assessments the ADI was lowered in three cases, i.e. for quinoline yellow, sunset yellow and Ponceau 4R. For these colours, the Panel found that exposure could go above the new ADI for both adults and children. The Panel also concluded that the existing ADI did not need to be changed for the other three colours that were assessed (tartrazine, azorubine/carmoisine and allura red AC). The re-evaluation of all food colours by EFSA is planned to be completed during 2011.

Now let us take a look at the two important groups of food colours in current use: the *azo colouring agents* and the *triphenylmethane colouring agents*.

Azo colouring agents

These colouring agents are strong, stable and dissolve easily in water, as the molecules used as colours contain two sulfuric acid groups (Fig. 24.7).

The compounds are not absorbed in the gastrointestinal tract but if they are decomposed to two amines these may be absorbed to some extent. The compounds (Table 24.1) are generally not toxic, mutagenic or carcinogenic. Several of these colouring agents can give rise to allergic reactions, however.

Tartrazine is reported to be able to cause an allergic-like response such as asthma after ingestion of a total dose of less than 1 mg, but this has not been proved by double-blind tests. Persons who are allergic to aspirin are also particularly allergic to tartrazine. It is not known why this occurs; as the compounds have very different structures it seems odd that they show this cross-allergic response.

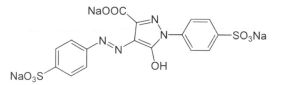

Fig. 24.7. The food colouring azo (R$_1$–N=N–R$_2$) compound tartrazine.

Table 24.1. ADI of selected azo food colourants.

Example	E-number	ADI (mg kg^{-1} BW)
Tartrazine	E102	7.5
Sunset yellow FCF	E110	1.0 (earlier 2.5)
Black PN	E151	1.0
Azorubin	E122	4.0
Amaranth	E123	0.5
Ponceau 4R	E124	0.7 (earlier 4.0)
Rubin pigment	E180	1.5

Table 24.2. ADI of selected triphenylmethane food colourants.

Example	E-number	ADI (mg kg^{-1} BW)
Brilliant Blue	E133	10
Patent Blue	E131	15
Green S	E142	5

No toxic response has been seen in tests where animals were dosed with tartrazine up to 5% by weight in feed. Tartrazine has a yellow colour and is one of the most used colourants, up to 200 mg kg^{-1} in certain products.

Sunset yellow can, like tartrazine, give rise to an allergic reaction. From experiments using dogs the NOAEL has been found to be 2% by weight of feed; higher concentrations (5%) gave rise to weight loss. The agent is yellow in colour as the name indicates and it is frequently used up to 200 mg kg^{-1}.

Black PN is not responsible for any allergic reaction. Pigs dosed with up to 900 mg kg^{-1} BW day^{-1} for 90 days showed no signs of toxic reaction except for cysts on the ileum because of the very high local concentration. It is a black colourant and may be used for a few food items such as marmalade, sweets and cheese rind.

Azorubin does not have any toxic effect in rats at up to 2% by weight of feed and the NOAEL was determined to be 400 mg kg^{-1} BW day^{-1}. The colour is red and the agent is frequently used up to 100 mg kg^{-1}.

Amaranth is a red colourant that was in frequent use, but has now been 'banned' because a Russian experiment demonstrated it to have carcinogenic and teratogenic effects. No other laboratory has been able to verify this, however. The compound can cause urticaria.

Ponceau 4R is a red colourant used for example in marmalade and alcoholic drinks. It has been shown not to be toxic but it can cause an allergy according to the literature.

Triphenylmethane colouring agents

Sulfuric acid derivatives of triphenylmethane are very stable and easily soluble in water. They are poorly absorbed from the gastrointestinal tract and excreted unchanged in faeces. No toxic symptoms have been seen using doses of up to 2% by weight of feed. The colours are blue and green and they are used for example in ice cream and alcoholic beverages (Table 24.2).

Preservatives

The preservation of food has been carried out for hundreds if not thousands of years – primarily to ensure a supply between growing seasons – using various means such as sun-drying, fermentation, or chemical methods such as salting and smoking. Today a number of chemical preservatives are officially approved for use, different compounds achieving the best results under different conditions.

Preservatives used in modern food production to prevent the growth of bacteria, yeast and moulds include a large number of very different compounds belonging to different structural classes, being of different origin. Examples are organic acids, sulfur dioxide and sulfites, nitrites and nitrates, alkyl esters of *p*-hydroxybenzoic acid (parabens), fungicides used on the surface of raw fruits such as bananas and citrus (diphenyl, *o*-phenylphenol, thiabendazole), the bacteriocin nicin from the dairy starter culture bacterium *Lactococcus lactis* subsp. *lactis*, and the antifungal compound natamycin from *Streptomyces natalensis*. Below we look at one or a few examples for each category.

Sorbic acid (E200) and sorbates (calcium, potassium; E202, E203)

Organic acids are present in a majority of foods to a greater or lesser extent. They can be present as natural food components, e.g. the acids present in fruit juices, or added artificially, as acidulants, preservatives, emulsifiers, antioxidants or flavours. As preservatives organic acids include sorbic acid, formic acid, benzoic acid and propionic acid.

For sorbic acid and sorbates:

- ADI = 0–25 mg kg^{-1} BW;
- LD$_{50}$ = 7.36 g kg^{-1} BW oral for the rat.

Concentrations often used are 1–2 g kg⁻¹ for foods (cheese, cakes, fruit, meat and fish) and 200 mg l⁻¹ for drinks.

In toxicity studies, rats fed a diet containing 5% sorbic acid by weight for 2 years showed no toxic reaction. Sorbic acid added to the drinking water (10 mg per 100 ml) induced no toxic effects after 100 weeks of dosing. Daily dosing in feed with 2–10% sorbic acid by weight can lead to increased liver weight, while 5 and 10% potassium sorbate by weight may lead to increased kidney size. Sarcomas may be induced at the injection site if administered by subcutaneous injection.

There may be a positive effect on lung infections as animals dosed with sorbates in long-term studies live longer than control animals.

Sulfur dioxide (SO₂) (E220) and sulfites (SO₃²⁻) (E221–E224, E226–E228)

These compounds are most effective at low pH; at pH 7 they are ineffective against yeast and mould and very high concentrations are necessary to inhibit the growth of bacteria. These compounds are also used to prevent fruit and vegetables from turning brown.

Concentrations used in certain European countries are, for foods, sodium sulfite 0.7 mg kg⁻¹, and for drinks (beer and wine), sodium thiosulfate 0.7 mg kg⁻¹.

The compound(s) are generally regarded as safe (GRAS) but several toxicity studies, especially mutagenicity studies, have shown that they may react with cytosine in DNA and RNA, giving rise to mutations. *Escherichia coli* incubated for 1.5 h with 3 M sodium sulfite at pH 5.6 exhibited mutations. Sulfite can break down thiamine, which to some extent is the cause of the effects seen after sulfite administration. Thus, decreased excretion of thiamine, was seen for rats dosed with $Na_2S_2O_5$ (E223) as a source of SO_2 by degradation. High doses of 1–2% by weight in feed gave rise to bloody faeces and stomach bleeding, and an enlarged spleen could also be observed. Human experiments showed that a dose of 400 mg kg⁻¹ BW day⁻¹ did not influence thiamine excretion.

Nitrite (NO₂⁻) (sodium, potassium; E250, E249)

These compounds also serve as preservatives as they inhibit especially the growth of *Clostridium botulinum*. Furthermore they give rise to the red colour of meat because they form nitromyoglobin in the form of nitrosylhaemochrome (see Chapter 22), and they also enhance the flavour of food. Nitrites were for a long time banned in Denmark, but from the year 2000 they may be added to bacon, for example, at 175 mg kg⁻¹ (residual).

The acute toxic effect of nitrite is caused by the oxidation of haemoglobin to methaemoglobin, which reduces the capacity for transport of oxygen. The acute toxic effects are therefore dyspnoea, cyanosis, increased pulse, and in severe cases loss of consciousness and death. Certain populations, such as: (i) people with low NADH-methaemoglobin reductase activity; (ii) pregnant women and older people with low gastric acid production; and (iii) small children because their haemoglobin is easily oxidized to methaemoglobin, are especially sensitive to nitrite. Rats dosed with nitrite (100 mg kg⁻¹ BW day⁻¹) in a chronic toxicity study showed reduced growth rate and decreased lifespan. No mutagenicity or teratogenicity was observed. However, nitrite can react with secondary amines and amides forming nitrosamines according to the reaction scheme shown in Chapter 22. Nitrosamines can be formed both in the body and in food containing amines and amides preserved with nitrite (pH optimum for the reactions is 2–3). The nitrosamines may also be formed at high temperatures, as when frying bacon in a frying pan. These nitrosamines are mutagenic, teratogenic and toxic to the liver. More than 130 different nitrosamines have been examined and more than 100 are carcinogenic in all species in which they have been tested. The nitrosamines are metabolized by the liver cytochrome P450 system giving rise to reactive metabolites that can alkylate the O(6) group in guanine; this alkylation correlates with the tumour formation.

The formation of nitrosamines can be inhibited or prevented by ascorbic acid, which reacts with nitrite forming one molecule of NO and one of dehydroascorbic acid, thereby reducing the nitrite concentration. It has been shown that ascorbic acid can inhibit the formation of nitrosamines by up to 90%. Cysteine, sodium sulfite and sorbic acid can also inhibit nitrosamine formation.

Nitrate (NO₃⁻) (potassium, sodium; E252, E251)

Nitrate is also a preservative and the mechanism by which it works is probably the same as for nitrite, i.e. it functions as a reservoir for the formation of nitrite.

- ADI = 0–5 mg kg^{-1} BW calculated as $NaNO_3$.

Examples of concentration in European food: cheeses, 50 mg kg^{-1}; fish foods, 200 mg kg^{-1}.

Toxicity studies have shown that vegetables are an important source of human nitrate intake, but the water in certain parts of a country may also contain high nitrate concentrations. Nitrate can be reduced to nitrite in the gastrointestinal tract, especially in very small children, accounting for their high sensitivity to nitrate. Rats ingesting 1% $NaNO_3$ (w/v) in the drinking water for 2 years did not show any toxic effect other than a reduced growth rate. The same experiment with dogs for 120 days did not result in toxic effects. A no effect level (NOAEL) was estimated to be 500 mg kg^{-1} BW day^{-1}.

Methyl-p-hydroxybenzoate (E218), ethyl-p-hydroxybenzoate (E214) and propyl-p-hydroxybenzoate (E216)

These three parabens are the ones most often used as preservatives in food products. However, heptyl-paraben, a more recently available long-chain paraben, may also be used in beer, ale, non-carbonated alcoholic drinks and fruit beverages in the USA. Parabens have limited solubility and a metallic bitter taste, which is why they are not widely used for food preservation. However, for non-acid foods, and for action against fungi in general, parabens are interesting compounds.

The parabens are esters of p-hydroxybenzoic acid and as such phenolic compounds. Phenol itself has a long medical history as an antibacterial agent. Also the weak acid benzoic acid (E210), the name of which is derived from gum benzoin that for a long time was the only source for benzoic acid, and its salts are used as food preservatives.

Methyl-, ethyl- and propylparaben are permitted in the EU as food additives in four categories of processed foods. Thus, they are authorized for use: (i) *quantum satis* (i.e. according to GMP based on the level required to achieve the desired technological effect) for the surface treatment of dried meat products; (ii) with a maximum permitted level of 1 g kg^{-1} in jelly coatings of meat products such as pâté; (iii) in confectionery, excluding chocolate, at levels of 0.3 g kg^{-1}; and (iv) in liquid dietary food supplements at 2 g kg^{-1}.

The former EC SCF evaluated the parabens in 1994 and allocated a temporary group ADI of 0–10 mg kg^{-1} BW for the sum of methyl, ethyl and propyl p-hydroxybenzoic acid esters and their sodium salts. In 2004 EFSA's AFC Panel re-evaluated the toxicology of these substances and the safety of their usage in foods taking into account findings from more recent studies.

A number of parabens have oestrogenic activity *in vitro*. No oestrogenic activity could be detected *in vivo* for methyl-, ethyl- or propyl-paraben in uterotrophic assays using oral or subcutaneous administrations of high doses to mice and rats, however. An *in vivo* uterotrophic effect was observed after subcutaneous injection of either butylparaben or isobutylparaben. These are not used as food additives, however, and the common metabolite of the parabens, p-hydroxybenzoic acid, was considered to be non-oestrogenic.

On this basis it was concluded that a group ADI of 0–10 mg kg^{-1} BW could now be established for methyl- and ethylparaben and their sodium salts. However, the Panel considered that propylparaben should not be included in this group ADI because this specific paraben, unlike the methyl and ethyl forms, had effects on sperm production at a relatively low dose in male juvenile rats. The Panel was unable to recommend an ADI for propylparaben because of the lack of a clear NOAEL for this effect.

This observation hints at the current very intense discussion in certain consumer circles about the use of parabens. It has become trendy – at least in certain population groups – to use products of different kinds that do not contain parabens. This does not target primarily food products, but rather cosmetic and toiletry products (see Box 24.2).

Not only EFSA but also for example FDA in the USA follow the development in knowledge concerning the effects of parabens. In 2009 FDA wrote:

> Although parabens can act similarly to estrogen, they have been shown to have much less estrogenic activity than the body's naturally occurring estrogen. For example, a research group in 1998 found that the most potent paraben tested in the study, butylparaben, showed from 10,000- to 100,000-fold less activity than naturally occurring estradiol (a form of estrogen).

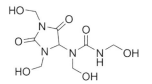
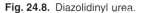
Diphenyl (E230), o-phenylphenol (E231) and thiabendazole (E233)

These three compounds are used for the surface preservation of fruits and vegetables.

Diphenyl (= biphenyl = phenylbenzene) is used predominantly against *Penicillium* fungi growing on citrus fruits. It is further used to disinfect containers and in impregnating the wrapping of citrus fruits. Sometimes fruits are dipped in a solution of diphenyl, which slowly penetrates the peel and may be present in low concentrations in the fruit itself. The ADI is up to 0.05 mg kg^{-1} BW. Sensitivity has been reported for people handling large consignments of citrus fruits (ships, trucks). Otherwise there are no side-effects reported.

Similarly, o-phenylphenol is used particularly against *Penicillium* fungi growing on citrus fruits, apples and pears. It slowly penetrates the peel and may be present in the fruit itself. No special adverse effects are known at the concentrations used. An ADI of up to 0.2 mg kg^{-1} BW has been set.

Finally, thiabendazole is widely used as a fungicide, particularly on fruits. It is mainly sprayed on fruits; it can also be a component of an aqueous solution, in which fruits are submerged. The ADI is approved as up to 0.1 mg kg^{-1} BW.

In Europe, fruits that have been surface-preserved should be labelled as such or a sign should be placed nearby to give this information. When cooking dishes including peels of citrus fruits, for example, it is preferable that non-surface-treated fruits are used.

One of the three surface preservatives is special. Besides its use for preservation, thiabendazole (a benzimidazole compound) is also used both as a broad-spectrum anthelmintic in various animal species and for the control of parasitic infestations in man. This means that exposure calculations must look at possibilities for exposure from different sources, including residues in animal tissues. CAC has derived the MRL for all such products to be 100 µg kg^{-1} (100 µg l^{-1} for milk).

Nisin (E234)

Bacteriocins are low-molecular-weight antimicrobial peptides produced by bacteria (particularly lactic acid bacteria) that are inhibitory to other bacteria, which are usually closely related to the producer bacteria. Nisin, the first bacteriocin to be discovered in the 1920s, has the broadest antibacterial spectrum of the many bacteriocins known today, a spectrum that extends to a wide variety of Gram-positive bacteria, including sporeformers.

Structurally nisin is a polypeptide consisting of 34 amino acids with a molecular mass of 3510 Da, produced by the bacterium *L. lactis* subsp. *lactis* normally used in cheese production. The nisin preparation, Nisaplin®, was developed by Aplin and Barrett in England around 1965. Nisaplin contains 2.5% nisin A (currently some structural nisin variants are known).

Toxicity studies carried out in a variety of animal species using levels far in excess of those used in foods indicate that nicin is non-toxic. Nisin is inactivated rapidly in the intestine by digestive enzymes, and cannot be detected in the saliva of humans 10 min after consuming a liquid containing nisin.

In 1969 JECFA recommended its acceptance for food use after a review of its toxicological profile. Nisin received GRAS status in 1988 by FDA in the USA. Nisin is currently approved as a food preservative in over 50 countries. In the EU nisin is authorized for food preservation by Directive 95/2/EC on food additives other than colours and sweeteners. Nisin is permitted in ripened cheese and processed cheese, certain puddings, clotted cream and mascarpone. The EU SCF derived an ADI for nisin of 0.13 mg kg^{-1} BW, a level that was confirmed by EFSA in 2006.

Natamycin (E235)

Natamycin obtained from *S. natalensis* – a microorganism found in 1955 in a soil sample from the province of Natal, South Africa – is a fungicide of the polyene macrolide group. The compound is very poorly absorbed from the gastrointestinal tract. The mechanism of action for this group of antibiotics is binding to sterols (principally ergosterol) in the fungal cell membrane. Bacteria are insensitive to polyene antibiotics since they lack sterols in their cell membrane. JECFA reviewed the safety of natamycin in 1968 and again in 1976 and 2002. An ADI of 0.3 mg kg^{-1} BW was assigned to this compound. In the EU natamycin was risk-assessed by SCF. SCF did not establish an ADI but considered that in relation to the uses of natamycin on cheese and sausages, this did not give rise to safety concern. Thus, natamycin was approved to be used for the surface treatment of semi-hard and semi-soft cheese and dry, cured sausage at a maximum level of 1 mg dm^{-2} in the outer 5 mm of the surface, corresponding to 20 mg kg^{-1}.

In 2006 EFSA re-evaluated natamycin, addressing also the issue of possible development of antimicrobial resistance to natamycin:

- Available toxicological studies interestingly showed reduced food intake and body weight loss for rats but the tendency for obesity in dogs. The dog study proved to be the most sensitive with an NOAEL of 6.25 mg kg^{-1} BW day^{-1}.
- Available genotoxic studies led to the following conclusions: (i) the induction of chromosomal aberrations observed was accompanied by cytotoxicity; (ii) *in vitro* studies on mutagenicity in bacteria and mammalian cells and on chromosomal aberrations in mammalian cells, which were performed in compliance with GLP, were negative; and (iii) no substance-related neoplastic effects were observed in the long-term studies.

On this basis the Panel considered that the available data do not raise concern with respect to genotoxicity of natamycin; moreover, the fact that bacteria are insensitive to polyene antibiotics because their membrane lacks sterols means that there was no concern for the induction of antimicrobial resistance. The Panel also found that the ADI established by JECFA is adequate.

Antioxidants

Antioxidants prevent the oxidation of fatty acids. The oxidation of fatty acids is a chain reaction that breaks down the fatty acids to aldehydes and acids, making the food rancid. Antioxidants also prevent fruit and vegetables from getting brown. Huge amounts of oil are used for deep-frying many food (including fast food) products. Deep-frying oils typically contain added antioxidants.

Butylated hydroxyanisole (E320) and butylated hydroxytoluene (E321)

BHA and BHT (Fig. 24.9) are widely used but mostly in dried products such as chips, cereals and powders for making puddings.

- Maximum = 200 mg kg^{-1} in total if both are used;
- ADI = 0.5 mg kg^{-1} BW.

In toxicity studies, rats fed BHA (500–600 mg kg^{-1} BW day^{-1} or 0.003–0.06% by weight of feed) showed no toxic effects. A 2-year study with rats fed 0.5% BHA by weight of feed resulted in decreased weight but no other side-effects. Liver

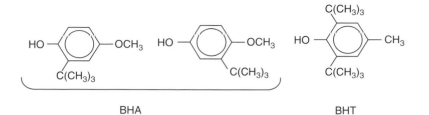

BHA   BHT

Fig. 24.9. The structure of BHA and BHT.

necrosis was seen in dogs fed BHA at 200 mg kg^{-1} BW day^{-1}, and an increased excretion of Na/K was seen in rabbits dosed with 1 g kg^{-1} BW day^{-1} for 5–6 days. The Na$^+$ was taken from the skeleton.

BHT fed to rats (0.2, 0.5 and 0.8% by weight of feed) for 2 years did not give any toxic effects, but feeding 1% led to increased weight, increased size of the liver, brain and other organs, and a dose-related increased level of serum cholesterol. Offspring from rats fed 0.1% BHT showed toxic signs such as liver enlargement, weight reduction and hair loss. However, these teratogenic effects could not be induced by other research groups using 250 mg kg^{-1} BW.

BHA is excreted quickly in humans. Doses of 0.5–0.7 mg kg^{-1} BW are reduced by 22–77% within 24 h.

Non-toxic effects are evident at lower doses (*in vivo* and *in vitro*): BHA and BHT reduce the carcinogenic effect of PAHs, diethyl nitrosamines and other carcinogens. This may be due to changes in microsomal enzyme activity that increases the activity of glutathione *S*-transferase. This results in lower levels of bioactivate metabolites that can form adducts with DNA, reducing the number of initiated cells. Apart from the inhibiting effect on cancer development, these compounds also protect against CCl$_4$ intoxication. CCl$_4$ is activated by cytochrome P4502E1, P4502B1 or P4502B2, and possibly cytochrome P4503A, to form the trichloromethyl radical, CCl$_4^{\cdot}$. This radical can bind to cellular molecules (nucleic acid, protein, lipid), impairing crucial cellular processes such as lipid metabolism, with the potential outcome of fatty degeneration (steatosis) primarily of the liver. In certain assays they also delay the ageing effect by decreasing the concentration of free radicals. Finally these compounds are also potent inhibitors of lipophilic viruses such as *Herpes simplex virus*.

Ascorbic acid (E300) (sodium salt, calcium salt; E301, E302)

Ascorbic acid is a natural water-soluble antioxidant that is present in especially fruit, berries, vegetables and mammalian liver. Man-made ascorbic acid is added to food because of the antioxidant effect.

- ADI – 15 mg kg^{-1} BW;
- LD$_{50}$ > 5000 mg kg^{-1} BW oral and 1000 mg kg^{-1} BW intravenous for rats.

These compounds are used mostly in oils and frozen vegetables.

In toxicity studies, experiments conducted on mice, rats and guinea pigs using doses up to 2500 mg kg^{-1} BW day^{-1} over a period of 1 week did not give any toxic effects. Chronic tests using rats dosed at 2000 mg kg^{-1} BW did not give any adverse effects. Teratogenicity tests and mutagenicity tests were also negative at a dose of 550 mg kg^{-1} BW. In humans, toxic effects such as nausea, diarrhoea, headache and disturbed sleep were seen after ingestion of 6 g kg^{-1} BW day^{-1} for 4 years. Children mainly get eczema after ingestion of ascorbic acid. The recommended daily dose is 30–100 mg.

Propyl gallate (E310), octyl gallate (E311) and dodecyl gallate (E312)

These three esters of gallic acid are all used as antioxidants.

- ADI = 1.4, 0.1 and 0.05 mg kg^{-1} BW for propyl, octyl and dodecyl gallate, respectively.

These compounds are used only in cereals, cakes and milk powder.

In toxicity studies, the following NOAEL levels were found from different *in vivo* experiments: propyl gallate 135 mg kg^{-1} BW day^{-1}, octyl gallate 17.5 mg kg^{-1} BW day^{-1} and dodecyl gallate 10 mg kg^{-1} BW day^{-1}.

Dodecyl gallate could give rise to pathological changes of the liver, kidney and spleen. Gallates may also cause dermatitis, especially among bakers, when it is added to the ingredients used for baking cakes.

24.4 Flavour Extracts and Aroma Compounds

Flavours and flavour carriers

Foods and their flavour

The flavour of a food product may be the result only of the ingredients meant to nourish, a mixture of this with new flavours formed as a result of the processing of these ingredients (e.g. compounds formed through Maillard reactions), or it may be modified by the addition of food flavours. The science, production and use of food flavours have their parallels to the perfume sector, and indeed the work of a flavourist remains akin to that of the perfumer, despite inroads made by sophisticated analytical technology. For example, use of gas chromatography/mass spectrometry enables the skilled analyst to identify most components of a competitor's flavouring or the minor ingredients of a natural extract. Despite this, the flavouring industry remains a unique blend of art, science and technology in which the experience and knowledge of the flavourist are vital.

The users of food flavours roughly can be grouped into the beverages, confectionery, baking and dairy industries. The different products – their production and matrices – mean different demands on the physico-chemical characteristics of a flavour product. An example is the baking process, which can be particularly hard on added flavouring. Thus, the effect of high temperatures and low moistures in biscuits amounts almost to steam distillation of the flavouring, with the loss of many of the highly volatile substances and degradation of some of the less volatile components. This can be seen most readily in the use of citrus oils in biscuits; the clean notes of the oil become musty and unpleasant.

If we focus on the composition of the product, i.e. the product as a matrix for the flavour to be dissolved in, we find more problems to overcome as a flavourist. Within each product group such as the beverages, one can make subdivisions of after-characteristics that govern the solubility and miscibility of flavours of potential interest when developing a new product (in this case a beverage). The following broad categories are often used:

1. Alcoholic beverages, subdividing into alcohol contents (by volume):

   ● lower than 20%; and
   ● higher than 20%.

2. Aqueous and aqueous sugar-containing beverages, subdividing into sugar contents (by weight):

   ● lower than 2.5%;
   ● higher than 2.5% and lower than 60%; and
   ● higher than 60%.

3. Mixtures of types 1 and 2, for example:

   ● liqueur;
   ● low-alcohol wine; and
   ● shandy or beer cooler.

Let us again take a look at the citrus essential oils, some of the most effective and readily available natural flavouring materials, released from the peel of citrus fruits during processing for juice extraction. The composition of both lemon and orange oil is dominated by a high content of water-insoluble terpenes. This makes them almost insoluble in aqueous and aqueous sugar-containing beverages; however, they are generally soluble in high-alcohol beverages and show a limited solubility (but greater miscibility) in aqueous beverages with sugar content higher than 60% by weight. The best beverage composition for such natural whole citrus oils, which have been neither solubilized nor processed, is thus a high-alcohol beverage with high sugar content. In accordance with this we actually do find many famous names within the liqueurs which have a strong, fresh, authentic citrus taste.

Flavouring products and compounds – the materials of the industry

The *flavouring compounds* can be grouped into *essential oils*, *natural extracts*, *fruit juices* and *synthetic ingredients*. The latter may be identical with compounds found in nature or artificial. Before we discuss the single groups it should be noted, however, that the total sensory perception of a food consists of different elements such as flavour, taste and mouthfeel (Table 24.3).

ESSENTIAL OILS. Essential oils are mixtures of *hydrocarbons*, which are made up almost exclusively of *terpenes* (monoterpenes, sesquiterpenes and diterpenes), and *oxygenated compounds*, which are mainly esters, aldehydes, ketones, alcohols,

Table 24.3. Classification of ingredients with regard to role in food perception.

Volatility	Organoleptic function	Molecular weight	Examples
High	Flavour, taste	<150	Esters, ketones, simple heterocyclics
Low	Taste, flavour	<250	Carbonic acids, amides, extended C-skeletons
None	Taste	50–10,000	Sugars, amino acids, monosodium glutamate, salt, nucleic acids, bitter agents, natural sweeteners

phenols and oxides, and can be of different biosynthetic origin. Essential oils are found in either glandular hairs on the surface of the plant (leaves and stems) or oil cavities (chambers). The first occur very much in species from the plant family *Labiaceae* such as *Salvia officinalis*, for which five distinct types of glandular hair with different secretory modes and secretions have been identified. In contrast, the many species of citrus all contain essential oil in cavities in the leaves and the outer yellow to green layer (the flavedo) of the mature fruits. The primary site of synthesis in this case is the oil gland, which develops within the tissue. The oil is emitted into and collects in an extracellular cavity, the chamber, which forms schizogenously through a separation of the walls of the central cells, which are pushed outward and flattened with the expansion and filling of the oil chamber. Examples of important essential oils are bergamot oil, cassia oil, cinnamon oil, clove oil, coriander oil, cornmint oil, dill oil, eucalyptus oil, garlic oil, ginger oil, grapefruit oil, lemon oil, lemongrass oil, lime oil, nutmeg oil, sweet orange oil, peppermint oil, rosemary oil, spearmint oil, star anise oil and tangerine oil. Production can be by steam or water distillation, expression or extraction. Further processing of an essential oil can be by simple redistillation, a procedure sometimes carried out for cassia oil to clean it from impurities such as iron, or by rectification, which means distillation where one selects the desirable fractions. Some of the first fractions of peppermint oil have undesirable harsh and vegetal odours, for example. For certain oils the process of rectification can be extended to cover the removal of a substantial part of the terpene hydrocarbons. Such terpeneless oils are produced by distilling under vacuum.

NATURAL EXTRACTS. As already mentioned, essential oils can be produced by extraction. However, a number of plants not very rich in essential oil still can be a starting material for the production of an extract for use as a flavouring component.

Extraction can be by water (water infusions), examples being cola nut infusion, tea, coffee and liquorice root extract, or by ethanol or other alcohols (alcoholic tinctures), e.g. quassia bark tincture. *Oleoresins* are generally produced by extraction with solvents such as ethanol, isopropanol, ethyl acetate, acetone, etc. However, these products have their extraction solvent removed. Commercially produced oleoresins include pepper (*Piper nigrum*), ginger (*Zingiber officinale*) nutmeg (*Myristica fragrans*) and capsicum, together with many others. Today oleoresins may be processed further and marketed as, for example, spread or plated on to salt or maltodextrin, as standardized emulsion oleoresins or as encapsulated (spay dried) standardized oleoresins.

FRUIT JUICES. Concentrated fruit juices are often used as a base to which other components are added.

SYNTHETIC INGREDIENTS. Synthetic flavour compounds have the great advantage of being available in the required quantity and quality irrespective of crop variation and season. The constant quality also permits better standardization of the flavourings. Furthermore, synthetically produced flavour compounds make it possible to vary the proportions of single components and thereby create new flavour notes. As for the natural flavours, synthetic flavour ingredients cover the whole range of organic substances. However, no obvious relationship has been established between structure and flavour properties, so although some components of similar structure have broadly similar odours, there still are many exceptions. One of the many possible ways to describe flavour substances or ingredients used in the process of flavour composition is to classify them in groups with parent flavour characteristics, as for example is done in a so-called *flavour wheel*. A commonly used edition of this wheel operates with the following 16 flavour notes: (i) green grassy; (ii) fruity ester-like; (iii) citrus terpenic; (iv) minty camphoraceous; (v) floral sweet; (vi) spicy herbaceous; (vii) woody smoky;

(xiii) roasty burnt; (ix) caramel nutty; (x) Bouillon hydrolysed vegetable protein; (xi) meaty animalic; (xii) fatty rancid; (xiii) dairy buttery; (xiv) mushroom earthy; (xv) celery soupy; and (xvi) sulfurous alliaceous. As an example of the structural variation found between the different compounds in a group we can look at the mushroom earthy flavour note. This includes compounds as different as 1-octen-3-ol and 2-ethyl-3-methylthiopyrazine.

The composition of a flavour

Many natural flavours contain a high number of molecules with significant influence on the overall perception. An example could be the natural flavour of raspberry, which has been shown to be dependent on at least 131 compounds, namely:

- 13 hydrocarbons including limonene and pinene;
- 36 alcohols such as ethanol, *cis*-3-hexenol, geraniol and menthol;
- 17 aldehydes like benzaldehyde and phenylacetaldehyde;
- 22 ketones including ionones, hydroxybutanone and camphor;
- 16 acids such as acetic, hexanoic and benzoic acids; and
- 27 esters like isoamyl acetate, benzyl acetate and methyl salicylate.

The job of the flavourist is to identify the substances present in the food that are the most important in producing its flavour and then to create a flavour profile which mimics the particular food in the most effective way. Today the average flavouring contains between five and 50 ingredients. A few flavourings contain many more.

The risk assessment of flavours and flavour components

Today's evaluation of flavours including essential oils concerning their safety as food additives in a certain way may be traced back to the story about the possible risk taken by drinking the French alcoholic beverage absinthe.

THE STORY OF ABSINTHE. The origin of absinthe may be traced back to the end of the 18th century. The French doctor Pierre Ordinaire used wormwood (*Artemisia absinthium*) together with anise, fennel, hyssop and other herbs distilled in an alcoholic base as a herbal remedy for his patients. Ordinaire's recipe eventually found its way to Henri-Louis Pernod, who established the Pernod Fils dynasty when he opened his first distillery in 1805. Soon 'Extrait d'absinthe' started on its route to becoming a national phenomenon in France. By the end of the 19th century over 2 million litres were consumed annually in France. Wormwood has a long history in folk medicine dating back to ancient Greece, where it was variously prescribed for rheumatism, jaundice, menstrual pains and as an aid in child birth.

The first published evidence for absinthe's harmful effects in animals dates from the 1860s with the appearance of two papers.[2,3] These reported that wormwood oil and alcohol produce a synergistic effect which leads to epileptiform convulsions. Magnan in his paper[2] extended his studies to acute alcoholics and concluded that absinthe produced symptoms in humans that were distinct from alcoholic delirium tremens and manifested themselves as epileptic convulsions. Gradually it became generally accepted that thujone, a terpene with a menthol odour found in wormwood, was responsible for absinthe's effects. Thujone occurs in nature as a mixture of α-(−)- and β-(+)-diastereoisomers, the proportions varying with the source. Synthetic α-thujone (Fig. 24.10) is also available commercially.

This led to regulations being implemented in different European countries, including France. Therefore, today's versions of the drink have to comply with an EU limit as found in Annex II to the Council Directive of 22 June 1988 on the approximation of the laws of the Member States relating to flavourings for use in foodstuffs and to source materials for their production (88/388/EEC). The maximum limits for thujone ($\alpha+\beta$) are as follows: 5 mg kg^{-1} in alcoholic beverages with not more than 25% alcohol by volume; 10 mg kg^{-1} in alcoholic beverages with more than 25% alcohol by volume; 25 mg kg^{-1} in foodstuffs containing preparations based on sage; and 35 mg kg^{-1} in bitters. The same Directive also contains the EU maximum limits for a number of other substances that a food or beverage product can obtain from flavourings, i.e. agaric acid, aloin, β-asarone, berberine, coumarin, hydrocyanic

Fig. 24.10. α-Thujone.

acid, hypericine, pulegone, quassine, safrole/isosafrole, nutmeg and santonin.

Thujone does indeed induce epileptiform convulsions also in rats and other animal species. Thus, the NOAEL for convulsions in subchronic toxicity studies in female rats was $5\,mg\,kg^{-1}$ BW day^{-1} but there are no long-term or reproductive toxicity data. In 1975 it was suggested that similarities between the reported mind-altering/hallucinogenic effects of absinthe and those of marijuana (*Cannabis sativa*) had to do with a similar molecular geometry of thujone and tetrahydrocannabinol. However, in 1999 Meschler and Howlett showed that thujone has no activity at the cannabinoid receptor. Rather, the compounds have now been shown to be rapidly acting modulators of the GABA-gated chloride channel. The effects seem to be due to the genuine compound, while metabolism leads to detoxification.

At the end of 2002 the EU SCF considered the available data on thujone and concluded that humans are at least as sensitive as rodents to the acute neurotoxic effects. Accordingly, the Committee did not consider it appropriate to use thujone as a chemically identified flavouring substance. The Committee also supported the continued application of the current upper limits (see above) to the occurrence of α- and β-thujone in foods and beverages.

However, some studies suggest that the adverse effects reported earlier for absinthe actually may not have been due to thujone, but rather to product adulterants in inferior brands. So let us take a look at this possibility.

These sources argue that it will take close to 60 litres of today's absinthe to reach the NOAEL for convulsions, and furthermore recent investigations using GC analysis on absinthe produced by the traditional recipe have shown that this probably had even lower thujone levels. Therefore, many believe that what is more likely to have caused harm to regular absinthe drinkers was the adulterants used in the cheaper products. Common adulterants were cupric acetate (to provide the valued green colour) and antimony trichloride (which provided a cloudiness when water was added in imitation of the milky appearance of diluted absinthe). The purity of the alcohol used for lesser brands would also have been questionable, and toxic levels of methanol from poor rectification would have been a real possibility.

RISK ASSESSMENT OF FLAVOURS TODAY AND IN THE FUTURE. As described in Chapter 11, the first system

for systematic evaluation of flavours was established in the USA: the FEMA GRAS list system. From 1997 onwards, JECFA has used the so-called *threshold of toxicological concern (TTC) method* in their then-initiated risk evaluation of chemical groups of flavouring substances. The method was developed mainly by Dr I.C. Munro (CANTOX Health Sciences International, Canada) with the aim of developing a methodology allowing:

- the evaluation a large number of flavouring substances in use;
- in a timely and consistent manner; and
- using sound toxicological principles.

In 1999 the JECFA procedure was acknowledged by the EU SCF as the most updated and systematic procedure for the evaluation of flavouring substances, and it has been applied since 2000 for the safety evaluation of flavouring substances in the EU (see also below). The main components of this JECFA evaluation process include chemical structure, human intake (exposure), metabolism to innocuous or harmless substances, and toxicity concerns consistent with JECFA principles. Schematically it may be presented as shown in Fig. 24.11.

In order to make such an evaluation, chemical groups must be defined. This is done as follows:

- Chemical groups are based on:
  - close structural relationships;
  - common pathways of metabolism; and
  - consistent patterns of toxicological potential.

JECFA operates with 47 chemical groups, while 34 chemical groups are recognized according to Regulation (EC) No. 1565/2000. In the EU system each flavouring substance is attributed a FLAVIS number (FL number). Substances within a group should have some metabolic and biological behaviour in common.

THE EU AND FLAVOURING EVALUATION. The regulatory framework is now harmonized through EU legislation on food flavourings. Thus, Regulation (EC) No. 2232/96 (Regulation of the European Parliament and of the Council of 28 October 1996 laying down a Community procedure for flavouring substances used or intended for use in or on foodstuffs) sets out the main rules on the use of flavourings in foods in the EU. Based on this legislation a procedure has been

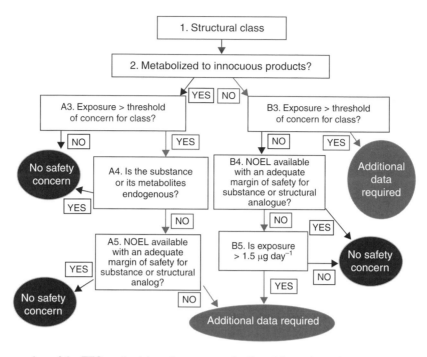

Fig. 24.11. An overview of the TTC methodology for group evaluation of flavouring substances. Adapted with permission of WHO.[4]

launched to establish an EU positive list of fla- vourings that may be added to foods. The positive list is to be set up after a comprehensive safety evaluation programme is completed. Member States have notified the Commission of about 2800 substances authorized at national level to be included in the programme. Among them are many substances which occur naturally.

In addition, Regulation (EC) No. 1331/2008 on a common authorization procedure for food addi- tives, food enzymes and food flavourings upgraded all existing EU rules in this area, including a simpli- fied common approval procedure for these sub- stances. The Regulation entered into force in 2009.

In Commission Decision 1999/217/EC, a list of some specified flavouring compounds to receive pri- ority in the evaluation programme – as based on safety concerns expressed by different Member States – was created. The list came to contain 43 fla- vouring substances including: quinine salts (for which JECFA in 1993 expressed no concerns up to a con- centration of 100 mg l^{-1} in soft drinks), glycyrrhizic acid, caffeine and theobromine, and vinylbenzene.

EFSA regularly adopts opinions on each chemical group, known as flavouring group evaluations.

If EFSA identifies data gaps – for instance on toxicity – it notifies the need for further data to the applicant and to the European Commission. In the course of its work EFSA has identified data gaps for approximately 300 substances.

The European Commission maintains a register of flavourings notified by Member States as present on the EU market. It may remove substances during the evaluation programme, particularly when EFSA identifies safety concerns.

Waxes for glazing and as carriers of flavours

A number of so-called *waxes* are approved for use as food additives. In fact the designation 'wax' covers two different types of complex mixtures. The first is the true waxes, which are made up mainly of esters between long-chain alcohols and fatty acids. Such waxes are biosynthesized by plants and used to cover leaves and other surfaces.

An example is carnauba wax (Brazil wax, palm wax) from the leaves of the palm *Copernicia pru- nifera* grown in north-east Brazil. Specific for car- nauba wax is the relatively high content of esterified fatty diols (about 20%), hydroxylated fatty acids (about 6%) and cinnamic acid (about 10%). In the EU carnauba wax was evaluated twice (1992, 2001) by SCF, which concluded that its use as a glazing agent up to a maximum level of 200 mg kg^{-1} food was acceptable.

Although produced by worker bees, beeswax has a quite similar composition, being a complex mixture of saturated and unsaturated linear and complex monoesters, fatty acids, fatty alcohols and hydrocarbons. Worker bees have eight wax-producing mirror glands on the inner sides of the sternites (the ventral shield or plate of each segment of the body) on abdominal segments 4 to 7. Beeswax is also authorized as a food additive worldwide including the EU (E901; glazing agents). As such it is used for the glazing of confectionery (excluding chocolate), fine bakery wares coated with chocolate, nuts and certain snacks. Furthermore, it is allowed for the surface treatment of certain fresh fruits such as apples, melons, peaches, pears and pineapples.

The second type of mixtures used widely for the same purposes in food and medicine comprise the class I mineral oils and the high-melting-point microcrystalline waxes, characterized by a high content of $\geq C_{25}$ hydrocarbons as defined by JECFA and SCF. An ADI of 10 mg kg^{-1} BW and 20 mg kg^{-1} BW was established by JECFA for class I mineral oils and microcrystalline waxes, respectively. In Europe SCF established a temporary group ADI of 4 mg kg^{-1} BW for white paraffinic mineral oils derived from petroleum-based hydrocarbon feed stocks and an ADI of 20 mg kg^{-1} BW for highly refined waxes.

With an opinion published in 2007 the EFSA AFC Panel concluded that allowing beeswax to furthermore be used as a carrier of flavours caused no toxicity concerns concerning the beeswax component.

24.5 Conclusion

Today both flavours and food additives of many different types have to be risk-assessed in most parts of the world in order to be approved for use.

Notes

[1] Damon, G.E. and Janseen, W.F. (1973) Additives for eye appeal. *FDA Consumer* July–August issue.
[2] Magnan, V. (1869) Epilepsie alcoholique; action spéciale de l'absinthe: épilepsie absinthique. *Comptus Rendu des Seances et Memoires de la Société de Biologie (Paris)* 5 (4th series), 156–161.
[3] Amory, R. (1868) Experiments and observations on absinthe and absinthism. *Boston Medical and Surgical Journal* 7(8), 68–71 and 83–85.
[4] WHO/FAO (2009) *Evaluation of Certain Food Additives. Sixty-ninth report of the Joint WHO/FAO Expert Committee on Food Additives. WHO Technical Report Series No. 952.* World Health Organization, Geneva, Switzerland; available at http://whqlibdoc.who.int/trs/WHO_TRS_952_eng.pdf

Further Reading

Smith, J. and Hong-Shum, L. (ed.) (2003) *Food Additives Data Book.* Wiley-Blackwell, Hoboken, New Jersey.

25 Food Allergies and Intolerances

- We define allergy as opposed to intolerance.
- We look at common food allergies.
- We look at intolerance to cow's milk and discuss PKU.

25.1 Allergy

Food allergy is a topic in itself when dealing with food safety. *Allergies* are caused by chemical compounds; however, the adverse effects are not seen as a result the first direct contact with these but rather at a later contact, i.e. if the immune system of the animal organism meanwhile has built up a defence to recognize and react when presented with the same chemical (the *allergen/antigen*). The allergic reaction(s) seen represent(s) a kind of over-reaction: a reaction going further than that of protecting the individual, instead causing adverse effects.

Symptoms of an *allergic reaction* are diverse depending on the body part involved and the severity of the reaction. Reactions to the same allergen may vary by individual and include: (i) the skin – redness, itching, swelling, blistering, weeping, crusting, rash, eruptions or hives (itchy bumps or welts); (ii) the lungs – wheezing, tightness, coughing or shortness of breath; (iii) the head – swelling of the face, eyelids, lips, tongue or throat, together with headache; (iv) the nose – stuffy nose, runny nose (clear, thin discharge), sneezing; (v) the eyes – red (bloodshot), itchy, swollen or watery; and (vi) the stomach – pain, nausea, vomiting, diarrhoea or bloody diarrhoea. A life-threatening situation termed *anaphylaxis* may also occur. Anaphylaxis is any combination of allergic symptoms that is rapid or sudden and potentially life-threatening. One sign is *shock*, where the organs of the body are not getting enough blood because of dangerously low blood pressure. Shock may lead rapidly to death. The person in shock may be pale or red, sweaty or dry, confused, anxious or unconscious; he/she may also show difficult or noisy breathing. The shock is caused by a sudden dilation of the large blood vessels.

Food allergies are reactions to proteins in foods. IgE specific to the protein in question is formed in huge amounts, causing an over-reaction the next time the body meets this protein. Some decades ago scientists began to realize that there exists an association between certain pollen allergies and certain (plant) food allergies, and a number of syndromes such as the 'celery–mugwort–birch pollen syndrome' and the 'apple–birch pollen syndrome' were described. New information then showed that pollen–food allergy syndromes are due to cross-reactivity of IgE antibodies to conserved plant proteins that are expressed in both related and unrelated plant species and in different plant tissues. By *conserved protein* we mean proteins that fulfil important biological functions and therefore are conserved in their sequence and structure. Important conserved proteins include the actin-binding protein profilin first described in birch pollen.

Allergy is seen for foods of animal as well as plant origin. An example of allergy to foods of animal origin is the allergy to fish proteins described in Chapter 22 as a differential diagnosis to scombroid (histamine) poisoning. While this allergy is relatively seldom seen with an overall prevalence (all age groups) of about 0.25%, others such as those towards eggs and milks occur more often, the overall prevalence for each being close to 1%. For both these a somewhat higher prevalence is normally reported for small children (0–4 years). While fish allergy is relatively infrequent the prevalence of allergy to shellfish seems to be a little more common, with the mean confirmed prevalence of symptomatically diagnosed and sensitized (IgE) people reported as about 0.75%.

When it comes to plant food allergies many sources of information are available; however, not all are equally reliable. Thus, it is fair to say that for decades there has been a great uncertainty regarding the prevalence of allergies to different plant foods. This prompted a large group of scientists to make a so-called *meta-analysis* including 36 studies with data from a total of over 250,000 children and adults, a study they published in 2008. Looking further into this study reveals the following conclusions:

- *Fruit.* Children below 3 years of age seem to show a relatively high prevalence of up to about 12% when it comes to allergy to any fruit, with apple (8.5%) and orange and/or lemon (6.8%) being the most important. In adults the prevalence of perceived allergic reactions to specific fruits was below 1% in all studies analysed.
- *Vegetables/legumes.* In adults, the highest prevalence was found in a Dutch study, i.e. 2.2% to any vegetable. The highest prevalence reported in the studies included was for Swedish children at 1.5 years of age (about 14% allergic to tomato).
- *Tree nuts.* In general hazelnut was reported as positive concerning perceived allergic reactions at a prevalence of about 4%. A Swedish study in addition showed that approximately 4% of all adolescents react to almond.
- *Groundnut* (= peanut; *Arachis hypogaea* L.). About 1% of the population showed allergy to groundnuts both when analysing the self-reported data and when looking at symptomatic and IgE confirmed allergies.
- *Wheat.* Wheat challenge tests performed in the UK as well as Germany showed a prevalence of wheat allergy of about 0.5% in children. Also a comparable fraction of the adult population was shown to be allergic. Wheat allergy may result in a wide range of symptoms, including hives, difficulty breathing and nausea. Wheat allergy can also cause a life-threatening anaphylactic reaction. Wheat allergy is different from a disorder known as *coeliac disease*, an immune system reaction that causes inflammation in the small intestines when a person eats any food containing gluten, one type of protein found in wheat.
- *Soy.* Most studies agree on an overall prevalence about or below 1% for this food item.
- *Nickel.* Nickel allergy is one of the most common causes of contact allergic dermatitis. As an example the prevalence of nickel allergy in the Danish population is 10% for women and 2% for men. In affected individuals, dermatitis (eczema) develops where nickel-containing metal is touching the skin. Common sites are the earlobes (from earrings), the wrists (from a watch strap) and the lower abdomen (from a jeans stud); the affected areas become intensely itchy and may become red and blistered (acute dermatitis), or dry, thickened and pigmented (chronic dermatitis). While no confirmed studies have shown that nickel allergy can be induced by eating foods with a high content of nickel, it seems relatively well established that individuals with severe nickel allergy should avoid such foods. Among dermatologists it is thus a general opinion that a flare of hand eczema can occur after peroral nickel exposure. The nickel intake from the Danish diet is estimated as $150\,\mu g\ day^{-1}$ on average. Vegetables and roots, grain and bread supply the average diet with nickel up to this amount. However, certain food items, e.g. cocoa (chocolate), soybeans, oatmeal, most nuts, almonds, and fresh and dried legumes, have very high nickel contents. Consumption of these items in larger amounts thus can increase nickel intake to $900\,\mu g\ day^{-1}$ or more. This is of interest because $600–5600\,\mu g$ of nickel, when given in a single oral dose as a nickel salt, has been shown to provoke hand eczema.

As already mentioned legumes and certain nuts in particular are well known to have a relatively high nickel content, the absolute concentration depending on the soil content. A recent investigation of different legumes and 56 samples of different nuts, which are widely consumed in Spain, reported the content in legumes to be in the range of $0.02–0.35\,\mu g\ Ni\ g^{-1}$ and that in nuts to be $0.10–0.64\,\mu g\ Ni\ g^{-1}$.

Until recently any kind of risk assessment within the area of food allergies was non-existent. However, recent studies have begun to shed light on the distribution of the individual threshold doses eliciting allergic reactions in a population with (an already acquired) allergy.

25.2 Intolerance

Having looked at food allergies as well as the scombroid poisoning caused by biogenic amines (notably histamine) that sometimes is misinterpreted as allergy, we also have to briefly discuss food intolerance.

Food intolerance is an adverse reaction to a food ingredient (a compound in the food) that occurs every time the food is eaten, particularly if larger quantities are consumed. Since the immune system is not activated we are not talking about a food allergy. Neither is it the same as food poisoning, which is caused by toxic substances that would cause symptoms in anyone who ate the food. It is very important to stress that food intolerance does not include psychological reactions to food either. So what is the cause of food intolerances, of which there are several different?

Food intolerance occurs when the body is unable to deal with a certain type of foodstuff. This is usually because the body does not produce enough of a particular enzyme that is needed for digestion of the specific component in the food to allow its subsequent absorption or its further normal metabolism.

One of the most common types is intolerance of cow's milk, which contains lactose. Many people have a shortage of the enzyme lactase, which is normally made by cells lining the small intestine. Without this enzyme the individual cannot break down the disaccharide lactose into galactose and glucose for absorption into the bloodstream. Lactose intolerance can cause symptoms very similar to irritable bowel syndrome. Another example is sucrose intolerance (also known as congenital sucrase-isomaltase deficiency (CSID) or sucrase-isomaltase deficiency), which occurs when sucrase is not secreted in the small intestine. With sucrose intolerance, the result of consuming sucrose is excess gas production and often diarrhoea and malabsorption. CSID seems to be especially widespread among Inuits.

Food intolerances also may be due to the lack (or reduced activity) of an enzyme essential for the conversion of a compound once absorbed into the bloodstream. This is for example the case for the several characterized intolerances to specific amino acids. The most well known and commonly occurring is PKU (also called Følling's disease/syndrome). PKU was discovered in 1934 by the Norwegian physician Ivar Asbjørn Følling, who noticed that hyperphenylalaninaemia (HPA) was associated with mental retardation. PKU is a human genetic disorder in which the body lacks phenylalanine hydroxylase, the enzyme that metabolizes phenylalanine to tyrosine. If left untreated, the disorder causes brain damage and progressive mental retardation as a result of the accumulation of phenylalanine and its breakdown products. The incidence of occurrence is approximately 1 in 15,000 births, but varies in different human populations from 1 in 4500 births among the Irish to fewer than 1 in 100,000 births in Finland. The disease is readily detectable within a few days after birth by analysing a small blood sample (the Guthrie heel prick test). Consequently, screening for PKU is done routinely today in most industrialized countries. An affected child can grow with normal brain development by eating a diet low in phenylalanine. Thus, foods high in protein, such as meat, nuts and cheese, must be restricted. Supplementary formulas are used to provide the protein and other necessary nutrients that would otherwise be lacking in a diet free of protein.

PKU is of special relevance when talking about chemical food safety. This is due to the fact that the intensively used artificial sweetener aspartame (NutraSweet®) is metabolized in the gut to release phenylalanine. Thus, PKU patients must avoid or restrict the intake of food and beverages containing this sweetener.

A number of other enzyme deficiencies are common; for example, lack of the enzyme alcohol dehydrogenase occurs particularly among Asian people, of whom about 50% are affected.

Further Reading

Rona, R.J., Keil, T., Summers, C., Gislason, D., Zuidmeer, L., Sodergren, E., Sigurdardottir, S.T., Lindner, T., Goldhahn, K., Dahlstrom, J., McBride, D. and Madsen, C. (2007) The prevalence of food allergy: a meta-analysis. *Journal of Allergy and Clinical Immunology* 120, 638–646.

Wensing, M., Penninks, A.H., Hefle, S.L., Koppelman, S.J., Bruijnzell-Koomen, C.A.F.M. and Knulst, A.C. (2002) The distribution of individual threshold doses eliciting allergic reactions in a population with peanut allergy. *Journal of Allergy and Clinical Immunology* 110, 915–920.

Zuidmeer, L., Goldhahn, K., Rona, R.J., Gislason, D., Madsen, C., Summers, C., Sodergren, E., Dahlstrom, J., Lindner, T., Sigurdardottir, S.T., McBride, D. and Keil, T. (2008) The prevalence of plant food allergies: a systematic review. *Journal of Allergy and Clinical Immunology* 121, 1210–1218.

26 Analytical Chemistry in Food Safety

- The preparatory steps such as extraction and pre-purification(s) are described.
- The major methods for elements/metals and for organic compounds are described.
- Speciation of metal and metalloid species is described.
- Bioassays are described with regard to their strengths and weaknesses.

26.1 Introduction

Having established a concentration beyond which an action should be taken in the form of a more detailed survey to disclose if there is a general problem of unacceptable contamination levels (action level) or a concentration which means withdrawal of the products from the market if exceeded (maximum accepted level), clearly a method of analysis for the contaminant in question must be at hand. The same is true of course for food additives with a maximum tolerated level, where the authorities also must be able to check if the rules have been followed.

Analysis includes everything from the analytic investigation of huge batches of raw or semi-processed food commodities (e.g. the occurrence of mycotoxins in cereals or of algal toxins in shellfish) to detailed analysis of highly processed single food products (or even complete dishes). Thus, the *sampling* must be standardized to ensure a representative and reproducible result. When dealing with processed foods these can vary a lot; most often are indeed very complex in both physical structure and chemical composition. This is why CEN, which has a technical committee dealing with methods of analysis in which both food additives and contaminants are discussed (TC 275), has established two different working groups when it comes to pesticides in foods. One group takes care of pesticides in fatty foods, the other of pesticides in non-fatty foods.

Actually a number of international organizations worldwide are involved in the development and validation as fit for purpose of analytical methods as well as of guidelines/legislative requirements concerning the accreditation and assessment of testing laboratories in the food sector. CAC through its Committee on Methods of Analysis and Sampling (CCMAS) was the first organization *working at the government level in the food sector* that laid down principles for the establishment of its methods. The 'Principles for the Establishment of Codex Methods of Analysis' require that preference should be given to methods of analysis the reliability of which has been established in respect of the following criteria:

- specificity;
- accuracy;
- precision – repeatability intra-laboratory (within a laboratory) and reproducibility inter-laboratory (within a laboratory and between laboratories);
- limit of detection;
- sensitivity; and
- practicability and applicability under normal laboratory conditions.

Today other international organizations that lay down procedures for the development of methods of analysis follow these principles to a great extent as they do concerning the principles for accreditation and assessment of testing laboratories. Among other reasons this has to do with the increasing importance of CAC because of the acceptance of the Codex Standards in the World Trade Organization agreements.

The EU started its attempts to harmonize both sampling and analysis procedures within the chemical analysis of foods for contaminants by issuing the directive on sampling and methods of analysis which contains a technical annex (Directive 85/591/EEC concerning the introduction of Community methods of sampling and analysis for the monitoring of food stuffs intended for human consumption of 31.12.1985). The EU during this process has placed emphasis on the fact that methods of analysis which are applicable uniformly to various groups of commodities should be given preference over methods which apply to individual commodities.

Other organizations involved in the development of different standards within the field of food analysis than those already mentioned include ISO (International Organization for Standardization), the world's largest developer and publisher of international standards. ISO is a network of the national standards institutes of 162 countries, one member per country, with a Central Secretariat in Geneva, Switzerland, that coordinates the system. Also AOAC – which was founded in 1884 as the Association of Official Agricultural Chemists, under the auspices of the USDA, to adopt uniform methods of analysis for fertilizers – is very important. By 1991 the Association had long ceased to be limited to regulatory ('official') analytical chemists in the USA and consequently, in that year, the name of the Association was changed to AOAC INTERNATIONAL. Finally one also must mention the Nordic Committee for Food Analysis (NMKL).

Within the area of analysis of drugs a number of organizations and guidelines also exist. However, one should mention that the discrepancies seen for decades between the requirements for getting a new drug (drug substance) approved in each of Europe, the USA and Japan meant that from the beginning of the 1990s a process of harmonization was started. As a result, in 1994 the International Conference on Harmonisation of Technical Requirements for Registration of Pharmaceuticals for Human Use (ICH) launched the first harmonized paper (the 'tripartite harmonised ICH core text'). This text identifies the validation parameters needed for a variety of analytical methods. An addendum was made public in 1996. The addendum extends the first guideline to include the actual experimental data required, along with the statistical interpretation, for the validation of an analytical procedure. The addendum was incorporated into the core guideline in November 2005 to give the document *ICH Harmonised Tripartite Guideline; Validation of Analytical Procedures: Text and Methodology Q2(R1)* (available online at http://www.ich.org/LOB/media/MEDIA417.pdf).

Laboratories analysing foods today, as a part of their general activities and most often actually as a compulsory component in their keeping one or more accreditations, participate in so-called *proficiency testing schemes*. A proficiency testing scheme can be defined as a system for objectively checking laboratory results by an external agency. At intervals comparison of the laboratory's results with those of other laboratories is made, the main objective being the establishment of trueness. Testing schemes are based on the regular circulation of homogeneous samples by a co-ordinator, analysis of samples by the laboratories included in the scheme, and an assessment of the results.

26.2 Methods Used to Analyse Food Contaminants: General Considerations

Sampling and sample preparation

In most cases the contaminant (a chemical compound from now on referred to as the *analyte*) must be extracted from the sample prior to its analysis, i.e. detection and quantification. Within food analysis (in contrast to pharmaceutical products), sample extraction has only in the past few decades or so been given the critical consideration it deserves as an important unit operation in obtaining reliable and robust analytical results. The *extraction*, i.e. the transfer of the analyte from the product (the matrix) into a solvent (or in rare cases, a gas) in which it can be detected, must of course be as quantitative as possible. This requirement actually includes two aspects: (i) that the compound is released quantitatively; and (ii) that it is kept chemically stable during and after this process (i.e. until the instrumental analysis can take place).

A liquid food product may be suitable for direct analysis or may be analysed after simple dilution with a proper solvent with which it is miscible. Alternatively the analyte may be extracted into another liquid phase by liquid–liquid partition with a non-miscible solvent or extracted on to a solid phase, e.g. by passing the original or diluted product through a column with a stationary phase that retains the analyte in a reversible manner. However, in most cases the food product is a solid or semi-solid. In solids and semi-solids the analyte may occur equally distributed throughout the product sample, but most often this will not be the case, which is why the sampling procedure is so essential. When the sample has been prepared the analyte must then be transferred to the chosen solvent, a process that depends on a number of factors such as:

- the solubility of the analyte in the solvent;
- the degree of contact between the analyte and the solvent;
- the temperature (a higher temperature facilitates diffusion); and
- the extraction time.

The degree of contact is a function of the solid surface area in contact with the solvent and, for analytes found in cells, also of the degree of cell damage to release the analyte. Hence comminuting the sample into smaller particles (by cutting and/or milling) is essential. This process can take place either prior to the extraction or as an integral part of this, e.g. by blending the sample directly in the solvent. Which of these two methods is chosen depends primarily on whether the sample, if not already totally dry, can be dried to allow milling, for example, without the risk of degradation of the analyte by oxidation, reduction, hydrolysis or other chemical reactions.

When extraction has taken place and the solid particles have been removed by filtration, centrifugation or other means, the analyte is often concentrated by solvent evaporation or freeze drying (lyophilized) as perhaps combined with liquid–liquid partition or solid-phase extraction on to a small column as already explained for liquid samples. The two latter methods of sample concentration include a component of purification, i.e. a number of compounds that are not of interest may be removed from the sample, making the subsequent analyses easier (Fig. 26.1). The mechanism behind the binding of the analyte to the particles of the stationary phase of the column can be adsorption, ion exchange, inclusion/exclusion depending on molecular size, binding to lectins present on the surface of the particles of the stationary phase (for sugars and glycosides) or binding to antibodies (affinity chromatography).

The choice of extraction medium and temperature for some analytes is even more delicate than already described. While many organic substances in general are relatively easy to extract quantitatively with different either hydrophilic or lipophilic

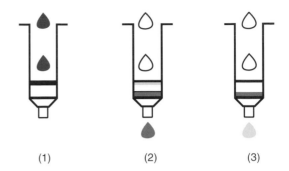

Fig. 26.1. Solid phase pre-purification of a sample: (1) add reaction mixture containing toxic solanine alkaloid from potatoes together with other organic and inorganic substances; (2) elute non-alkaloids; (3) elute alkaloids.

media, others may give rise to more complicated considerations.

An example is gossypol, a polyphenolic compound (Fig. 26.2) occurring naturally in the seeds, foliage and roots of most cotton plants. In 1957 it was reported that there were no births in one village in Jiangsu Province in China between the 1930s and 1940s. However, the villagers were fecund before and after that period. This infertility incident was shown to be due to a contamination of cottonseed oil for human consumption with gossypol. A large-scale study involving more than 8000 Chinese men on the use of gossypol as an anti-contraceptive was carried out with daily doses of 20 mg (±)-gossypol. The study revealed that the drug was efficient. However, a side-effect (hypokalaemia) affected about 10% of users. Gossypol can be found in 'free' or 'bound' forms, with the bound form being less toxic orally than the free form. In the seeds, almost all the gossypol is found in the free form. Heat and moisture during food and feed processing convert the free form into the less toxic, bound form. Free gossypol is readily extractable with solvents while the bound gossypol mostly represents covalent adducts of gossypol to proteins, from which free gossypol can be (partially) liberated by heating with acids.

When it comes to toxic metals and metalloids again there are delicate considerations to make when extracting samples. The usual specimen preparation method when analysing toxic elements such as arsenic, chromium, lead, selenium or tin using FAAS (flame atomic absorption spectroscopy), GFAAS (graphite furnace atomic absorption spectroscopy) or other methods such as NAA (neutron

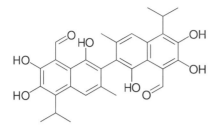

Fig. 26.2. The structure of gossypol.

activation analysis) and ICPMS (inductively coupled plasma–mass spectrometry) is digestion with strong mineral acid, what we measure being the total concentration of the element present in the sample. However, for some metals the *state of oxidation* is essential for the toxicity as seen for example with chromium. By the oral route Cr^{3+} has a low toxicity due to low absorption while Cr^{6+} is highly toxic due to its high absorption and easy penetration of the cell membranes. For other metals and metalloids the form in which they occur also means something for their toxicity. This is the case for mercury, arsenic and selenium for example, where inorganic and different organic forms may show very different toxic profiles. For such elements the so-called *molecular speciation* may indeed be essential when analysing a food product. Hence, the method of extraction must preserve the elements in their genuine forms and the method of analysis must be able to separate and quantitatively detect the different molecular species.

Analysis

Methods of analysis depend of course on the nature of the analyte and may even include the use of bioassays as seen for toxins involved in shellfish poisoning. Before we move to such bioassays, however, let us first look briefly at the chemical and biochemical techniques used most often in the analysis of organic compounds and metals and other elements.

26.3 Organic Compounds (Additives and Toxicants)

Organic additives and toxicants found in food (and feed) may include a large number of purely organic low-molecular-weight compounds, macromolecules such as proteins (e.g. ricin) or polysaccharides (gum arabic) and different metallo-organic compounds. The latter are discussed below in section 26.4.

Very often when we analyse for organic toxicants we are actually looking for a possible content of a number of different members within a group of compounds. Such a group may be either: (i) a group of chemically related compounds, e.g. a mixture of dioxins (see also section 26.6), a group of related mycotoxins such as the trichothecenes from species of the genus *Fusarium*, or a group of natural toxic plant constituents such as glucosinolates present in food and feed plants from the plant family *Brassicaceae*; or (ii) it may be a mixture of chemically unrelated compounds (typically compounds used for the same purpose), an example being analyses made to monitor the occurrence of pesticide residues in different commodities.

To identify and quantify the individual components in such mixtures we need to separate them, which today we typically do by using chromatographic procedures coupled with one or more suitable detectors.

Gas chromatography

In gas chromatography (GC) the sample is injected into a chromatographic column packed with or its wall covered with (only capillary columns) an adsorbent – the *stationary phase* – that has variable affinity for the components to be separated. The sample, including all of its different compounds and the solvent in which it is dissolved, must be gaseous when injected or have boiling points that allow it to become fully volatilized within the liner of the injector. Once injected and volatilized the sample is entrained by a moving *carrier gas*. While travelling through the column the individual components of the sample interact with the stationary phase, being delayed to different degrees as they partition between the moving gas and the stationary phase. The components eventually reach the end of the column (*elute*) after different periods of time (called the *retention time*), i.e. they are separated. Now they enter the detector, which monitors the progress of the run and the elution of each substance (Fig. 26.3).

The detection step is of course crucial. GC detectors are devices that detect the presence of solute vapours as they are eluted from a gas chromatographic column. In general, traces of vapour modify the properties of a gas far more extensively than traces of solute modify the properties of a liquid. As a consequence, the detection of vapours in gases is easier than the detection of traces of solutes in liquids. Thus, GC

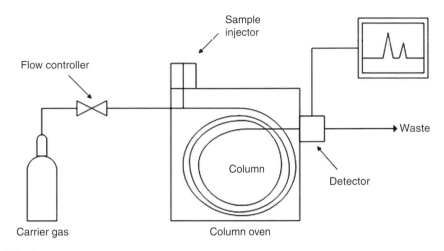

Fig. 26.3. A GC setup.

detectors are normally more sensitive than liquid chromatography (LC) detectors (discussed below under HPLC) and there are more of them.

The first detectors developed for GC were the gas density balance detector (responds to the change in density of the gas), the thermal conductivity detector (TCD) (responds to the change in specific heat and thermal conductivity of the gas) and the flame thermocouple detector (responds to the heat of combustion of the gas). These showed sensitivities of about 5×10^{-7} g ml^{-1} at a signal-to-noise ratio of 2. Gradually more sensitive GC detectors were developed. The first high-sensitivity detector was the flame ionization detector (FID) (responds to the ion current produced in the flame during the combustion of carbon-containing solutes). This detector had a sensitivity of about 5×10^{-12} g ml^{-1} for *n*-heptane at a signal-to-noise ratio of 2. A further development based on this detector, the nitrogen phosphorus detector (NPD), shows selectively to nitrogen- and phosphorus-containing compounds.

The argon detector (developed at about the same time as the FID) provides sensitivities about an order of magnitude greater than the FID. A further development of the argon detector, the electron capture detector (ECD), again exhibits a sensitivity nearly an order of magnitude greater than the argon detector but is highly specific, only giving a significant response to electron-capturing substances (e.g. halogenated compounds).

Despite giving rise to a peak the height or area of which can be related to the amount of the substance in question, the detectors mentioned above in general give very little information concerning the nature (structure) of the compounds that elute from the column. This changed dramatically when the mass spectrometer (MS) was introduced as a GC detector. With the GC/MS setup the compounds could be identified by means of a combination of their retention time and the mass spectrum of the analyte peak. The development with regard to the limit of detection of GC analysis is illustrated in Table 26.1.

Further developments soon followed with the so-called GC/MS-MS (tandem MS) in which two mass spectrometers are coupled in a series, i.e. after each other. This setup can be run in different modes, one possibility being that a selected ion produced in the fragmentation of the parent compound in the first mass spectrometer is selected for further analysis in the next, which then produces a mass spectrum of this ion (whether this is the molecular ion or a fragmentation ion). Today

Table 26.1. Historical development of the GC technique and its sensitivity.

Year	Instrumental GC technique	Limit of detection (pg)
1967	GC-FID (packed column)	500
1973	GC/MS (packed column)	300
1977	GC/MS (capillary column)	5
1992	GC/HRMS (capillary column with double focusing magnetic sector detector technology)	0.005
2006	GC×GC/HRMS	0.0003

MS-MS techniques, which are very powerful, are used a lot in food contamination trace analysis. An example of ions and derived mass spectra for food-relevant mycotoxins is shown in Table 26.2.

General limitations do exist for GC and GC/MS analysis, however. Most compounds with a molecular weight above ~450 cannot be brought into the gaseous form without degradation, and even further restrictions exist. For example if we look at an analysis for the quantitative occurrence of alkaloids in plants from the genus *Galanthus*, from which we have the cholinesterase inhibitor galanthamin used in the treatment of Alzheimer's disease, we find that the quaternary alkaloids cannot be analysed, the molecules being positively charged and hence non-volatile. The same goes for the alkaloid N-oxides present in these and many other alkaloid-containing plants, such as those containing pyrrolizidine alkaloids (see Chapter 15). Some compounds can be stabilized and made volatile by derivatization such as silylation or acylation. Thus, trimethylsilyl (TMS) ethers are a convenient way to derivatize a variety of functional groups prior to GC analysis, as shown in Fig. 26.4.

Table 26.2. Examples of parent and product ions used for confirmation and MS-MS determination of selected mycotoxins.

Mycotoxin (derivative)	MS-MS mode, electrospray ionization	
	Parent ion (m/z)	Product ions (m/z)
Patulin-TMS	136	108, 98, 104, 85
Deoxynivalenol-tri-TMS	512	393, 333, 392, 496
Deoxynivalenol-tri-TMS	393	333, 259, 260, 305
Nivalenol-tetra-TMS	510	407, 317, 361, 289
T-2 toxin-TMS	290	259, 274, 275, 257
T-2 toxin-TMS	244	229, 214, 173
HT-2 toxin-di-TMS	466	287, 303, 284, 288
HT-2 toxin-di-TMS	185	142, 157, 141

TMS, trimethylsilyl.

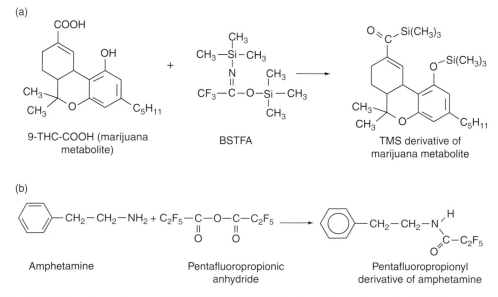

Fig. 26.4. (a) Silylation of a marijuana metabolite (9-THC-COOH, 9-carboxytetrahydrocannibol; BSTFA, bis(tetramethylsilyl)trifluoroacetamide); (b) acylation of amphetamine with pentafluoropropionic anhydride.

The most recent development within GC analytical techniques is the development of the so-called GCxGC methodology. In this technique two columns (two gas chromatographs) are coupled in a series, so that selected eluted peaks from the first column enter the next column, which shows different separation characteristics (e.g. a polar column as opposed to the first which was apolar). The heart of any GCxGC system is the modulator, which is the interface between the two columns. It controls the flow of analytes from the first column to the second column, acting as a gate that performs these injections in a consistent and reproducible fashion. Common commercial modulators are based on jets of cold gas applied to a segment of capillary between the two separation columns. This creates a cold spot where analytes are trapped through partitioning or freezing. Applying a heating pulse while turning off the cold jet remobilizes the trapped material and injects it as a narrow plug into the second column. Due to the narrow nature of GCxGC peaks, the detector must be capable of acquiring data at a high rate. Common detectors that are used include the FID, ECD and a special kind of mass spectrometer called a time-of-flight mass spectrometer. In TOF-MS (time-of-flight (TOF) mass spectrometry) ions are accelerated by an electrical field to the same kinetic energy, with the velocity of the ion depending on the mass-to-charge ratio. Thus, the time of flight determines the mass-to-charge ratio.

High-performance liquid chromatography

As in GC, the sample in high-performance liquid chromatography (HPLC) is injected into a chromatographic column packed with an adsorbent – the stationary phase – that has variable affinity for the components to be separated. The mobile phase (the *eluent*) is a solvent, normally made up by mixing a number of different liquids to obtain the best eluent strength and perhaps even with a component added for the control of pH or to form an ion-pair with the analyte (see later for more details). While travelling through the column the sample is separated into its components as already described for GC. A typical HPLC setup is illustrated in Fig. 26.5.

High-pressure liquid chromatography, as the method was called in the beginning, was developed in the mid-1970s. Quickly it was improved with the development of column packing materials and the additional convenience of a selection of online detectors. While the first generation of HPLC used silica gel columns (later called normal phase or straight phase columns), in the late 1970s new methods including the so-called *reverse-phase liquid chromatography* allowed for improved separation between very similar polar compounds. Reverse-phase columns typically are columns where the stationary phase is made up of hydrophobic alkyl chains ($-CH_2-CH_2-CH_2-CH_3$) that interact with the analyte and are bound to and cover the surface of silica particles (Fig. 26.6). There are three common chain lengths, C4, C8 and C18. C4 is generally used for proteins and C18 is generally used to capture peptides or small molecules.

The beads or particles are normally characterized by their particle size and pore size. Particle sizes generally range between 3 and 50 μm, with 5 μm particles being the most popular for peptides. Larger particles will generate less system pressure and smaller particles will generate more pressure. The smaller particles generally give higher separation efficiencies. The particle pore size is measured in angstroms and generally ranges between 100 and 1000 Å. A pore size of 300 Å is the most popular for proteins and peptides and 100 Å is the most common for small molecules. Since silica dissolves

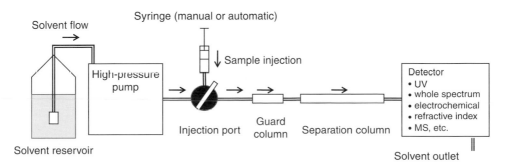

Fig. 26.5. Illustration of a basic HPLC setup.

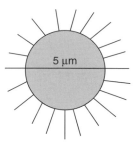

Fig. 26.6. A silica particle covered with hydrophobic alkyl chains. To give an idea of scale, a 5 μm silica particle is 50,000 Å across. In total 166 pores of diameter 300 Å could be fit across the equator of this particle. As can be seen the C18 chains are not to scale.

at high pH, in most cases it is not recommended to use solvents that exceed pH 7.

By the 1980s HPLC was commonly used for the separation of chemical compounds. For compounds that are charged/non-charged depending on the pH, in the past the approach used to separate such analytes was *ionic suppression*. This technique was based on the pH adjustment of the mobile phase to result in a non-ionized analyte. However, this requires extensive method development and is suitable only for single compounds or simple mixtures where the pK_a values of the analytes lie close together. Furthermore, the silica support used in bonded reverse-phase columns is stable only within a pH range of 2 up to about 8. The limitations of this method led to the development of *ion-pair chromatography* (IPC). IPC is a more general and applicable approach that allows the separation of complex mixtures of polar and ionic molecules. The selectivity is determined by the mobile phase: the organic eluent is supplemented with a specific *ion-pairing reagent*. The IPC reagents are large ionic molecules having a charge opposite to the analyte of interest, as well as a hydrophobic region to interact with the stationary phase. The counterions combine with the ions of the eluent, becoming ion-pairs, which can interact with the stationary phase. This results in different retention, thus facilitating separation of the analytes. IPC is now an established and reliable technique.

The detection in HPLC may be based on many different principles such as:

- the absorption of light (visible and ultraviolet, Vis and UV);
- fluorescence of the sample;
- the refractive index of the sample being different from that of the solvent;
- radioactivity of the analyte; and
- electrochemical reaction.

Detection by absorbance may be based on the absorbance of light of a fixed wavelength, such as the very often used wavelength of 254 nm. UV detectors have a sensitivity of approximately 10^{-8} to 10^{-9} g ml^{-1}. One may also measure an absorption spectrum as is possible when using a so-called *photodiode array (PDA) detector*, which measures a spectrum of wavelengths simultaneously. PDA detectors were introduced commercially in the 1990s. While they showed lower performance at the beginning, today's PDA detectors have sensitivity performance close to the benchmark level of $\pm 1 \times 10^{-5}$ AU (absorbance units) for UV-Vis detectors.

A PDA detector (often just called a *diode array detector* and abbreviated as DAD) consists of a number of photosensitive diodes place side by side and insulated from one another in the form of a multi-layer sandwich. Each diode is only a few thousandths of an inch thick. The output from each diode can be scanned, stored and subsequently processed by a computer in a number of different ways. The light source is usually polychromatic (e.g. light from a deuterium lamp) and, after passing through the cell, the light is dispersed by a quartz prism or a diffraction grating on to the surface of the diode array. Thus, each diode receives light of a slightly different wavelength compared with that received by its neighbour. The wavelengths most useful in LC range from about 210 to 330 nm (i.e. UV light), and thus a sufficient number of diodes must be incorporated in the array to (at least) cover this spectral range. Since many organic compounds have characteristic spectra in the UV region, the PDA can be used to help identify the substance passing though the detector cell. The principle in a PDA detector is illustrated in Fig. 26.7.

The *fluorescence detector* is a specific detector that senses only those substances that fluoresce. The flow cell is used as the sensor through which the excitation light passes axially. At the side of the cell a photocell is situated to receive radially emitted light. To prevent the excitation light (usually UV light) from reaching the photocell, the cell wall may be made of Pyrex glass. When a solute that fluoresces in the excitation light is situated in the cell, the fluorescent light passes through the walls of the cell on to the photocell, the output of which is electronically processed and the output passed to

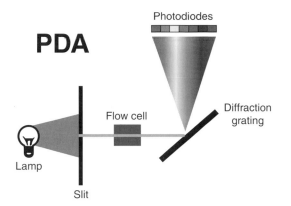

PDA

Photodiodes

Diffraction grating

Flow cell

Lamp

Slit

Fig. 26.7. The principle behind the PDA-HPLC detector.

a computer. The excitation light may for example be light of any wavelength selected from the light produced by a deuterium lamp using a monochromater. A monochromater can also be used to analyse the fluorescent light, and hence a fluorescence spectrum can be produced for excitation light of any specific wavelength and an excitation spectrum produced for fluorescent light of any specific wavelength. For non-fluorescing compounds a fluorescent derivative of the substance of interest may be prepared.

Refractive index (RI) detectors measure the ability of sample molecules to bend or refract light. The RI detector is one of the least sensitive HPLC detectors. Also it is very sensitive to changes in ambient temperature, pressure and flow rate, and so cannot be used for gradient elution. Nevertheless the RI detector is useful for the detection of compounds that do not absorb in the UV-Vis region and do not fluoresce. Thus, the RI detector provides solutions for analytical applications including substances such as alcohol, sugar, saccharides, fatty acids and a number of polymers.

The designation *electrochemical detector* covers several different principles. However, mostly one is thinking of one of three different so-called voltammetric detector principles, namely the amperometric, the coulometric and the polarographic. Initially neuroscientists used amperometric HPLC-ECD to measure labile neurotransmitters such as catecholamines in brain tissue extracts. Here we do not go further into the theory behind the different electrochemical detectors but instead illustrate one application developed for the selective detection of toxic cyanogenic glycosides found in different food and feed products. These glycosides can, after their separation, be hydrolysed online while passing through a column with immobilized β-glycosidases to form cyanohydrins, which can be split into an oxo compound and cyanide by online addition of an alkaline solution. The cyanide in turn can be determined by using an electrochemical detector equipped with a silver electrode (Fig. 26.8).

In the case of LC/MS the scale is usually smaller than seen for normal analytical HPLC with respect to the internal diameter of the column and even more so with respect to flow rate, since it scales as the square of the diameter. Recently 300 μm and even 75 μm capillary columns have become the state-of-the-art. At the low end of these column diameters, the flow rate approaches 100 nl min⁻¹. LC/MS came later than GC/MS because the interface between a liquid-phase technique which flows liquid continuously and a gas-phase technique carried out in a vacuum was difficult to develop. The invention of *electrospray ionization* (ESI) changed this. The primary advantage LC/MS has over GC/MS is that it is capable of analysing a wider range of components. Compounds that are thermally labile, exhibit high polarity or have a high molecular mass may all be analysed using LC/MS.

In ESI the analyte solution flow passes through an electrospray needle that has a high potential difference (with respect to the counter electrode) applied to it (normally in the range of 2.5–4 kV). Charged droplets are formed with a surface charge of the same polarity as the charge on the needle. The droplets are repelled from the needle towards the source sampling cone on the counter electrode. As a droplet traverses the space between the needle tip and the cone, evaporation of the solvent occurs. This is shown in Fig. 26.9a and enlarged in Fig. 26.9b. As the solvent evaporates, the droplet shrinks until it reaches a point at which the surface tension can no longer sustain the charge (the 'Rayleigh limit'), at which point a 'Coulombic explosion' occurs and the droplet is ripped apart. This produces smaller droplets that can repeat the process, as well as naked charged analyte molecules. These charged analyte molecules can be singly or multiply charged. ESI is a very soft method of ionization since very little residual energy is retained by the analyte upon ionization. It is the generation of multiply charged molecules that enables high-molecular-weight components such as proteins to be analysed: the mass range of the mass spectrometer is greatly increased since it actually measures the mass-to-charge ratio rather than mass per se. A disadvantage of the technique is that

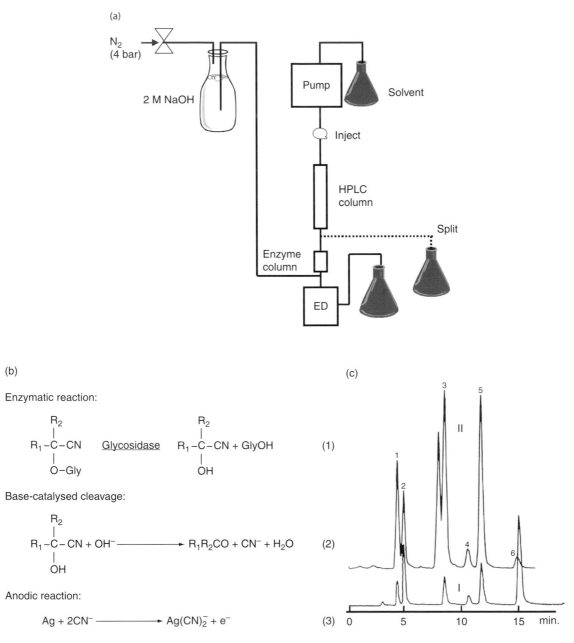

Fig. 26.8. (a) HPLC system for the separation and specific detection of cyanogens. Immobilized β-glycosidases hydrolyse the glycosides prior to the detection of CN^- by means of a silver electrode (ED = electrochemical detector). (b) The reactions taking place during the online detection of separated cyanogenic glycosides. (c) Reverse-phase HPLC separations of cyanogenic glycosides and cyanohydrins. (I) Chromatogram obtained with *Acacia sieberana* var. *woodii*. Fresh leaves frozen in liquid N_2 and lyophilized prior to cold (2°C) extraction with dry ethylether. (II) Standards: 1,3-hydroxyheterodendrin; 2, corresponding α-hydroxynitrile; 3, proacacipetalin; 4, heterodendrin; 5, α-hydroxynitrile corresponding to proacacipetalin; 6, α-hydroxynitrile corresponding to heterodendrin. Mobile phase 15% (v/v) methanol in water; electrochemical detection. With permission from Wiley from Brimer (1998).[1]

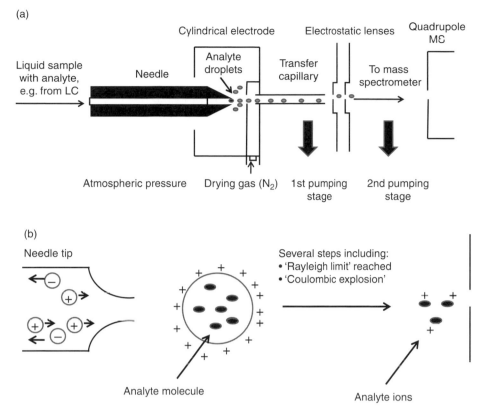

(a)

Cylindrical electrode   Electrostatic lenses   Quadrupole MS

Liquid sample with analyte, e.g. from LC

Needle

Analyte droplets

Transfer capillary

To mass spectrometer

Atmospheric pressure   Drying gas (N_2)   1st pumping stage   2nd pumping stage

(b)

Needle tip

Several steps including:
• 'Rayleigh limit' reached
• 'Coulombic explosion'

Analyte molecule

Analyte ions

Fig. 26.9. (a) Schematic illustration of an ESI interface; (b) schematic illustration of the mechanism of ion formation. Adapted from a University of Bristol web page.[2]

very little fragmentation is produced although this may be overcome through the use of tandem mass spectrometric techniques such as MS-MS.

26.4 Metals and Other Elements

When talking about chemical food safety and analysis of elements we think mainly of the metals and a few metalloids, although we must not forget selenium and fluorine. For the metals, the food-relevant toxic metalloids (boron, arsenic) and selenium, we can be interested in both the total content and the speciation, i.e. the oxidation state (e.g. chromium) and/or the total structure of the organic compound of which the element is part.

Historically metal analysis began with *colorimetric methods* as for example with arsenic, for which a test was introduced into forensic practice during the 19th century. In 1873 so-called *flame photometry* was introduced for the detection of sodium. Gradually the method was developed to become quantitative and flame photometry (an atomic emission method) became the routine method for a number of metals, principally sodium, potassium, lithium, calcium and barium. Quantitative analysis of these species is performed by measuring the flame emission of solutions containing the metal. The solution is aspirated into the flame. The flame evaporates the solvent, atomizes the metal and excites a valence electron to an upper state. Light is emitted at characteristic wavelengths for each metal as the electron returns to the ground state. The emission wavelength monitored for the analyte species is selected by optical filters. A comparison of emission intensities of unknowns with that of either standard solutions or an internal standard allows quantitative analysis of the analyte metal in the sample solution.

In 1928 the method of (flame) atomic absorption spectroscopy was introduced. In AAS, elements in the analyte are transformed into the free atomic state in an atomization device by input of thermal energy. Now the atoms are able to absorb element-specific radiation. To this end, an element-specific lamp with a hollow cathode made of the element to be investigated is introduced into the ray path of the spectrometer with the atomization device and a detector. In FAAS, the liquid sample is sucked into a burner so that analyte elements can be atomized in a flame of a fuel gas, such as acetylene, and an oxidation gas, usually air (Fig. 26.10). Two photomultipliers measure the intensity of the non-attenuated radiation and the radiation after leaving the atomization device during the supply of a sample solution. The element concentrations in the sample are calculated from the difference in the two intensities.

In 1959 the flame was for the first time replaced with a graphite furnace, a technical change that extended the sensitivity to the parts per billion range. Graphite furnace atomic absorption spectroscopy was born. In GFAAS, the sample is deposited in a small graphite tube (or pyrolytic carbon-coated graphite tube) which is then heated to vaporize and atomize the analyte. A droplet of the sample is pipetted into the graphite tube, where it dries through electrical heating, and the residues are ashed. In a subsequent heating step at very high temperatures, elements present in the residue are atomized. During this phase, the attenuation of the lamp radiation by the atomization in the narrow volume of the graphite tube can be measured with very good sensitivity.

The sample needs to be in liquid form, whether an aqueous solution or a solution containing organic solvents. A number of samples thus can be analysed directly or after simple dilution. Examples of this are fresh water, seawater, wine, urine and serum. Elements described to be successfully analysed by GFAAS in this way include arsenic, cadmium, chromium, copper, iron, germanium, nickel, lead, antimony, silicon and zinc. In the case of non-liquid samples extraction must take place. Such extractions (often termed *decompositions* or *wet ashing*) are typically done by heating the sample in, for example, a mixture of nitric acid and sulfuric acid (1:1 v/v; soil), or 65% (v/v) nitric acid and 30% aqueous hydrogen peroxide (2:1 v/v; hair). Food samples such as potato chips often are wet-ashed in a two-step procedure by heating in nitric acid followed by hydrogen peroxide. Heating may be done in digestion blocks at about 175°C or in closed autoclaves as heated in microwave ovens.

Element speciation

Element speciation is, as already mentioned, sometimes relevant when we talk about toxicology/chemical food safety.

When an extraction method can be developed that retains the different species unchanged, one can quite often use a more general method – such as *ion chromatography* (IC) – to detect them. IC is close to HPLC in its setup, the major difference being that the separation column – by means of ion exchange based on Coulombic (ionic) interactions – retains the charged analyte molecules. The stationary phase surface displays ionic functional groups (R–X) that interact with analyte ions of opposite charge. This type of chromatography is further subdivided into *cation-exchange chromatography* and *anion-exchange chromatography*. The detection can be of different natures, the electrochemical detector invented by A.J.P. Martin in 1944 being important, although other detectors such as the UV

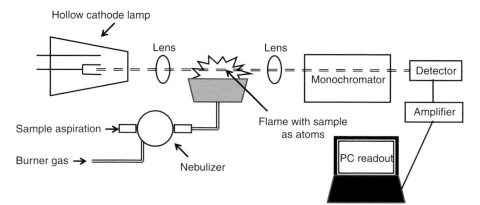

Fig. 26.10. Sketch of an atomic absorption setup (flame version).

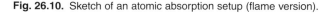

detector and in certain instances the fluorescence detector can also be used.

A great breakthrough was the coupling of IC (and later also GC) with detection by means of ICPMS, which was developed in the late 1980s. ICP technology builds upon the same principles used in atomic emission spectrometry. Samples are decomposed to neutral elements in a high-temperature argon plasma and analysed based on their mass-to-charge ratios. ICPMS can be seen as four main processes, comprising sample introduction and aerosol generation, ionization by an argon plasma source, mass discrimination and the detection system. An example of an analysis of arsenic species by IC/ICPMS is shown in Fig. 26.11.

However, the analytical problems faced are often indeed very complex and difficult to solve. A few examples are now discussed to illustrate the subject.

- *Arsenic*. In the case that one wants to determine acute exposure to arsenic relevant to its toxicity, one can determine arsenic in urine using the so-called *hydride technique*. This technique detects only inorganic trivalent and pentavalent arsenicals, and the mono- (MMA; monomethylarsonic acid) and dimethylated species (DMA; dimethylarsinic acid) of arsenic. It does not detect arsenobetaine and arsenocholine, arsenicals from seafood which leave the human body unchanged and are regarded as non-toxic. The more chronic exposure of health relevance can be estimated by analysis of

scalp hair using the method of GFAAS after wet ashing as described above.

- *Chromium*. Chromium exists in trivalent Cr(III) and hexavalent Cr(VI) oxidation states, the latter being much more toxic than the former. Cr(VI) exists as the chromate ion in basic solutions and as dichromate in acidic solutions. A traditional method for determining Cr(VI) uses diphenylcarbohydrazide (DPC), which forms a coloured complex with Cr(VI). The complex is measured quantitatively by its visible absorption at 520 nm. However, this test is sometimes subject to positive interference from other coloured materials in the sample as well as from other elements that form coloured complexes with DPC. A more specific and much more sensitive method free from interference couples the separation of Cr(VI) by IC with the colorimetric detection of DPC post-column.

- *Mercury*. The high toxicity and penchant for bioaccumulation of mercury make it of particular concern among heavy metals, as well as in a food context. There are several ways of determining total mercury in different samples. However, speciation of mercury is much more difficult. Different mercury species can be converted metabolically to methylmercury (MeHg$^+$), a highly toxic form which can accumulate in tissues. This is especially true in fatty fish. Thus, measurement of methylmercury is of vital importance in accurately assessing risk. Previous methods of determining methylmercury involved

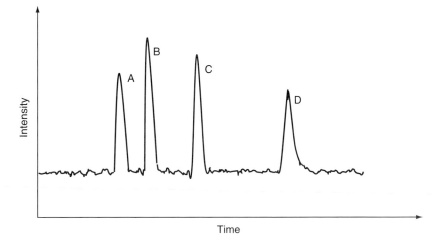

Fig. 26.11. An example of an IC/ICPMS chromatogram of a sample containing different arsenic species: A, As^{3+}; B, dimethylarsinate; C, monomethylarsonate; D, As^{5+}.

GC analysis of the poorly behaved methylmercuric chloride (CH$_3$HgCl). A new method improves our possibilities. Biological tissue samples are extracted into a mixture of L-cysteine and 2-mercaptoethanol by microwave digestion. Mercury compounds are separated by HPLC on a C8 column using the same mixture of L-cysteine and 2-mercaptoethanol. An ICPMS system is used as the HPLC detector. This method, when applied to the National Research Council of Canada Reference Material DORM-1 (dogfish muscle), gave concentrations of 0.70±0.03 µg g^{-1} for methylmercury and 0.12±0.03 µg g^{-1} for inorganic mercury, in good agreement with the certified value for total mercury of 0.800±0.074 µg g^{-1} and for methylmercury of 0.721±0.033 µg g^{-1}.

- *Selenium.* Many different molecular species of selenium exist (see Table 3.2) and knowledge about the distribution of total selenium over these may be essential for judging the fate of selenium ingested through food and/or health products. The field of selenium speciation has received increasing attention in recent decades. Research and routine analysis of selenium have been developed for and undertaken in soils, plants, nutritional supplements and biological samples (urine, etc.). Hence a number of different setups presently exist each with its own strengths and weaknesses. Thus, commercial companies can determine selenite (Se^{4+}) and selenate (Se^{6+}) together with SeMet and other selenoamino acids (important forms in selenized yeast supplements) and selenocyanate (SeCN$^-$), a major species found in petroleum refinery wastewater, by LC/ICPMS. Others use reverse-phase HPLC (C18 column) with a quaternary ammonium compound such as didodecyldimethylammonium bromide (DDBA) as eluent modifier for the separation. This is followed by post-column online UV/heat compound degradation and a hydride generation (HG) unit to allow detection of five selenium species – SeCys, selenite, SeMet, selenosugar and selenate – as selenium hydride by atomic fluorescence spectrometry (AFS).

26.5 Immunological Methods for the Determination of Organic Compounds

Quantitative determination of a number of different unwanted organic contaminants in food and feed today can also be achieved using methods based on recognition of the contaminant (or the derivatized contaminant) by a pre-prepared antibody. It all started in the 1950s when Rosalyn Yalow and Solomon Aaron Bernson working together at the Mount Sinai School of Medicine of New York University developed a *radioimmunoassay* (RIA) for insulin. Dr Yalow later received the Nobel Prize in Medicine for this development.

In a RIA, a known quantity of the compound to be measured (the antigen) is made radioactive, often by labelling it with γ-radioactive isotopes of iodine attached to tyrosine. The labelled antigen is then mixed with a known amount of antibody for that antigen, resulting in the two binding chemically to one another. Then the sample to be analysed, e.g. a sample of serum from an animal or person containing an unknown quantity of that same antigen, is added. This causes the unlabelled (or 'cold') antigen from the serum to compete with the radiolabelled antigen for antibody-binding sites. Thus, the 'cold' antigen displaces some of the radiolabelled variant, reducing the ratio of antibody-bound radiolabelled antigen to free radiolabelled antigen. Now the bound antigens are separated from the unbound ones, and the radioactivity of the free antigen remaining in the supernatant is measured. Using known standards, a binding curve is generated that allows the amount of the compound (the antigen) in the sample to be derived.

The RIA technique is extremely sensitive and specific; however, it requires specialized equipment as well as special precautions, since radioactive substances are used. Also it is very costly in general. Therefore, it has largely been supplanted today by the so-called *ELISA method*. In this method the antigen–antibody reaction is measured using the formation of colour instead of a radioactive signal.

The enzyme-linked immunosorbent assay, abbreviated ELISA (or sometimes just EIA for enzyme immunoassay), has now been developed into several different subtypes such as: (i) the direct ELISA; (ii) the indirect ELISA; (iii) the sandwich ELISA; and (iv) the competitive ELISA. Each has its own advantages and disadvantages. The direct ELISA is applied mainly to detect and quantify large molecules with multiple antigenic sites, usually a protein, in a sample. A typical general protocol for a direct ELISA analysis is as follows:

1. Apply a sample containing the antigen to a surface, often the well of a microtitre plate. The antigen is fixed to the surface to render it immobile.
2. Coat the plate well (or other surface) with a blocking buffer.
3. Apply detecting antibody, usually diluted in blocking buffer, to the plate for binding to the antigen coated on the plate.
4. Wash the plate, so that unbound antibody is removed. After washing, only the antibody–antigen complexes remain attached to the well.
5. Now add the second type of antibody, which will bind to any antigen–antibody complexes, to the well. These second antibodies are coupled to the substrate-modifying enzyme needed for the final quantification by colorimetric or fluorimetric methods or by chemiluminescence.
6. Wash the plate, so that excess unbound antibodies are removed.
7. Add the substrate, which is converted by the enzyme to elicit a signal, e.g. a chromogenic or fluorescent signal.
8. Measure the result using a spectrophotometer or other optical device.

As another example let us look at the sandwich ELISA. Here the compound (the antigen) of interest is quantified between two layers of antibodies: the capture and the detection antibody. These antibodies must bind to non-overlapping epitopes on the antigen. Either monoclonal or affinity-purified polyclonal antibodies are used as the capture and the detection antibodies, respectively, depending on cost, the dynamic range and the sensitivity of the final assay. The principle is shown in Fig. 26.12.

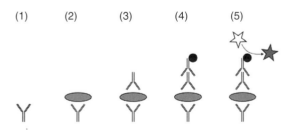

(1)   (2)   (3)   (4)   (5)

Fig. 26.12. A sandwich ELISA: (1) the plate is coated with a capture antibody; (2) sample is added, and any antigen present binds to the capture antibody; (3) detecting antibody is added, and binds to the antigen; (4) enzyme-linked secondary antibody is added, and binds to the detecting antibody; (5) substrate is added, and is converted by an enzyme to a detectable form. Adapted from a University of Manitoba (2008) web page.[3]

Important (groups of) food contaminants for which commercially available, ready-to-use ELISA kits have been developed include: the mycotoxins – aflatoxins total amount, AFB_1, AFM_1, fumonisin and OTA together with vomitoxin (DON, deoxynivalenol), T-2 toxin and zearalenone. Histamine, the major causative agent in scombroid poisoning, can also be analysed this way, as can now (recently developed) semicarbazide (SEM). The latter was considered concerning its possible negative public health effects by WHO. Concerns arose from the finding of SEM in food products packaged in glass jars with metal lids that have foamed plastic seals. SEM was detected at low levels in a number of such food products, including baby foods. The origin of SEM has been linked to the permitted use of azodicarbonamide in the plastic seals. The presence of SEM raised concern since it has weak carcinogenic activity when fed to laboratory animals at high doses. Based on levels reported in food, the health risk, if any, to consumers, including infants, appears generally to be very small, however. Still, since the relatively high consumption of products in glass jars by infants can result in higher exposure compared with other consumers, the presence of SEM in baby foods is considered particularly undesirable. Therefore, WHO now recommends, as a priority, that alternative materials be evaluated for their suitability, including their microbiological and chemical safety, and introduced as rapidly as possible for baby foods, and subsequently other foods.

26.6   Bioassays

Algal toxins and the standard mouse bioassay

Shellfish, such as oysters, scallops and blue mussels, live by filtering plankton including algal plankton. Some micro-algae can produce toxins that shellfish can take up and concentrate, especially during blooms of such algae. The shellfish show no apparent ill effects from large amounts of toxin and such marine algal toxins can occur in shellfish in all seasons. The algal toxins do not affect the taste of the shellfish, and are in general not destroyed by freezing or cooking. People therefore have no possibility of checking whether the shellfish are toxic on their own.

The groups of algal toxins of potential importance as food poisons include (see also Chapter 17): (i) the PSPs (paralytic shellfish poisons) including STX (saxotoxin); (ii) the DSTs (diarrhoetic shellfish toxins) including OA (okadaic acid); (iii) the ASTs (amnesic shellfish toxins) including DA (domoic acid); and (iv) the AZA (azaspiracid) toxins, together with; (v) PTX (pectenotoxin); and (vi) YTX (yessotoxin) toxins.

Many countries worldwide have established regulations for PSP. Most are set for PSP toxins as a group. Some countries indicate specific regulations for one of the PSP toxins, mostly STX (Fig. 26.13). A limit of 400 MU (mouse units) per 100 g or 80 μg STX equivalents per 100 g is the level most commonly seen now. The standard mouse bioassay (MBA) of AOAC INTERNATIONAL is most often the method of analysis for official purposes. However, in the EU a directive came into force in January 1993 (Council Directive 91/492/EEC of 15 July 1991) stating that the total PSP content in molluscs has to be determined according to the 'biological testing method in association, if necessary, with a chemical method for detection of STX. If the results are challenged, the reference method shall be the biological method'.

Today all six groups of marine biotoxins listed above are regulated within the EU. The MBA is the officially prescribed method for the detection of the OA, AZA, YTX, PTX and STX groups of toxins; however, it has two main protocols, one for lipophilic toxins (OA-, AZA- YTX- and PTX-group toxins) and one for STX-group toxins. The ability of the MBA to detect OA-group toxins at the current EU regulatory limit value is, however, inadequate, leading to false-negative results in official controls. At the time of writing, intense work is ongoing worldwide to try to establish more specific as well as more sensitive methods not only for STX (PSP toxins), but also for compounds making up the other groups of algal toxins which may be found in shellfish and shellfish-based food.

Many countries have defined so-called *action levels*. In Canada as an example, molluscan shellfish with a PSP content of less than 80 μg per 100 g of meat are permitted to be harvested, processed and sold; and for 'roe-on' scallops, PSP levels must be less than 80 μg per 100 g of roe. However, harvesting of

molluscan shellfish for canning purposes is permitted in areas where levels are between 80 and 160 μg per 100 g and the canned packs are tested before release for sale. On the Pacific Coast, butter clam canning has been permitted up to 300–500 μg PSP per 100 g, where it is done under permit and the neck has been removed and discarded.

The MBA for STX and other PSP toxins is run as shown briefly in Fig. 26.14.

Dioxins and the DR-CALUX bioassay

In order to analyse chemically in a meaningful way for the toxicity stemming from contamination of a food product with dioxins and dioxin-like compounds, in general it is necessary to analyse for at least 17 different PCDDs (2,3,7,8-chlorinated dibenzo-*p*-dioxins) or PCDFs (furans) at the pg g^{-1} level. After the analysis, which requires gas chromatography coupled with high-resolution mass spectrometry (GC/HRMS), the result has to be transferred to so-called TCDD equivalents (TEQs) per gram of sample. This is done by multiplying the concentration found for each compound by the compound's TEF (toxic equivalence factor) and finally summing the products. The TEFs range from 1 to 0.0001 and express the toxicity of each compound relatively to the toxicity of the most toxic dioxin congener, TCDD.

Such an analysis can be laborious and expensive, especially when faced with the need for large-scale surveys, as was the case during two food scandals with unacceptably high levels of dioxins: (i) the 'Citrus pulp incident' where milk in Germany was high in dioxins due to the use of contaminated citrus pulp from Brazil as feed for milking cows; and (ii) the 'Belgian dioxin incident' where chicken feed was contaminated. Therefore, the so-called DR-CALUX bioassay was developed and has been in use for the screening of a number feed and food products in the Netherlands.

The DR-CALUX assay is a cell assay based on the binding of dioxins to the cytosolic Ah receptor. The assay is performed using a specially developed rat hepatoma cell line (H4IIE). Following binding of the dioxin (an Ah agonist) to the receptor, the complex is transported to the nucleus and binds to the so-called dioxin-responsive element (DRE). This event results in increased transcription of the gene encoding the enzyme luciferase and therefore in a dose-dependent synthesis of this enzyme. The gene for luciferase has been engineered into this cell line

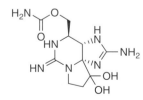

Fig. 26.13. The structure of STX.

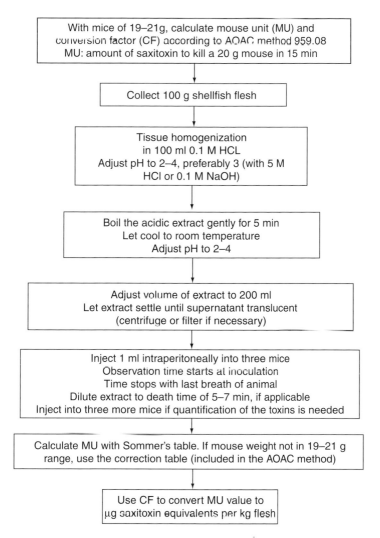

Fig. 26.14. AOAC method 959.08 for sample preparation and extraction methods of shellfish flesh for the mouse bioassay (MBA). Adapted with permission from EFSA (2009).[4]

and put under control of the murine DRE. When the compound luciferin and ATP are added to the incubation mixture, the luciferase produced emits light as part of an enzymatic reaction (Fig 26.15). The light production is measured quantitatively and the test can be performed in a microtitre plate.

26.7 Quick Assays for Continuous Control in the Production

Deep-frying is widely used especially in the restaurant and fast food sector. As discussed in Chapter 22, a number of toxic chemical components are formed during the process of heating the

frying oil. This – together with unwanted changes in the olfactory characteristics of the oil, and thereby of the fried products – is the reason why the oil in the fryer must be changed regularly.

In most countries including the USA no national legislation exists concerning the quality of a deep-frying fat or oil acceptable for use. However, in the USA a guideline concerning the deep-frying of meat and poultry is available which defines criteria regarding when to discard/change the oil. Hungary has recommendations concerning the maximum time of use and concerning filtering of deep-frying media. The EU has no legislation or common guidelines; however, a number of EU countries such

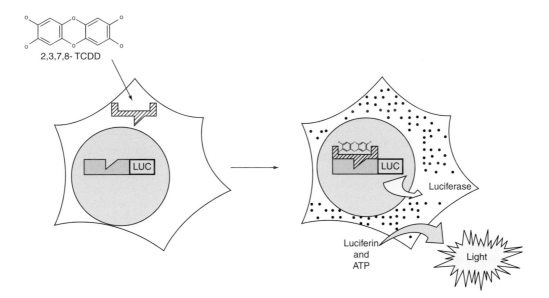

Fig. 26.15. Principle behind the CALUX bioassay for Ah-receptor agonists. Following binding of the agonist to the Ah receptor, the complex will be transported to the nucleus and bind to a so-called dioxin-responsive element, resulting in increased transcription of the gene encoding luciferase and thus the production of luciferase. Following incubation this enzyme can subsequently be measured in cell lysates by a light production reaction. Adapted from Watson (2001).[5]

Table 26.3. Guidelines for deep-frying and the quality of oils and fats used in deep-frying.

	Austria	Belgium	France	Germany	Italy	Netherlands	Portugal
Frying temperature (max, °C)	180	180	180		180		180
Smoke point (min, °C)	170			170			
Free fatty acids (max, % by weight)		2.5					
Acid value (max)	2.5			2			
Polar components (max, % by weight)	27		25	24	25		25
Oxidized acids (max, % by weight)	1			0.7			
Dimers/polymers (max, % by weight)		25				16	
Viscosity at 50°C (max, mPa s)		37					

as Austria, Belgium, France, Germany, Italy, the Netherlands and Portugal have launched national guidelines for the quality of oils and fats, how to fry and/or when to change the oil (Table 26.3).

To help operators and quality managers in this sector, the industry has developed a number of *rapid tests for the quality of used frying fats and oils*. Some of these are based on the chemical properties of the oil while others measure the oil's physical properties. Examples are the following:

- *Fritest* – a colorimetric test from Merck sensitive to carbonyl compounds. The colour formed in a mix between the oil sample and a reagent is compared against a colour scale with four colour intensities: light yellow = good, yellow = acceptable, yellow-orange = to be changed and orange = spoilt.

- *Oxifritest* – a colorimetric test from Merck based on a redox indicator which responds to the total content of oxidized component in the sample. After the mixing of two reagents the sample is added. The colour formed is compared against a colour scale with four colour intensities: blue = good, blue-green = acceptable, green = to be changed and olive-green = spoilt.

- *Viscofrit* – the test measures the time it takes for a standard funnel to empty itself by gravity, i.e.

it measures the viscosity. The test is calibrated in two different ways for the analysis of oils predominantly monounsaturated and polyunsaturated with respect to fatty acids, respectively.

- *Food oil sensor* – a portable electronic instrument (Northern Instruments Corp.) which measures the dielectric constant in the used oil sample versus a fresh (unused) sample of the same oil.

The Finish authorities have launched a national guideline for food inspectors concerning how to analyse deep-frying oils/fats. The test criteria include among others a sensory evaluation and the use of either *Fritest* or *Oxifritest*.

Notes

[1] Brimer, L. (1998) Determination of cyanide and cyanogenic compounds in biological systems. In: *Cyanide in Biology, CIBA Foundation Symposium No. 140.* Wiley, Chichester, UK, pp. 177–200.

[2] University of Bristol (not dated) High performance liquid chromatography mass spectrometry (HPLC/MS), Gates, P. (ed.). University of Bristol, NERC Life Sciences Mass Spectrometry Facility, Bristol, UK; available at http://www.bris.ac.uk/nerclsmsf/techniques/hplcms.html

[3] University of Manitoba (2008) Antibodies in transgenic plants. PLNT4600 Issues in Agricultural Biotechnology, Mini Report 3, part 1 of 1. University of Manitoba, Winnipeg, Canada; available at http://home.cc.umanitoba.ca/~umguerri/PLNT4600/mini3/mini3.1.html

[4] EFSA (2009) Scientific opinion of the panel on contaminants in the food chain on a request from the European Commission on marine biotoxins in shellfish. *EFSA Journal* 1019, 1–76.

[5] Watson, D.H. (ed.) (2001) *Food Chemical Safety*, vol. 1: *Contaminants.* CRC/Woodhead Publishing Limited, Cambridge, UK.

Further Reading

Pic, Y. (ed.) (2008) *Food Contaminants and Residue Analysis. Comprehensive Analytical Chemistry, 51.* Elsevier, Amsterdam.

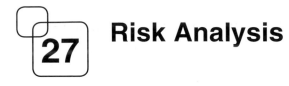

27 Risk Analysis

- General dose–response curves and determination of the NOAEL and Benchmark Dose are described.
- The calculation of ADIs, RfDs and MRLs is described.
- Withholding and withdrawing periods are touched upon.

27.1 Introduction

Risk analysis covers risk assessment, risk management and risk communication.

- *Risk assessment* includes the *identification of a hazard* (e.g. ingestion of methylmercury), the investigation of the *qualitative effects of the hazard* (e.g. poisoning with symptoms of neurotoxicity including mild (mainly of sensory symptoms), moderate (sensory symptoms accompanied by cerebellar signs) and severe (gross ataxia with marked visual and hearing loss which, in some cases, progresses to akinetic mutism followed by coma)) and a *quantitative study of the dose–effect relationship(s)*. It may further include the derivation of, for example, an ADI and an analysis of the exposure for different groups of individuals.
- *Risk management* takes over, transforming the ADI to *recommendations or legislation* concerning MRLs of, for example, pesticides in different food commodities.
- *Risk communication* covers *the activities to spread the knowledge about the risk management decisions and their background*.

27.2 Risk Assessment and Management – Use of the Toxicological Data Set Created for a Substance

When a toxicological data set for a substance has been created it is ready to be used for the intended purpose. This can, for example, be the derivation of an ADI in mg kg^{-1} BW for a food additive or a pesticide (in US legislation, ADI is referred to as Reference Dose abbreviated as RfD) or of a TDI for a contaminant such as a mycotoxin, toxic metal or POP (such as a dioxin). The two are derived in the same way. From the ADI or TDI subsequently an MRL can be set for a pesticide, as can a 'Maximum Level' (for a food additive).

An MRL is the maximum concentration of a substance, expressed in milligrams per kilogram (parts per million, ppm) or in micrograms per kilogram (parts per billion, ppb), that is legally permitted in a food commodity. An MRL is typically applied to a veterinary drug or a pesticide and is established for particular food commodities such that potential consumer exposure to residues is judged to be toxicologically acceptable. The MRL set for a substance may *differ for different food commodities*, reflecting the contribution of the particular food to a 'standard' diet. Normal intake of food containing a residue of a substance at its MRL is not expected to result in the ADI being exceeded.

27.3 NOAEL, LOAEL and Benchmark Dose

For each toxicity test contributing to the data set we start with the determination of the so-called NOAEL or – if not possible – the LOAEL. Both of these are actual data points from the experimental animal studies as illustrated in Fig. 27.1. Alternatively, the so-called Benchmark Dose (BMD) can be determined for each individual test. The BMD is the dose that, on the basis of the dose–response curve, produces a predetermined (low) change in the rate of an adverse response (designated the benchmark response or BMR) compared with the background level. This change is usually in the range of 5–10%. Determination of a BMD requires that the statistically best-fitting curve derived from the experimental results is determined, which is not necessary for the determination of an NOAEL. A BMD is conceptually superior to an NOAEL because of being less determined by experimental design, because it is a precisely defined entity and because its precision can be estimated. For further use in the derivation of, for example, an ADI in the case of a BMD procedure, the lower confidence bound of the BMD (the BMDL; Fig. 27.1) is used. As an example within chemical food safety it can be mentioned that a number of BMDLs were determined recently for different neuropsychological deficits in Faroese children at the age of 7 years, deficits that are associated with prenatal methylmercury exposure. The lowest BMDLs averaged approximately 5 μg l^{-1} cord blood, which corresponds to a maternal hair concentration of approximately 1 μg g^{-1}.

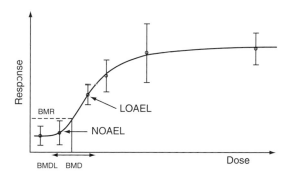

Fig. 27.1. Illustration of the determination of NOAEL, LOAEL and BMD on the basis of a test with six data points. The dotted horizontal line is the benchmark response (BMR) line, which defines the Benchmark Dose (BMD). The double-sided arrow indicates the confidence interval (usually 95%) of the BMD. The lower confidence limit on the dose that would result in the defined response is the BMDL. In addition, the No Observed Adverse Effect Level (NOAEL) and the Lowest Observed Adverse Effect Level (LOAEL) of this test are illustrated. Adapted from Filipsson *et al.* (2003).[1]

27.4 Calculation of ADI/RfD and MRL

As an introduction to the usual procedures for deviation of an ADI/RfD, it must be emphasized that we cannot determine precisely what total exposure a person can tolerate throughout his/her life without any adverse effect. What we can derive is our best judgement.

For this purpose we start to look at the data set and the NOAEL/BMD for each of the tests performed. These will all be measured in mg kg^{-1} BW day^{-1} for the animal species, organ or cell type used in the test in question. As an example let us imagine we have performed five different tests and obtained the following NOAELs: 0.3 mg kg^{-1} BW day^{-1} (rat subchronic study – peroxisome proliferation in liver), 2 mg kg^{-1} BW day^{-1} (rat subchronic study – inhibition of germ cell development), 4.5 mg kg^{-1} BW day^{-1} (rat subchronic study – testis weight reduction), 16.3 mg kg^{-1} BW day^{-1} (mouse repeated dose 28 days – hepatitis) and 17.8 mg kg^{-1} BW day^{-1} (rat second-generation reproduction study – reduced F2 generation). First analysis of the data set indicates the effect of *peroxisome proliferation in liver* to be the risk seen at the lowest dose and hence the effect on which the derivation of an ADI for the compound should be based. However, since a general consensus has been agreed among toxicologists that rodents are extremely sensitive to the phenomenon of peroxisome proliferation and that this particular effect should not be used for human risk assessment, the relevant NOAEL is 2 mg kg^{-1} BW *rat* day^{-1}.

The generally accepted method for the derivation of an ADI (RfD), i.e. the maximum dose (in mg kg^{-1} BW *human being* day^{-1}) that we believe a person can ingest throughout his/her life without any adverse effects, is based on the division of the NOAEL selected from the data set by one or more factors. These factors are introduced to minimize the risks taken by basing an accepted exposure level in animal studies, using small dosing groups consisting of genetically very similar (inbred) individuals. In the USA these factors are termed Standard Uncertainty Factors (UFs) while the UN System (FAO/WHO – Codex Alimentarius) names them Safety Factors. Table 27.1 describes the background for and generally accepted numerical value for some such factors.

Table 27.1. Standard Uncertainty/Safety Factors. Adapted from Anon. (1993).[2]

Factors
a. Use a tenfold factor when extrapolating from results involving small groups of genetically similar individuals. This factor is intended to account for the uncertainty involved in extrapolating to a huge population with genetically different individuals
b. Use a tenfold factor when extrapolating from results of long-term studies on experimental animals. This factor is intended to account for the uncertainty involved in extrapolating from animal data to humans. The animal species in question may be either more or less sensitive to the compound tested than are human beings
c. Use an additional tenfold factor when extrapolating from less than chronic results on experimental animals when there are no useful long-term human data. Such a factor is intended to account for the uncertainty involved in extrapolating from a less than chronic NOAEL to a chronic NOAEL
d. Use an additional tenfold factor if deriving an RfD/ADI from an LOAEL instead of an NOAEL. This factor is intended to account for the uncertainty involved in extrapolating from an LOAEL to an NOAEL

Thus, in cases considered uncomplicated most often we derive an ADI from a data set based on animal experiments as follows:

$$\text{ADI (mg kg}^{-1}\text{ BW } human\ being\text{ day}^{-1}) =$$

$$\frac{\text{lowest NOAEL (mg kg}^{-1}\text{ BW } animal\text{ day}^{-1})}{10 \times 10}$$

Retrospective analysis of the actual existing differences in sensitivity of species to toxic effects of different compounds has shown that, in most cases, these are to be found within the tenfold factor accounted for by Safety Factor b in Table 27.1. However, we do see exceptions. For example, the reported acute oral toxicity (measured as LD_{50}) of the mycotoxin AFB_1 (Fig. 27.2) varies from 0.55 mg kg^{-1} BW in the cat to 10 mg kg^{-1} BW in the hamster, i.e. a factor of 18. Also within the POPs we have interspecies differences greater than a factor of 10, an example being the most toxic dioxin TCDD (Fig. 27.2), for which LD_{50} (oral in mg kg^{-1} BW) is hamster/dog=1.2/0.001=1200.

Limited publications on the application of uncertainty factors to BMDs suggest uncertainty factors to account for within-human and animal-to-human variability, the severity of the modelled effect and the slope of the dose–response curve. A recent paper also suggests that the BMD at 10% will frequently be near the LOAEL.

27.5 MRL and Withholding/Withdrawing Periods

When an ADI (RfD) has been derived and approved, risk managers take over and begin the process of ensuring (to the extent it is possible) that individuals of the population are exposed only to a level that does not exceed this value. This is done by setting maximum accepted levels for use of the different approved food additives, maximum levels of occurrence in foods for different toxic contaminants (heavy metals, POPs, etc.) and MRLs for pesticides and veterinary drugs. In the latter cases we talk about 'residue limits' owing to the fact that we deliberately use these chemicals in our food production to protect our plants or our animals and hence maximize the yield. When spraying (or at drug delivery)

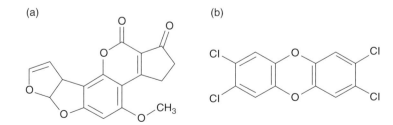

(a)   (b)

Fig. 27.2. AFB$_1$ (a) and TCDD (b).

Table. 27.2. MRLs for amitraz as proposed by Codex Alimentarius (2010).

Commodity	Maximum Residue Limits	
	MRL (mg kg⁻¹)	Note
Cattle meat	0.05	The MRL accommodates external animal treatment
Cherries	0.5	
Cottonseed	0.5	
Cottonseed oil, crude	0.05	
Cucumber	0.5	
Edible offal of cattle, pigs and sheep	0.2	The MRL accommodates external animal treatment
Milks	0.01	The MRL accommodates external animal treatment
Oranges, sweet, sour	0.5	
Peach	0.5	
Pig meat	0.05	The MRL accommodates external animal treatment
Pome fruits	0.5	
Sheep meat	0.1	The MRL accommodates external animal treatment
Tomato	0.5	

the farmer typically uses the dosing recommended by the producing chemical company or by the agronomist/veterinarian functioning as the farmer's extension officer. After the administration the concentration of the compound in the plant/animal typically declines due to environmental degradation and/or metabolism and excretion by the organism treated. At the time of harvest or slaughter (milk or egg collection) the concentration must be below the MRL value approved for the product/tissue in question. In order to ensure that this normally is the case, national and international authorities have established and published so-called withholding and withdrawing periods for different pesticides and veterinary drugs.

- The *withholding period* is the time that must be allowed to elapse after application of a pesticide before the crop can be harvested and eaten.
- The *withdrawal period* is the time from the last administration of the medicine during which products from the production animal concerned may not be used as foodstuffs. For fish, the withdrawal period is established using a combination of time and water temperature.

Thus, an MRL is the maximum concentration of a compound (e.g. a pesticide or a veterinary drug) that is permitted in a given food commodity, thereby ensuring that the total exposure of consumers to the compound is toxicologically acceptable. The MRL

may *differ for different food commodities*, reflecting the contribution of the particular food to a 'standard' diet. Normal intake of food containing a residue of a substance at its MRL is not expected to result in the ADI being exceeded.

When setting MRLs (or other maximum limits) to control exposure, the total situation must be considered. If either the general population or a special subgroup (e.g. as a result of their work situation) is exposed to the compound in question from sources other than food, this should be taken into account when deciding on MRLs, although this is often not done. For the daily food production it is crucial to ensure (by information as well as control) that farmers stick to the recommended dosing regimes and the approved withholding/withdrawal periods, i.e. they adhere to GAP.

Table 27.2 presents the MRLs derived and recommended by CAC for the compound amitraz, which is interesting from the point of view that it is used both for crop protection (mites on fruits and cotton) and as a veterinary drug. Amitraz (Fig. 27.3) is an amidine, known as a tick-detaching agent used in cattle production. It is also effective against mange mites on pigs.

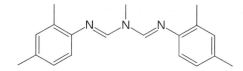

Fig. 27.3. Amitraz.

27.6　Risk Assessment of Mixtures

As described in this chapter we normally assess the risk from each compound individually. However, over about the last 10 years scientists and risk managers have become increasingly aware of the fact that sometimes we may have to consider the effect of mixtures. This started with the recognition that many insecticides occurring as residues in food commodities share the same mechanism of action, namely the inhibition of acetylcholinesterase. Hence, it was only natural to ask the question whether these compounds, when occurring in a mixture, could give an unexpected result concerning the overall risk. In particular, it was asked if a number of such residues – all of which were below the detection limits for each of the compounds in question – together could add up to give rise to an effect that would correspond to a residue level above the detection limit for one such compound.

The development continued and resulted in the situation discussed in Chapters 20 and 26 for POPs, where the dioxins and the dioxin-like PCBs are today risk-assessed as a mixture using the WHO-TEFs for each compound.

Today the most discussed problem is whether a mixture (cocktail) of compounds with different mechanisms of action but affecting the same function/hormone/organ should be risk-assessed as a cocktail, a situation which, however, will be very complicated. The newest research within this field has focused on whether concurrent exposure to several endocrine-disrupting substances in small doses can increase the frequency of malformations such as hypospadias even though the doses are harmless individually.

Notes

[1] Filipsson, A.F., Sand, S., Nilsson, J. and Victorin, K. (2003) The benchmark dose method – review of available models, and recommendations for application in health risk assessment. *Critical Reviews in Toxicology* 33, 505–542.

[2] Anon. (1993) *Reference Dose (RfD): Description and Use in Health Risk Assessments. Background Document 1A; March 15, 1993*. US Environmental Protection Agency, Washington, DC; available at http://www.epa.gov/iris/rfd.htm

Further Reading

Tenant, D.R. (1997) *Food Chemical Risk Analysis*. Blackie Academic & Professional, Chapman & Hall, London.

Food Safety (Quality) Assurance and Certification of Production

- The history behind the HACCP concept is outlined.
- The seven steps in establishing a HACCP plan are presented.
- Management systems to develop and assure production of a chemically safe food are introduced.
- Full quality assurance cycles including the HACCP plan as a key component are described.

28.1 Introduction

As already discussed the process of assuring a good and constant quality of a food product involves a large number of aspects of the production from plant to plate or meat to meal. When it comes to product quality with respect to food safety, in many countries today including the EU countries it is an obligation for food businesses to establish a traceability system. Full traceability from the primary producer to the final (marketed) product is often followed by obligations to also implement a quality assurance system following the HACCP concept. Indeed, many bigger producers and processors/food product handlers do not stop there but also on their own initiative undergo one or more certifications following one of the existing international certification systems, perhaps including regular audits from external quality assurance/certification companies.

Actually a food business that does not produce safe products will not survive long on the international market. Worldwide, the need for highly effective self-evaluation and control systems gradually has increased, which is why many companies look to a certified food safety company management system such as, for example, ISO 22000. However, let us start with an introduction to the HACCP concept.

28.2 The HACCP Concept

The National Aeronautics and Space Administration (NASA) in the USA developed a standard procedure to be enforced on the producers of food products for astronauts in order to ensure food safety and satisfactory nutritional quality of the products. In general the products were canned foods based on meat, poultry and seafood. Obviously an incident of food-related illness – as, for example, caused by *Salmonella* in chicken meat or by too high a concentration of histamine in a fish product – among astronauts in space would give rise to serious problems. HACCP is an acronym of Hazard Analysis and Critical Control Points. HACCP is a framework to produce food or food products safely and to prove that they were produced safely. In more detail, it can be said that HACCP is a systematic preventive approach that is set up to identify potential food safety hazards so that certain predefined actions can be taken to reduce or eliminate the risk of the hazard being realized.

Once developed this new proactive standard soon spread to the food industry in general. Some of the first products for the general market to be produced under an established HACCP protocol were low-acid canned meat products. The programme was a success with only very few recalls of products being seen after its implementation. It is the food business operators themselves who must analyse their own processes in order to put a HACCP system in place themselves.

In short, HACCP is a system built on seven principles that one can often see described in different wording, an example being the following.

The HACCP system encompasses the following seven steps:

- identifying any hazards that must be prevented, eliminated or reduced to acceptable levels;

- identifying the critical control points at the steps at which control is essential to prevent or eliminate a hazard or reduce it to an acceptable level;
- establishing critical limits at critical control points which separate acceptability from unacceptability for the prevention, elimination or reduction of identified hazards;
- establishing and implementing effective monitoring procedures at critical control points;
- establishing corrective actions when monitoring indicates that a critical control point is not under control;
- establishing procedures that shall be carried out regularly to verify that the measures outlined above are working effectively; and
- establishing and implementing recording-keeping procedures that document the HACCP system, enabling the company/institution to prove the product was produced in a safe manner.

Today HACCP systems are used in many industrial sectors apart from that of food producing and processing. In a food production context the hazard analysis part includes a systematic study of ingredients, processing, handling, storage, packing, distribution and consumer use for potential physical, chemical or microbiological hazards. For potential problems identified one explores how they could be prevented. *Critical control points* (CCPs) are points anywhere in the process at which control can be applied and a food safety hazard can be prevented, eliminated or reduced to an acceptable level.

As a basis for a good and – as discussed below – *internationally certified production and internal product quality control programme*, most industries today take their outset in existing protocols for GMP and GLP, which describe the process of effective organization and the conditions under which production/laboratory investigations are properly planned, performed, monitored, recorded and reported. However, a production still may end up producing unsafe food products. As an example, if samples to go for chemical analysis are taken at a wrong point in the production, contamination with, for example, plasticizers diffusing into the product from the packaging material during storage may lead to unacceptable high levels in the product, when purchased from the retail shop by the consumer. Obviously the development of a HACCP plan in this case should have identified a CCP for the analysis of the end product's concentration of plasticizers after, for example, 2 months of storage.

28.3 Developing a HACCP Plan – Ensuring an Acceptable Level of Mycotoxins in Plant Products

In 2001 FAO published the very informative and operational *Manual on the Application of the HACCP System in Mycotoxin Prevention and Control*. The manual clearly demonstrates that HACCP systems can be used as tools for ensuring product safety at all technical levels of production, ranging from the relatively simple on-farm production of dried coconut flesh for later production of coconut oil and copra cake/meal to the technically advanced industrial production of pasteurized and aseptically packed apple juice.

From coconut to coconut oil and copra cake for animal feed

Coconut oil is produced by extraction from copra, which the dried coconut's flesh. If the oil is expelled mechanically the residue is called copra, while a subsequent solvent extraction to increase the yield of oil leads to the by-product copra meal. The two by-products are used as sources of protein for dairy cattle. The main production takes place in South-East Asia. During the 1990s the EU gradually started to tighten the mycotoxin regulations. Among others the maximum level of AFB_1 in dairy feed was lowered to $5 \mu g\ kg^{-1}$ and that for copra by-products in general to $20 \mu g\ kg^{-1}$. This meant the loss of a market worth US$80 million to one south Asian country alone. A HACCP approach was developed and introduced to reduce the content of aflatoxins in the copra and copra meal.

An analysis of the whole production chain soon showed that the aflatoxin contamination occurred during drying of the split coconuts on the farm. Levels of aflatoxin were almost zero after harvest and prior to splitting and drying. However, it was found that aflatoxin was produced and accumulated in the flesh within about the first 10 days of on-farm drying when the water activity was higher than 0.82. The subsequent production steps towards the two end products of coconut oil and coconut cake/meal in general did not give rise to any further aflatoxin contamination. Controlled drying and storage trials have shown that direct smoke drying protected copra from aflatoxin contamination, i.e. drying to a moisture content of $\leq 16\%$ enabled the copra to be stored safely until transport and further processing.

From apples to apple juice in South America

Apple juice products as produced in many Latin American countries are different from those produced in, for example, many parts of Europe. For example, products from Chile and elsewhere often have added sucrose and water and are preserved by adding sodium metabisulfite. A survey carried out in 1996 in Chile found that approximately 30% of the products exceeded the globally most often seen regulative limit for the mycotoxin patulin of $50 \mu g \ kg^{-1}$.

An analysis of the production (a HACCP process flow diagram) gave the following result:

(1) farm growing – (2) farm harvesting – (3) farm bulk storage – (4) bulk transportation to factory – (5) factory procurement – (6) sorting – (7) washing – (8) – bulk storage of whole apples – (9) pressing – (10) filtration – (11) pasteurization – (12) adding sugar/sodium metabisulfite solution – (13) aseptic filling – (14) storage and dispatch.

Patulin contamination is likely to be produced in the apple orchard during growing and during bulk storage. There is little risk of further contamination during transport, but damage to the fruits can increase the risk of subsequent contamination. Postharvest patulin contamination can be reduced by storage at <10°C, and by minimizing storage times at the orchard as well as the factory.

Contamination of the final juice product can in general be reduced at steps where rotten apples can be rejected from the process, either in the orchard or during sorting in the factory. Washing (and in particular pressure spraying) has been demonstrated to be effective in removing patulin from those apples that are selected for production. Actually, studies have shown that more than half of the patulin present can be removed in this way. The control measure is washing using high-pressure spraying. The critical limits for this CCP will be related to the pressure of the spray treatment and the duration. The water pressure thus must be monitored using pressure gauges and the washing step must be timed.

When the juice has been pressed, a further reduction of the patulin content can be achieved by filtering. Thus, research has shown that conventional clarification by means of a rotary vacuum pre-coat filter can reduce the patulin level by up to about 40%. Patulin is to quite an extent bound to particles held in suspension in the crude juice.

28.4 Certification Systems – ISO 22000 as an Example

Many recently developed systems of certification relevant for food producers and processors include as part of their compulsory components more than the implementation of GMP, GLP and a HACCP plan. The ISO (International Organization for Standardization), set up in 1947 and located in Geneva, Switzerland, has as its purpose the development of standards that facilitate international trade. ISO 22000 is a generic Food Safety Management System (FSMS) standard. It is designed to be used for certification (registration) purposes. Once a company has established an FSMS that meets ISO's requirements, it can ask a registrar to audit its system. If the registrar agrees that the ISO 22000 requirements are met, it will issue an official certificate that states the company's FSMS meets the ISO 22000 food safety requirements. However, a company does not have to be certified (registered) (see Box 28.1). ISO does not require certification (registration). A company can be in compliance without being formally registered by an accredited auditor.

Looking at 'ISO 22000:2005 Food safety management systems – Requirements for any organization in the food chain' reveals that development of the HACCP plan for the production is coupled with a quality circle including steps called *validation*, *monitoring* and *verification*, respectively. Validation in this connection is a systematic, documented investigation of whether the overall production process (with its HACCP system) established actually results in safe food products. In the monitoring phase the established CCPs are monitored over time to ensure that they constantly are working effectively. Finally the verification step controls that the monitoring has taken place, that the results have been evaluated and that the original result of the validation therefore is still valid. The new validation step is found as a component in both ISO 9001 (quality) and ISO 22000 (food safety).

Box 28.1. Certification, registration and accreditation[a]

In the context of ISO 9001:2000 (and ISO 9001:2008) or ISO 14001:2004, *certification* refers to the issuing of written assurance (the certificate) by an independent external body that it has audited a management system and verified that it conforms to the requirements specified in the standard.

Registration means that the auditing body then records the certification in its client register. So, the organization's management system has been both certified and registered.

Therefore, in the ISO 9001:2000 (and ISO 9001:2008) or ISO 14001:2004 context, the difference between the two terms is not significant and both are acceptable for general use.

Certification is the term most widely used worldwide, although registration is often preferred in North America, and the two are used interchangeably.

On the contrary, using accreditation as an interchangeable alternative for certification or registration is a mistake, because it means something different.

In the ISO 9001:2000 (and ISO 9001:2008) or ISO 14001:2004 context, *accreditation* refers to the formal recognition by a specialized body – an accreditation body – that a certification body is competent to carry out ISO 9001:2000 (and ISO 9001:2008) or ISO 14001:2004 certification in specified business sectors.

In simple terms, accreditation is like certification of the certification body. Certificates issued by accredited certification bodies may be perceived on the market as having increased credibility.

[a] Adapted from the ISO web page 'Certification' (http://www.iso.org/iso/iso_catalogue/management_standards/certification.htm).

28.5 Conclusion

A number of nationally and internationally developed protocols and systems of protocols linked with pre-described management systems exist. National and international (such as the EU) food legislations have to some extent adapted these as part of the requirements for producer approval and registration within the sector. However, all food producers and handlers – no matter if such demands are part of their legislative environment or not – can improve the safety quality of their products by implementing such systems or elements thereof.

Further Reading

Paster, T. (2007) *The HACCP Food Safety Training Manual.* John Wiley & Sons, Hoboken, New Jersey.

29 GMOs and Food

Mette Tingleff Skaanild

Associate Professor of Toxicology, Department of Veterinary Disease Biology, Faculty of Life Sciences, University of Copenhagen, Denmark

- How to produce GMOs.
- Examples of GMOs are given.
- We discuss safety testing of GMOs with regard to consumers.
- Environmental risks and benefits of GMOs are discussed.

29.1 Introduction

GMOs (genetically modified organisms) are organisms that have had their genes modified, either by introducing a new gene or by altering the genes already present in their genome. These alterations could include a change in the expression of already existing genes. GMOs most often are bacteria, which are used for the production of enzymes for washing powders and of medicines for patients with diabetes and haemophilia. However, in this chapter the focus is on GMOs used for food (feed), such as different crops. Feeding the world's increasing population will require an increase in food production and thereby increased agricultural production, and this will mean greater exploitation of the Earth. This could have negative consequences for the environment such as loss of biodiversity and increased emission of greenhouse gases. Cultivation of genetically modified (GM) crops is increasing; according to the International Service for the Acquisition of Agri-biotech Applications (ISAAA) the increase from 2008 to 2009 was 7% from 125 million ha to 134 million ha. The predominant crops involved are soy, maize and rape, and they are currently grown in 25 different countries. This chapter reviews the following aspects of GMOs:

- how they are produced;
- safety testing with regard to consumers; and
- environmental risks and benefits.

29.2 GM Crop Production

The first stable transgenic plant was produced in 1980, and several more transgenic plants have been produced since then. The process is a complex multistage procedure including: (i) delivery of exogenous DNA to the host cell; (ii) stable integration of the exogenous DNA; and (iii) recovery of viable transgenic plants. When producing transgenic plants different gene delivery systems can be used, which may be either:

- biological; or
- non-biological (physical or chemical).

The most used *biological transformation system* is based on the bacterium *Agrobacterium tumefaciens*, as this organism contains a plasmid that naturally transfers DNA located on the plasmid into the nucleus of the host plant cell and stably incorporates it into the plant's DNA. Despite the development of non-biological systems this *transfection* system remains popular and among the most effective, and can be used to transfer several genes at one time. Different plant viruses have also been used for gene transfer; although these systems provide a high expression level, the transformation is not stable.

Of the *non-biological systems* used for gene transfer in plants, particle bombardment (or *biolistics*) is by far the most widely used procedure both in research and commercially. This method was first described in 1987 where it was used to transform cereals. In the biolistic procedure small gold or tungsten particles are covered with the DNA coding for the gene that is going to be transferred to the plant. The particles are then fired into the plant cell. Transformation with gold particles 0.7–1.0 μm in diameter gives the highest transformation efficiency. The disadvantages of using biolistics are the random intracellular targets and that the DNA is not protected from damage, which may cause it to break down before it enters the plant nucleus. Several other non-biological systems have been tried such as *electroporation*, where strong electrical field pulses are applied to the cell membrane resulting in a temporary increase in porosity and providing a local driving force for ionic and molecular transport through the membranes. One of the more recently developed methods for the transfer of genes into plants is *silicon carbide-mediated transformation* (SCMT). The physical and chemical characteristics of silicon carbide fibres make them capable of puncturing the cells without killing then. The advantages of this system are that it is rapid, inexpensive and easy to set up, being effective in a wide variety of cells. However, the transformation efficiency is low and inhalation of the fibres may be a health problem for those working with the process.

After introduction of the gene modification, the plants are grown and tested for normal growth and normal expression of both all of the normal genes and the gene modification. Most of the *first-generation GM crops* (i.e. those currently in or close to commercialization) have been modified to increase yield or to facilitate crop management and this has been done by making plants:

- resistant to insect pests;
- tolerant to herbicides; or
- resistant to viral, fungal and bacterial infections.

Crops are made resistant to insects by transferring a gene from *Bacillus thuringiensis* (*Bt*) coding for an insecticidal protein (δ-endotoxin). This protein is activated by proteinases in the gut of the insect, whereupon it binds to receptors in the gut lining and damages it. As this receptor is specific for insects the protein is specifically insecticidal and no toxicity towards mammals is seen. *Bt* produces different toxins that affect different insects, such as caterpillars that destroy maize.

Many different crops (Table 29.1) have been made tolerant to broad-spectrum herbicides such as glufosinate and glyphosate, which are the most commonly used. These herbicides normally inhibit the amino

Table 29.1. Examples of first-generation GM crops and their genetic modifications.

Crop	Genetic modification
Maize	Insect protection
	Herbicide tolerant
Oilseed rape	Herbicide tolerant
Papaya	Virus resistant
Potato	Insect protection
	Virus resistant
Soy	Herbicide resistant
Squash	Virus resistant
Sugarbeet	Herbicide resistant
Tomato	Virus resistant
	Delayed ripening

acid synthesis in plants, but the transformation of the plants makes them resistant to this inhibition and they will continue to grow although sprayed.

Although resistance to viral, fungal or bacterial infection is known for some plants it has not been possible to transfer these genes from one plant species to another by traditional cross-breeding. The new gene modification techniques have now made it possible to transfer such resistance genes, however, these genes coding for proteins or enzymes that interfere with the growth of the infective agents.

Some of the so-called *second-generation GM crops* have been made to enhance human health, such as rice with a higher concentration of pro-vitamin A, soy with an increased level of vitamin E and cassava with a reduced level of cyanogenic glucosides.

29.3 GMOs – Safety Testing with Regard to Consumers

Before a GM crop can be used as a food component it has to go through several tests with regard to safety and commonly raised concerns such as:

- toxicity of the new gene;
- toxicity/allergenicity of the new protein;
- possible unintended effects; and
- possible alteration in nutrient composition.

Insertion of a foreign DNA sequence in a food commodity could cause concern because of direct toxicity or transfer of the gene. However, the foreign DNA in itself should not cause any toxic effect because all food contains significant levels of DNA and the composition of the DNA is the same; moreover, all DNA is metabolized in the same way in the gastrointestinal tract. Risk of transfer of the gene to either microbial cells in the gut or mammalian endothelial cells is considered extremely low, as the genes would have to survive the nucleases in the gut and the cells would have to be competent for transformation.

The new protein expressed in the cells of the transformed plant may be a cause for concern, however, as it could have a potentially toxic effect if it is not digested in the gastrointestinal tract and if it is absorbed. The protein is therefore tested in standard mammalian oral acute toxicity tests; if the protein shows no toxicity in these tests it is concluded that it presents no hazard to humans.

The identification of hazard with regard to possible allergenicity of the protein is done according to the FAO/WHO decision tree (Fig. 29.1).

The first step focuses on the source of the gene and the sequence homology of the protein compared with known allergens. If there is homology then the protein is regarded as a potential allergen; however, if there is no homology the protein is tested in a specific serum screen. In this test it is determined whether there are IgE antibodies in sensitized subjects

that can react with the protein. If the test is positive the protein may be an allergen. If there is no homology and no reaction with IgE, the protein is further tested for resistance to pepsin, i.e. to determine if the protein can or cannot be degraded by pepsin. The test for pepsin resistance and the test in animals may give positive and negative responses with regard to being a possible allergen. In the animal test it is possible to rank the allergenicity of the protein compared with other known allergens.

Unintended effects may arise if the new gene is inserted into a DNA sequence encoding another protein, thereby altering the 'normal' protein: reducing the enzymatic activity or changing the protein in this way may lead to a toxic or allergenic response. Insertion of foreign DNA can also result in changed expression of a 'normal' protein by either increasing or decreasing the expression of its gene. This could potentially again result in an allergenic or toxic response towards the GM crop. If the regulation of normal genes is changed, this can have also an impact on the nutritional balance of the GM crop compared with the normal crop. The toxicity and allergenicity of the GM crop is tested in laboratory animal feeding studies

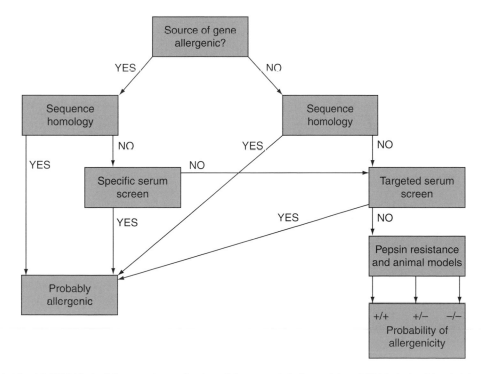

Fig. 29.1. The FAO/WHO decision tree for evaluation of the potential allergenicity of GMO-derived food. Adapted with permission from FAO.[1]

using rats or mice. The nutritional balance is also studied using smaller 'doses'; the animals getting the GM crop are compared with animals fed the same crop but unmodified. In this experiment it is possible to evaluate the nutritional level of the GM crop versus the normal unmodified crop. Lately crops have also been analysed using *metabolomics*, a method that compares all of the metabolites (small molecules) in the GM crop with those in the unmodified crop. This analysis will give an idea of the changes of metabolism and changes in metabolite profiles that the gene modification may cause.

Foods that have been derived from GM crops have to be labelled (Council Regulation (EC) No. 1139/98) and to enforce the legislation different methods for detection have been developed. Gene modifications can be detected at either the DNA level using PCR or the protein level using different immunological methods.

29.4   GMOs – Environmental Risks and Benefits

The potential risk of growing these GM crops may be development of resistant pests. After having grown pest-resistant crops such as *Bt* maize for a long time the pests may suddenly become resistant and that will make it necessary to develop either new insecticides or new GM crops, which again may have an impact on non-target species. The benefits will be a reduction in the usage of pesticides and reduction in carbon dioxide emissions from the tractors used for spreading the pesticides.

The risk of growing herbicide-resistant crops may be transfer of the gene to weeds, making them 'superweeds' that tolerate herbicides, and this may cause loss of biodiversity. Genes may be transferred by cross-pollination between the crop and the weed. However, this can be avoided by making the crop sterile or ensuring that the crop does not flower at the same time as the weeds which they can cross-pollinate. Again the benefits of growing these crops are lower usage of herbicides and lower carbon dioxide emissions.

As already stated, the new second generation of GM crops are made to increase the nutritional level of food such as rice by increasing the level of iron or vitamin A. It is thought that about half the world's population suffers from lack of iron; thus, rice with increased iron content will have a beneficial effect. Especially in the non-developed countries many children go blind because of a lack of vitamin A. Therefore, in these parts of the world rice (Golden Rice) with an increased level of pro-vitamin A will be beneficial.

29.5   Conclusion

Different GM crops are grown and used for food and feed. They are evaluated for their toxicity, allergenicity and nutritional levels before they are released, and no GM crop is released that can cause any toxicity or allergenicity according to these tests. Furthermore, they are evaluated with regard to their possible environmental and ecological effects. With regard to the environment, GM crops may cause changes in biodiversity by decreasing the number of different pests, as non-target pests may die as well as target pests. The transfer of genes from herbicide-tolerant crops to weeds is of great concern; this may produce 'superweeds' tolerant to herbicides that will then be able to invade more land, killing other weeds and crops.

Note

[1] FAO/WHO (2001) *Evaluation of Allergenicity of Genetically Modified Foods. Report of a Joint FAO/WHO Expert Consultation on Allergenicity of Foods Derived from Biotechnology, 22–25 January 2001.* Food and Agriculture Organization of the United Nations, Rome; available at http://www.who.int/foodsafety/publications/biotech/en/ec_jan2001.pdf

Further Reading

König, A., Cockburn, A., Crevel, R.W., Debruyne, E., Grafstroem, R., Hammerling, U., Kimber, I., Knudsen, I., Kuiper, H.A., Peijnenburg, A.A., Penninks, A.H., Poulsen, M., Schauzu, M. and Wal, J.M. (2004) Assessments of the safety of foods derived from genetically modified (GM) crops. *Food and Chemical Toxicology* 42, 1047–1088.

Ruse, M. and Castle, D. (eds) (2002) *Genetically Modified Foods: Debating Biotechnology.* Prometheus Books, New York, New York.

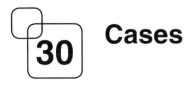

30 Cases

Sometimes a group of people suddenly are poisoned because of the occurrence of poisonous substances in their food. At other times – due to the implementation of modern systems of risk identification and management – the presence of toxins is realized and products are withdrawn in time. In this chapter we briefly describe a few incidents: their individual background, what happened and what was done to minimize the damage (if anything). The purpose is to illustrate the variability and (in certain cases) unpredictability of such situations, whether they are a result of a failure/accident, limited economic possibilities of the victims or deliberate fraud by producers or distributers.

30.1   The Spanish Toxic Oil Syndrome

The ingestion of a toxic oil fraudulently sold as olive oil in 1981 caused an outbreak of a previously unknown condition. In the early phases of the outbreak the clinical picture suggested the condition was an acute infectious pneumonitis caused by either *Legionella* or *Mycoplasma*. Indeed, many of the patients were treated with erythromycin and/or tetracycline antibiotics, but without any effect, however. Gradually theories took over that it had to do with some source of food. Contamination of tomatoes and perhaps other vegetable products grown in Andalusia with pesticides of an organophosphorus nature was discussed; particularly the compounds isofenphos and fenamiphos were under suspicion.

By 10 June 1981 most agreed that the condition, which was seen in Madrid and the north-west provinces of Spain, was due to intake of food oil and the condition acquired the name 'toxic oil syndrome' (abbreviated TOS). Today nearly 30 years later we know that some 20,000 people were affected and over 300 died within the first 20 months. Among the survivors the prevalence of some chronic conditions such as sclerodermia and certain neurological changes is high. But what was the problem?

Despite intense investigations – chemical as well as biological, involving the Spanish state as well as WHO – definitive proof concerning the causative agent(s) still has not been presented to date. However, the following is known.

By 1987 – yes, it took that long – epidemiological evidence was strong that TOS was causally associated with ingestion of a food-grade rapeseed oil containing aniline derivatives and sold for human consumption by itinerant street vendors. What seems to have happened was that cheap rapeseed oil originating from France, and denaturized with 2% aniline to make it suitable only for industrial use, was refined illegally in Spain to remove the aniline. Afterwards it was mixed with other edible oils and sold at a clear profit for the people involved in the operation.

Epidemiological studies integrated with chemical analysis of case related oils have shown that the disease is strongly associated with the consumption of oils containing fatty acid esters of 3-(N-phenylamino)-1,2-propanediol(PAP). Whether PAP esters are markers of toxicity or possess the capability to induce TOS still remains to be established.

30.2   The Belgium Dioxin and PCB Food Incident

In February 1999 some Belgium laying hens were reported to be showing signs resembling chick oedema disease. The signs comprised a marked drop in egg production followed a few weeks later by the observation of reduced hatchability of the eggs and increased mortality among the resulting chicks. It was not until May that it became obvious that this was not chick oedema disease, rather symptoms of a poisoning.

In January 1999 a tank of recycled fats used to produce animal feeds had accidentally been contaminated with about 100 litres of a mixture of two oily commercial PCB products (Aroclor 1260 and 1254) heavily contaminated by dioxins from thermal degradation of the PCBs during use.

In May the stock of about 60 tonnes of contaminated fats had been sold to a total of nine different manufacturers of animal feeds. These in turn had distributed their potentially contaminated feed products to around 2500 farms. Calculations made when the incident was clarified showed that dioxins equal to approximately 1 g of TCDD toxic equivalents (WHO-TEQ) and no less than an additional 2 g of toxic equivalents of a mixture of different dioxin-like PCBs were present in the contaminated fat stock used to produce these feedstuffs, the more specific distribution of the dioxin-like PCBs being unknown, however.

The toxic effects of dioxins include dermal toxicity, immunotoxicity, carcinogenicity, and reproductive and developmental toxicity. The toxicity is related to the amount accumulated in the body during a lifetime, the so-called body burden. Within the EU a TWI of 14 pg WHO-TEQ kg^{-1} BW was established in 2001 by SCF.

A delay in making this incident public resulted in a major political and food control crisis, causing much concern in the population, in Belgium and elsewhere. Luckily, calculations later showed that the incident was too limited in time and scale to have increased the PCB/dioxin body burden of the general population at large. Only farmers in poultry farms actually affected by the incident (i.e. facing intoxication of their hens) and having regularly consumed their own products could have increased their PCB/dioxin body burden. These farms were 30 in number. Even when looking at these farmers it was concluded unlikely that their body burden due to this incident should have increased beyond levels found in the 1980s in the general population or the present levels found in persons from communities that regularly consume seafood.

30.3   The Irish Dioxin Food Incident

Routine monitoring by the Irish authorities found elevated levels of PCBs in pork. Since this could be an indicator for unacceptable dioxin contamination (see above), further investigations were immediately started to analyse for the dioxin content. The use of contaminated animal feed was identified to be the source. Preliminary evidence indicated that the contamination problem was likely to have started in September 2008.

The contaminated feed had been provided to ten pig farms, which were producing about 7% of the total supply of pigs in Ireland. The analysis showed levels of dioxins (about 100 times the legal maximum limit) in certain pork and pork products produced in the country.

EFSA was asked to make a risk assessment on the basis of the information available. In December 2008 this was published. EFSA had defined a number of different scenarios concerning the spread of the contaminated products and the intake of these by different groups within the European population. EFSA concluded among other things:

> In very extreme cases, assuming a daily consumption of 100% contaminated Irish pork, for a high consumer of pork fat during the respective period of the incident (90 days), at the highest recorded concentration of dioxins (200 pg WHO-TEQ/g fat), EFSA concludes that the uncertainty factor embedded in the TWI is considerably eroded. Given that the TWI has a 10-fold built-in uncertainty factor, EFSA considers that this unlikely scenario would reduce protection, but not necessarily lead to adverse health effects.

30.4   The Melamine Incident in China

An increased incidence of kidney stones and renal failure among infants was publicly reported in China from early September 2008 onwards. On 9 September 2008, *The Shanghai Daily* reported that 14 infants from Gansu Province were suffering from kidney stones after drinking a particular brand of powdered infant milk formula. While the exact onset date for symptoms remains unknown, the first sick babies with discoloured urine were seen in hospitals and at clinics as early as December 2007 and the first child died on 1 May 2008. Up until 12 September 2008 the State Council of China reported 432 cases and one death. All of the infants identified with kidney stones had consumed infant formula produced by the Sanlu Group.

The source of the illness was traced to the contamination of infant formula with melamine. Investigations showed that the melamine had been added deliberately to diluted raw milk to boost its apparent protein content. Previous outbreaks of renal failure related to melamine, a molecule with a high nitrogen content, had been reported in pets in 2004 in the Republic of Korea and in 2007 in the USA when the substance was added deliberately to pet food ingredients. But why did this happen?

The short answer is because commonly used methods for protein analysis of these products do not distinguish between nitrogen from protein and from non-protein sources. A wide investigation into the extent of melamine contamination of dairy products in China soon revealed that no less than 22 manufacturers of infant formulas were selling melamine-contaminated products. In the Sanlu products, melamine levels were found to be as high as $2500\,mg\,kg^{-1}$.

Soon after, as a result of further investigations, melamine was also found in liquid milk, yoghurts and frozen desserts. As the incident developed, updates on the affected children were provided by the Chinese Ministry of Health. Today it seems fairly well established that a total of six deaths and close to 50,000 hospitalized cases associated with the consumption of melamine-contaminated milk and milk products were seen.

30.5 An Outbreak of Aflatoxin Poisoning in Eastern and Central Kenya

In 2004 an outbreak of jaundice with a high case-fatality rate was reported in the districts of Makueni and Kitui, Eastern Province of Kenya. In May a group of specialists from WHO and other organizations started investigating this incident. As of 20 July, a total of 317 cases had been reported with no less than 125 deaths. Suspicion soon concentrated on a food poisoning of some kind. Food samples collected from household visits during May included maize flour and grains, millet, sorghum and beans. Owing to the symptoms of jaundice indicating liver failure the samples were analysed among other things for their possible content of the aflatoxin group of mycotoxins. A total of 182 samples representing more than 50% of the collection showed a content higher than 20 ppb (the maximum US level at that time); however, a substantial number of samples had really scary contents higher than 1000 ppb ($\mu g\,kg^{-1}$). The Kenyan government thereafter advised residents in the affected geographical region to avoid consumption of especially maize but also in general foods that were mouldy or discoloured. Furthermore, this incident meant that the government for a period had to provide replacement food to around 1.2 million people in the two districts.

30.6 The 'Ginger Jake Paralysis'

During the 1930s a federal ban on alcohol sale and use was in place in the USA. However, certain medicinal remedies containing ethanol were still allowed. Thus, the Prohibition Bureau permitted sale of the so-called 'Jamaica Ginger Extract' as a means of treating headache and digestive troubles. Quickly the remedy became popular owing to its composition of about 70% ethanol content. People mixed it with soda water to make a kind of cocktail.

The Jamaica Ginger Extract production of one unscrupulous producer hit trouble, however, when he ran out of ginger oleoresin, the normal flavouring agent. In one large batch he substituted the oleoresin with the synthetic organic compound tri-o-cresyl phosphate (TOCP), which conveyed a taste relatively similar to the customary taste of the extract. About 50,000 adults were struck by what was soon termed 'Ginger Jake paralysis': they developed a permanent or only slowly reversible partial paralysis resulting in difficulty walking, the so-called 'Jake leg' or 'Jake walk'. Studies showed that TOCP caused an axonal neuropathy that affected primarily large muscle groups. The mechanism is not totally clear but was speculated to be related to the known OPIDN (see Chapter 20).

30.7 The Sudan III Scare

Sudan I, II, III and IV are non-ionic, fat-soluble dyes used as additives in gasoline, grease, oils and plastics. The compounds are classified by IARC as Category 3 carcinogens. This is due to the fact that they have been demonstrated to induce some forms of liver and bladder cancer in animals. In Europe Sudan dyes are banned as food additives for humans.

Chemically the Sudan colours belong to the azo dyes, a class of synthetic organic colorants (characterized by a chromophoric azo group) that are typically used in different industrial applications including the coloration of solvents, oils, fats, waxes, plastics, printing inks and floor polishes. Their widespread usage is due to their colourfastness and low price. However, azo colorants are biologically active through their metabolites and have in general been associated with increased occurrence of bladder cancer, as seen after occupational exposure of textile and leather dyers and painters.

In 2004 UK food inspections found that a number of food products such as Worcestershire sauce contained Sudan colours. This was traced back to chillies and chilli products imported from India, chillies making up a part of the recipe of this traditional English product. Further investigations disclosed that the chilli products had had Sudan III added to improve their colour. A subsequent investigation showed that a number of products on the shelves in Europe had contents of Sudan III; these were withdrawn from the market. The addition of Sudan III was at that time not illegal in the countries where the chilli products were produced.

30.8 Conclusion

Earning more money from producing or selling food adulterants may attract certain individuals no matter where in the world one lives, no matter the developmental state of the community and the legislation within the area of foods. Likewise, poverty may lead to situations where one has to live from sources of food that one would reject under more optimal conditions. No matter the situation, the cases described above illustrate that when incidents occur rapid intervention by multi-disciplinary expert teams is the most important measure.

Index

safety of food 76–79, 81, 265–268
    GMOs 270–272
safety pharmacology 81
safflower (*Carthamus tinctorius*) 124
salt-cured meat 199–200, 203, 227
sampling procedures 242–244, 252
saponins 35–36, 65, 124–126
sarin 172
saxitoxin (STX) 63, 130, 256
scombroid poisoning 212–213, 214
seafood *see* fish; shellfish; whale meat
seaweed 9, 133
secondary metabolites 97–98
    alkaloids 100–101, 103–8, 246
    fluoroacetic acid 64, 99, 102
    furanocoumarins 108
    gossypol 26–27, 109, 243
    mono- and sesquiterpenes 109
    non-protein amino acids 102–103
    phytic acid 17, 99
    proteins 97, 98, 99
    tannins 99
    see also glycosides
secondary producers 5
selenium 18–19, 64–65, 134, 146–149, 254
selenomethionine 65, 146
semicarbazide 255
Seveso incident 186
sewage treatment 188–189
shellfish 6, 11
    algal toxins in 27, 65, 129–130, 255–256
    allergy to 239
    metals in 135, 139
silicon carbide-mediated
    transformation 270
silylation 246
simmondsin 121–122
skatole 17
skin irritation/corrosion
    photodermatitis 108
    tests for 84, 93
small intestine 33–36
smallholders 9–10, 10
smoking (curing process) 207–209
smoking (tobacco) 137, 207
α-solanine 120–121
sorbic acid/sorbates (E200/E202/E203) 226–227
sorbitol (E420) 223–224
sorghum (*Sorghum bicolor*) 99, 118, 159
soy sauce 214
soybean (*Glycine max*) 8, 98, 123, 127, 239
    epoxidated soybean oil 193
Spain, toxic oil syndrome 273
speciation (of elements) 138–139, 244, 252–254
stainless steel 139
Standard Uncertainty Factors (UFs) 261, 262
standards *see* regulations

steroids 189
    growth promoters 11, 217
    see also endocrine disrupters
stevioside 224
stomach, absorption of toxicants 32–33
storage containers 136, 149, 191–193, 255
STX (saxitoxin) 63, 130, 256
subsistence farming 9, 10
sucralose (E955) 224
sucrose intolerance 240
Sudan III dye 275–276
sulfites (E221-E224, E226-E228) 227
sulfur dioxide (SO_2)
    air pollution 8
    as a preservative (E220) 227
sulfuric acid 164, 179
sunset yellow 225, 226
sweeteners 35, 220–224

2,4,5-T (2,4,5-trichlorophenoxyacetic acid) (agent
    orange) 21, 180–181, 187
T-2 mycotoxin 157, 158
tannins 99
target organs/molecules 61–65
tartrazine 225–226
TCDD (2,3,7,8-tetrachlorodibenzodioxin) 185–187
TDE (1,1-dichloro-2,2-bis(*p*-chlorophenyl)ethane) 166–167
TDI (Tolerable Daily Intake) 260
tea 105, 150
teeth 150
tempeh 8
TEPP (tetraethylpyrophosphate) 172
teratogenicity
    potato alkaloids 121
    tests for 93, 95
testis, blood–testis barrier 38
tetraethyl lead (TEL) 2, 21, 142
tetrodotoxin 130–131
theobromine 105
theophylline 105
thiabendazole (E233) 229
thiaminases 17, 97
thiocyanate 120
threshold of toxicological concern (TTC) 235
thujone 234–235
tin 149–150
tobacco use 137, 207
Tolerable Daily Intake (TDI) 260
tonic water 106
toxaphene 184
toxic oil syndrome 273
toxicity testing 80–82
    acute toxicity 85–87, 92–94
        brine shrimp test 88–90
    general assays 82, 85–87
    of GMOs 271–272